Nursing Care of Children and Young People with Chronic Illness

This book is dedicated to all children and young people
with chronic illness and their families

Nursing Care of Children and Young People with Chronic Illness

Edited by

Fay Valentine
RGN, RSCN, MA, PGDip. HSSM, ENB998
Director of Children and Young People's Directorate, School of Nursing and
Midwifery Studies, Cardiff University, UK

Lesley Lowes
RGN, RSCN, PGCHPE, DPSN, M.Sc., Ph.D.
Research Fellow/Practitioner, Nursing, Health and Social Care Research Centre,
School of Nursing and Midwifery Studies, Cardiff University, UK

Foreword by
Simon Weston, OBE

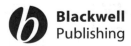
Blackwell
Publishing

© 2007 by Blackwell Publishing Ltd

Blackwell Publishing editorial offices:
Blackwell Publishing Ltd, 9600 Garsington Road, Oxford OX4 2DQ, UK
Tel: +44 (0)1865 776868
Blackwell Publishing Inc., 350 Main Street, Malden, MA 02148-5020, USA
Tel: +1 781 388 8250
Blackwell Publishing Asia Pty Ltd, 550 Swanston Street, Carlton, Victoria 3053, Australia
Tel: +61 (0)3 8359 1011

The right of the Author to be identified as the Author of this Work has been asserted in accordance
with the Copyright, Designs and Patents Act 1988.

First published 2007 by Blackwell Publishing Ltd

ISBN: 978-1-4051-4402-5

Nursing care of children and young people with chronic illness / edited by Fay Valentine,
Lesley Lowes; foreword by Simon Weston.
p. ; cm.
Includes bibliographical references.
ISBN-13: 978-1-4051-4402-5 (pbk. : alk. paper)
1. Chronic diseases in children–Nursing.
2. Chronic diseases in adolescence–Nursing.   I. Valentine, Fay.   II. Lowes, Lesley, 1950-
[DNLM: 1. Chronic Disease–nursing.   2. Adolescent.   3. Child.   4. Holistic Nursing.
5. Patient Participation.   WY 152 N97436 2007]
RJ380.N868 2007
618.92′044 – dc22
2007002025

A catalogue record for this title is available from the British Library

Set in 10/12pt Palatino
by Graphicraft Limited, Hong Kong
Printed and bound in Singapore
by Fabulous Printers Pte Ltd

The publisher's policy is to use permanent paper from mills that operate a sustainable forestry
policy, and which has been manufactured from pulp processed using acid-free and elementary
chlorine-free practices. Furthermore, the publisher ensures that the text paper and cover board
used have met acceptable environmental accreditation standards.

For further information on Blackwell Publishing, visit our website:
www.blackwellpublishing.com

Contents

Foreword

Simon Weston OBE

When approached to write this foreword, I felt I needed to examine my qualifications for addressing the need for a book relating to the nursing requirements of children and young people with chronic illness. I realised that as the son of a nurse, the father of a child with asthma and eczema and the survivor of 48% burns (80% body scarring) whilst only 20 years old, I am more than qualified to speak from a layperson's perspective.

In today's ever moving and multicultural society, this book is long overdue. The task set for the authors has been to create an all encompassing book that will deal not only with the issues of chronic disease in children and young people, but also with a whole catalogue of situations that the modern nurse will have to deal with when faced with their care.

Having examined the premise for this book, it is clear that it will alleviate the need to wade through heavily jargoned and complicated texts, spread over numerous manuals, thus using up student nurses' valuable study time. This book provides a quality tool that will raise the awareness and effectiveness of not just student nurses but all health professionals working with children and young people with chronic illness.

The material collated spans the knowledge and experiences of several renowned and articulate professionals whose combined talents form an interlaced understanding of the total need of children and young people with chronic illness. It gives a holistic view of illness, emotions, cultures and religions, all of which may impact on the ability of the child and family to cope with a chronic condition.

I firmly believe that this book, with its compilation of informative and insightful data, will help ensure the empowerment of children and young people with chronic illness and their families through increased awareness and understanding by those involved in their care.

Contributors

Siân Bill RGN, RSCN, BN, MN (Melb.), Grad. Dip. Adolescent Health (Melb.), Grad. Dip. Education & Training (Melb.), Grad. Dip. Nsg (Infant Child and Youth Health) (UWS)
Siân is a lecturer within the Children and Young People's Directorate at the School of Nursing and Midwifery Studies, Cardiff University. Her main interests are in adolescent chronic illness, in particular cystic fibrosis, and in transitional care. Siân has worked extensively with young people in both the acute care and community setting.

Mandy Brimble RN, Dip. HE (Child), B.Sc. (Hons) Community Health Studies (Public Health Nursing/Health Visiting), PGCE
Mandy is a lecturer in the Children and Young People's Directorate, School of Nursing and Midwifery Studies, Cardiff University. She has worked as a children's nurse in general medicine, day surgery and at a special children's centre. She has an interest in a wide range of medical and surgical conditions as well as a specific interest in all aspects of child protection. Her training and work as a health visitor has fostered a keen interest in public health and health promotion, particularly childhood accident prevention. Mandy has recently commenced an MSc in Education, with an aim towards gaining a deeper insight into strategic teaching, learning and educational management issues.

Maggie Furness SRN, RSCN, RNT, RCNT, WNB(6), ONC, MA (Ethics)
Maggie is a lecturer within the Children and Young People's Directorate at the School of Nursing and Midwifery Studies, Cardiff University. She has worked in a wide range of clinical settings including orthopaedics, theatres and general paediatric areas. She has a wide range of interests, including ethical issues in children's nursing and the history of nursing.

Suzanne Hazell RSCN, RGN, BA, MN, PGCE

Having qualified as a general nurse in 1967, Suzanne has many years' experience of children's nursing, mainly in the field of neonatal nursing in several UK hospitals. Subsequently, she undertook the RSCN and neonatal nursing courses and a Master's in nursing. It was while nursing neonates that she developed an interest in genetics and the aetiology of conditions affecting children and young people. For the last 11 years, Suzanne has been lecturing in children and young people's nursing and has continued to develop this interest.

Beverly Hodges M.Sc. in Clinical Practice (Child), PGCE, B.Sc. (Hons), Dip. Asthma, Dip. Allergy and Immunology, L/PE, RSCN, RGN

Beverly is a lecturer in the Children and Young People's Directorate at the School of Nursing and Midwifery Studies, Cardiff University. She has worked in a variety of settings caring for children and young people. Her specialist interest areas are respiratory health, allergic disease, pain management and management of change. Beverly was a member of the external working group for the children and young people specialist services project, for the All-Wales Standards for Paediatric Respiratory Services, with the Welsh Assembly Government. She has represented the Royal College of Nursing in responding to appraisals for the National Institute of Health and Clinical Excellence.

Yvonne Knight RSCN, EN(G), B.Sc. (Hons), PGDip. (Professional Health Care Education), ENB 147, 820, 998

Yvonne is a lecturer in the Children and Young People's Directorate, School of Nursing and Midwifery Studies, Cardiff University. Her clinical experience and research interests are in the acute and chronic nursing needs of children. She is currently studying for a Master's in child health.

Lesley Lowes RGN, RSCN, PGCHPE, DPSN, M.Sc., Ph.D.

Lesley is a research fellow/practitioner at the Nursing, Health and Social Care Research Centre, School of Nursing and Midwifery Studies, Cardiff University. She is an experienced qualitative researcher, whose research interests include childhood chronic illness (diabetes in particular), theories of loss, grief, adaptation and change, and the involvement of service users in health and social care research. She has an extensive clinical and academic publication portfolio, particularly in the field of paediatric diabetes. In addition to her academic work, she has a 50% clinical remit as a paediatric diabetes specialist nurse with Cardiff and Vale NHS Trust.

Peter Mcnee RGN, RSCN, ENB (415), BA (Hons), PGCE, M.Sc.

Peter is a lecturer in the Children and Young People's Directorate, School of Nursing and Midwifery Studies, Cardiff University. His clinical background is predominantly within paediatric critical care. His main interests include the acquisition of clinical skills, bereavement care, child protection and children's participation in care decisions.

Martina Nathan RSCN, RGN, B.Sc. Professional Practice, PGCE
Martina is currently on secondment to the Children and Young People's Directorate from the position of Paediatric Chemotherapy Nurse Trainer, Cardiff and Vale NHS Trust. She has spent nine years working in the acute paediatric oncology setting, in Ireland, Singapore and Cardiff.

Melda Price B.Sc. (Hons) RGN, RSCN, PGCHPE, Dip. DN
Melda is currently a lecturer in Children's Nursing in the Children and Young People's Directorate, School of Nursing and Midwifery Studies, Cardiff University. Her teaching expertise is in the care of children with chronic illness and complex conditions in the community, with an emphasis on inter-professional collaboration in care. Her research interests are community children's nursing, paediatric oncology and paediatric palliative care.

Sian Thomas RGN, RSCN, M.Sc.
Sian is a Nurse Consultant in Community Child Health at Caerphilly Local Health Board. Prior to this post, she was the manager of the Community Children's Nursing Service at Cardiff and Vale NHS Trust. During this time she had the opportunity to undertake a secondment to the Welsh Assembly Government as Project Manager for the Children and Young People's Specialist Services Project.

Julia Tod RGN, RM, RSCN, ENB405/998, B.Sc. (Hons) Psychology, PGCE
Julia's clinical nursing practice was mainly in neonatal care in North and South Wales, Glasgow and Nottingham. A joint post (Gwent NHS Trust/UWCM) as children's nursing clinical teacher led to her current role as nurse lecturer at Cardiff University. Currently studying for a Master's in health psychology, her research interests include health behaviours, the role of young carers and application of psychology in health care.

Fay Valentine RGN, RSCN, MA, PGDip. HSSM, ENB998
Fay is Director of the Children and Young People's Directorate in the School of Nursing and Midwifery Studies, Cardiff University. She has a long history of working with children and young people with chronic illness. Her specialist interests are leadership, adolescence and chronic illness. She is the Welsh representative on the RCN Children and Young People's Advisory Panel, a member of the All-Wales Senior Children's Nursing Forum and committee member for the Welsh Nursing and Midwifery Council.

Simon Weston OBE
Following his injuries (48% burns) while a Welsh Guardsman on the *Sir Galahad*, which was destroyed in the Falkland Islands' Bluff Cove, Simon has been active in a number of successful ventures, including the establishment of the Weston Spirit, a Liverpool based but UK-wide young people's charity. He has worked tirelessly for the Royal Star and Garter Home and his charitable work earned him an OBE in the 1992 Queen's Birthday Honours. In 2005, Simon was awarded an honorary fellowship from the School of Nursing and Midwifery at Cardiff University.

Introduction

Fay Valentine and Lesley Lowes

There are currently limited books available that analyse the context, theory and practice of nursing children and young people with chronic illness. This book provides a comprehensive and up-to-date resource for nursing students and post-registration children's nurses on assessing health needs and delivering care and services holistically within and across a variety of care settings in order to meet the changing needs of children and young people with chronic illness and their families.

Although each chapter can be read independently, the book is designed to encompass a broad perception of the changing health care needs of children and young people with chronic illness and the implications for delivering nursing practices and services to children and young people of several age groups, cultural backgrounds, with differing conditions and in a variety of care settings.

In each of the chapters, individualised case scenarios and reader activities are used to apply theoretical principles and current evidence to the realities of nursing practice. In addition, readers are able to gain a greater understanding of the clinical conditions used in the case scenarios in relation to age development issues and associated care needs.

Chapter 1 revisits the aetiology of chronic illness, examining the generic basis of children and young people's chronic conditions and certain disabilities as a consequence of hereditary influence, providing an overview of chromosomal anomalies and genetic pathways of inheritance. The latter half of this chapter explores the differing onsets of chronic illness, considering prenatal, neonatal and late onset, and their implications for practitioners and care delivery.

Chapter 2 examines some of the current political, economic and social policies that are shaping the context and service delivery for children and young people with chronic illness, and the issues and challenges these bring to managers, practitioners and service users. Particular points discussed include workforce changes, patient engagement and commissioning. Examples of service models and nursing roles are analysed to apply these issues and challenges to nursing practice and demonstrate the changing boundaries of clinical practice, multidisciplinary working and service delivery.

Chapter 3 provides a theoretical basis for the impact of chronic illness on the child and family, examining in detail some classic and contemporary theories relating to grief, loss, coping and adaptation. Suggestions are made concerning effective care strategies and practices to support and help parents adapt to their child's diagnosis of chronic illness. A clinical case scenario of a girl with type 1 diabetes is used to apply the key principles outlined in the chapter.

Chapter 4 explores these issues further by examining the particular care needs of a girl with eczema, focusing on the implications for children, young people and their families in their adaptation to chronic illness and addressing the practical implications of assessing and meeting their physical, psychological and social needs. Interesting discussions include issues around ethnicity, culture, spirituality, social isolation and the use of complementary therapies.

Chapter 5 provides insights into the general principles for the need to inform, educate and promote health to children and young people with chronic illness and their families as an effective means of empowering them to be 'experts' in their care. Using an asthma case scenario, challenges that may arise due to the receptiveness of children, young people and their families, or their intellectual or resource ability to change behaviour, are considered.

Chapter 6 reviews ethical, legal and professional aspects of nursing children and young people with chronic illness. Scenarios from other chapters are analysed within a framework of ethical principles to identify potential ethical debates and difficult decision making that practitioners may encounter. The ethical discussions are applied to the practice situation.

Chapter 7 presents a partnership approach between theory and practice, examining changing service boundaries, nursing roles and relationships with parents in the provision of continuing care for children and young people with chronic illness and their families in the community. To explore this from a practice perspective, multidisciplinary working, discharge planning and respite care are considered using the case scenario of a Welsh speaking rurally isolated family with a child with the neuromuscular disorder of Batten's disease.

Chapter 8 recognises the importance of acute emergency care, resulting from illness or an unrelated admission, for children and young people with chronic illness, and the need to ensure effective services and communication processes. Using an oncological haematological condition, current debates and care practices are explored including the need for alternative admission settings.

The last two chapters of the book are especially devoted to teenagers, an increasingly important issue for nurses to consider due to the increasing life expectancy of children with chronic illnesses. Chapter 9 provides a critical analysis of the impact of chronic illness upon development transitions of adolescence and the possible health associated risks and longer-term consequences of these. The implications for practitioners in particular focus on communication, body image, compliance and resilience. Chapter 10 builds upon some of the themes raised in Chapter 9 by exploring further a number of aspects of adolescent development in relation to the planning and delivery of effective transition from child to adult services.

This edited book brings together contributions from a team of experienced lecturers in the Children and Young People's Directorate at the School of Nursing and Midwifery Studies, Cardiff University, along with the only consultant children's community nurse in Wales.

1 The Definition and Aetiology of Chronic Illness

Fay Valentine and Suzanne Hazell

Introduction

The intention of this chapter is to help the reader further develop their knowledge and understanding of the genetic basis of children and young people's chronic conditions and certain disabilities, as a consequence of hereditary influences. Following an overview of chromosomal anomalies, genetic pathways of inheritance will be defined and illustrated via examples of both sex-linked and autosomal recessive and dominant disorders. This chapter does not intend to provide an in-depth critique on the current ethical debates, research and practice controversies surrounding genetic engineering and modification. For this the reader is guided to nursing anatomy and physiology books.

The latter half of the chapter focuses on examining the differing onsets of chronic illness, considering prenatal, neonatal and late onset. To provide the reader with a practice focus, case studies will be used as examples to examine the professional and care implications of nursing children, young people and their families whose chronic illness has been diagnosed at various stages of their development. To allow these issues to be further developed and explored, the same case studies will be used in subsequent chapters.

Aim of the chapter

To enhance the genetic knowledge and understanding of nurses, including the aetiology of chronic illness in children and examine how this genetic competence can be implemented in their practice to:

- Lead to a reduced risk of conditions occurring, or a reduction in severity for those where a condition has been identified

- Enable them to fully participate in the relevant debates and ethical discussions that can have implications for children, young people and their families.

Intended learning outcomes

- To examine the hereditary influences upon the genetic basis of chronic diseases in childhood
- To determine patterns of genetic inheritance
- To investigate the origins of chronic disease
- To explore the role of the children's nurse during the period leading to, and at the time of, diagnosis

Genetic knowledge

This chapter is written on the assumption that the reader comprehends the basic foundations and principles of genetics. These being: the biology of chromosomes, the structure and role of deoxyribonucleic acid (DNA) in coding genetic information, its ability to replicate and the mechanisms for protein synthesis. In particular, knowledge of the nitrogenous bases and the mechanisms of transcription and translation are required. A good grasp of the cell cycle and its governing control system, along with knowledge of the distinct stages of mitosis and the two divisions, 1 and 2, of meiosis and their resulting products, is also assumed. It is important that the reader has knowledge and understanding of these basic units relating to normal DNA development and of the processes undertaken for the production of sperm and oocytes. Without this knowledge, the reader may find it difficult to comprehend how DNA mutations can cause disease and how errors within the processes of mitosis and meiosis can result in chromosomal abnormalities.

Test your knowledge

- What are the two major phases of a somatic cell cycle?
- What are the four stages of mitosis?
- What are the subdivisions of meiosis 1?
- What are the products of meiosis 2?
- What are the three parts of a DNA nucleotide?
- What are the four nitrogenous bases in DNA?
- In what way does RNA differ from DNA?
- Cells contain three different kinds of RNA. What are they and what is their function in carrying out the instructions encoded in DNA?
- Do you understand the following terms? Haploid and diploid germ cell, homologous chromosomes, allele, heterozygosity and homozygosity?

If the reader wishes to refresh their knowledge on these areas following this test they are advised to refer to a nursing anatomy and physiology text.

The need for genetic knowledge

Several authors have argued that children's nurses need genetic knowledge to maintain currency of practice (Skirton & Patch, 2002; Edgar, 2004; Skirton *et al.*, 2005; Burke & Kirk, 2006). This is regarded as essential if they are to provide appropriate information and advice to families, and be able to engage in policy decisions and relevant genetic debates. The genetics White Paper *Our Inheritance, Our Future* (DoH, 2003) supports this premise, emphasising that education for health professionals is vital to enable advances in genetics to be translated and applied to everyday clinical practice. To support this White Paper, the Department of Health commissioned the development of guidelines for use across the UK for genetic education programmes for nurses, midwives and health visitors. This resulted in the publication of a competence based education framework containing seven competency standard statements and associated learning outcomes (Kirk *et al.*, 2003). In 2005, a series of seven papers were published by the Royal College of Nursing (RCN) outlining the framework and application of the seven competency standards to nursing, midwifery and health visiting practice (Kirk, 2005). The RCN in collaboration with the Progress Educational Trust (PET) have also produced a guide to genetics for nurses, which provides a good basic overview of genetics (PET/RCN, 2006).

For children's nurses, this genetic education would be required to impart several key areas of practice when delivering care and education to children and young people with chronic illness and their families. Sex education and genetic advice may be required for the teenager with a genetic chronic illness, for example sickle cell anaemia, who may be considering commencing a sexual relationship. Alternatively, parents may require support, advice and guidance following the diagnosis of their child with a genetic disorder. Parents who already have a child with a genetic condition and are considering future pregnancies may also require genetic counselling and advice.

If children's nurses are to deliver sensitive, informed, evidence based information, education and support to children, young people and their families, they must ensure that they have a current knowledge base upon which to draw. They must also be professionally aware of their limitations in this field and have a good knowledge of, and guide their patients to, local resources and expertise. This could be a hospital's local genetic department or a genetic specialist nurse.

The ethical, legal and social implications in the screening, testing and recording of genetic information

Along with technological advances, our enhanced knowledge and understanding of the human genome and the role of genes in body processes has enabled the mechanisms for genetic screening and testing to be realised for a number of genetic disorders. This new ability to predict the potential for, or to identify, disease-related genes in individuals long before they can be clinically detected, has brought both positive advantages and some practice challenges. For example, knowing from birth that a child has Duchenne muscular dystrophy provides the opportunity for prophylactic treatment regimes and health education strategies to commence immediately. This potentially reduces the complications that can negatively impact upon a child's quality of life. However, this new knowledge has also resulted in some ethical dilemmas and debates that need to be considered, for example issues such as consent, confidentiality, and the management of situations where the child or young person, their family and the professional's views are not in unison.

Other areas of debate and controversy include, who should be tested? What should be the availability of testing? Is mandatory prenatal testing and neonatal screening required or ethical? What are the predictive values of the genetic test and the appropriateness of testing for diseases where there is no treatment or intervention available, as in the case of Huntington's chorea? For those children and families that are tested, there are concerns about possible stigmatisation or discrimination and the role of family counselling within this process (Edgar, 2004; Kenner & Moran, 2005). Barr and McConkey (2006) support this point when discussing the support parents require during the referral and process of genetic investigations. They highlight that parents view this process as part of a 'longer journey' when obtaining information, advice and support about their child's condition or disability via services that have established protocols for effective collaboration between primary care, secondary care and regional genetic services.

This chapter, however, wishes only to draw the reader's attention to these growing ethical dilemmas and the legal and social issues related to genetic screening and the identification of a genetic disease. Although there is no absolute guide to good action, there are frameworks and models for resolving ethical decision making. For further information regarding these ethical frameworks, the reader is directed to Chapter 7, where ethical frameworks are used to guide the reader through decisions. Bradley (2005) also outlines some example scenarios in relation to the utility and limitations of genetic testing and information.

◁▯━▱▯   Key points

Children's nurses need genetic competence to implement this knowledge and understanding into their practice in order to:

- Lead to a reduction of risk of conditions occurring, or a reduction in severity for those where a condition has been identified
- Enable them to fully participate in the relevant debates and ethical discussions that can have implications for children, young people and their families

The determinants of genetic disease

Due to the intricate nature of DNA formation that occurs during embryological and foetal development, chance mutations or damage can easily alter DNA, producing abnormal sequences of base molecules. There are natural processes within the cell to monitor, recognise and repair defects produced in DNA base sequencing. However, if these internal mechanisms do not detect or repair this damage, expression of the dysfunctional gene can either cause a congenital problem in that child or become part of the genome to be passed on to future generations (hereditary).

Environmental insults to DNA material caused by chemical (carcinogenic), physical (heat) and ionising radiation (X-ray) processes may also produce damage to the genetic material. Damage to somatic cells, by radiation, carcinogenic chemicals and ultraviolet light may cause mutations, particularly in cells that are constantly regenerating and can lead to tumour growth in that individual (Jones, 2004). However, damage to the sex cells that go on to produce the gametes for fertilisation means that the mutation will not affect the individual but could be passed on to future generations.

The term 'multi-factorial inheritance' is used to describe the origin of diseases where there are multiple genetic and environmental factors involved in determining the phenotype, such as leukaemia, where there is familial clustering, and asthma. Some writers believe, however, that the environment has a role to play in all genetic conditions (Thurmon, 1999).

Later in the chapter, prenatal onsets of genetic disorders are discussed in more detail including potential permanent effects caused to the developing foetus by the prenatal intrauterine environment.

⏲ Time out

- Before you get to that section write a list of teratogens, agents that cause birth defects.

Chromosomal abnormalities

In humans, each cell, except the germ cells (ova in girls, sperm in boys), contains 46 chromosomes, which are further classified as 22 pairs of autosomes and one pair of sex chromosomes (XX in girls, XY in boys). Located throughout the chromosome are genes, intricate chemical units made up of DNA. As chromosomes are inherited from both parents, individuals have a copy of genes from both the maternal and paternal line. In homologous chromosomes, each gene sequence inherited from the father will have a corresponding gene sequence inherited from the mother (Jones, 2004). Depending on inheritance factors, the gene sequences may be identical or different.

Chromosomes are numbered according to size and centromere position. Chromosome number 1, for instance, is the largest pair of chromosomes and number 22 the smallest pair of autosomes. The centromere, a constriction on the chromosome either in the centre or close to one end, divides the chromosome into a shorter arm (p) and a longer arm (q). The relative centromeric position allows the morphological classification of chromosomes: metacentric (p and q in equal lengths), submetacentric (q slightly greater than p), acrocentric (q much greater than p), or telocentric (the centromere terminal).

Where a chromosomal anomaly is detected, it can be present in all or just a certain set of cells within the body, demonstrating what is termed a 'mosaic pattern'. Chromosomal anomalies are usually categorised into three discrete areas:

(1) Numerical abnormalities, where there is an excess or deficit in the normal complement of 46 chromosomes
(2) Structural abnormalities of the chromosomes
(3) Uniparental disomy, caused through non-disjunction of a chromosome pair

Numerical abnormalities

If a haploid gamete or a diploid cell lacks the expected number of chromosomes, aneuploidy exists. Monosomy is the term used to depict where there is a deficit in the expected chromosomal numbers. Although autosomal monosomy is usually lethal (e.g. 45XY) in Turner syndrome, monosomy (45X) is not always lethal.

The term 'trisomy' identifies the presence of an additional chromosome. Autosomal trisomy usually occurs as a result of meiotic non-disjunction, with the most common autosomal trisomy being Trisomy 21 (Down syndrome). Other common trisomy syndromes include Trisomy 18 (Edwards syndrome) and Trisomy 13 (Patau syndrome). The term 'polysomy' is frequently applied if the additional chromosome is a sex chromosome, for example 47XXY (Klinefelter syndrome).

The most common reason for abnormalities in chromosome number is a process called non-disjunction during cell division. Non-disjunction is a failure of separation of the homologous chromosomes during meiosis 1, or of sister chromosomes during meiosis 2. If non-disjunction occurs at meiosis 1, the gamete will have too few chromosomes, or too many if non-disjunction occurs at meiosis 2. Non-disjunction can involve both autosomes and sex chromosomes.

Translocations

Translocations are structural abnormalities where one or more chromosomes break and there is an exchange of genetic material between two or more chromosomes. Translocations are classified into two main types, a Reciprocal translocation and a Robertsonian translocation. In a Reciprocal translocation, the broken fragments of two different chromosomes exchange places. A Robertsonian translocation, however, occurs in acrocentric chromosomes where the centromere is situated near one end, with one arm much longer than the other. Acrocentric chromosomes are Group D (13, 14, and 15) and Group G (21, 22). In these trans-locations two whole chromosomes merge together through the fusion of their centromeres. One of the most important Robertsonian translocations involves chromosomes 14 and 21.

Translocations are important in heredity, disability and chronic illness depend-ing on whether they are balanced or unbalanced. Where infants are phenotypic-ally normal and the translocation is referred to as balanced, it is assumed that during the translocation no genetic material was lost or gained and infants are not themselves affected. However, as they are carriers, in adulthood they should carefully consider their decision to have children, as their children could inherit what is termed an unbalanced form of the translocation. However, if infants are phenotypically abnormal, an unbalanced arrangement, either deficiency or duplication of genetic material, is assumed and the translocation is referred to as unbalanced (Simpson & Elias, 2003). The degree of disability for a child will depend upon which chromosomes are affected and the extent of genetic material lost or gained. There will, unfortunately though, always be some degree of dis-ability in an unbalanced translocation.

Deletions and duplications

Partial chromosome abnormalities involve a deletion (missing) or duplication (extra) segment of a chromosome. A classic deletion syndrome is Cri du chat, where there is a deletion of the short arm of chromosome 5. Contiguous gene syn-drome has been used to identify smaller sections of chromosome abnormalities, such as microdeletions and duplications. The end result is an altered, normal gene dosage, which leads to a specific and complex phenotype that, in some cases, is recognised as a generic syndrome (Skirton & Patch, 2002). Some major contiguous gene syndromes include DiGeorge syndrome and Prader-Willi syndrome, both occurring as a result of microdeletions. DiGeorge syndrome involves chromo-some 22 and children with this syndrome tend to have cardiac defects, learning difficulties, feeding and speech problems due to a cleft palate or weakness of the palate. Other medical problems can be kidney abnormalities, poor immune systems, and neurological and endocrine abnormalities. Prader-Willi syndrome involves a microdeletion on chromosome 15. Classic features of this syndrome include floppy muscles and, initially, poor feeding and weight gain. However, by three years of age, children with Prader-Willi syndrome develop large appetites and suffer from obesity. There is also associated pubertal delay along with learn-ing and behavioural challenges.

Chromosomal nomenclature

At a certain stage during cell division, chromosomes form into visible structures and can be detected by photography, producing a picture known as an ideogram.

This picture represents the complete diploid number of chromosomes in a cell called the karyotype.

An official chromosomal nomenclature exists (ISCN, 1995) and designates the chromosomal complement in the following manner:

- The total number of chromosomes (e.g. 45, 46 or 47)
- A comma
- The sex chromosome complement (XX in normal females; XY in normal males)
- The specific abnormality, if any

A + or − sign indicates the addition or absence of autosomes in a complement. This is followed by the specific chromosome responsible.

Examples of official nomenclature include:

46, XY	Normal male karyotype
46, XX	Normal female karyotype
45, X	Monosomy X
47, XXX	Polysomy X
47, XXY	Polysomy X
47, XY+21	Trisomy 21 Down syndrome
46, XX, Sp-	Cri du chat syndrome (caused by a deletion on the short arm of chromosome S)

Single gene (Mendelian) disorders

Single gene disorders occur as a result of a mutation or defect, usually involving only a single genetic locus, rather than a partial or total chromosomal abnormality. These disorders normally follow a simple, definite inheritance pattern. However, the transmission of mutant genes within families is dependent upon whether the gene is dominant or recessive in nature and also whether the mutant gene is located on an autosome or sex chromosome. This leads to the possibility of five transmission patterns:

- Autosomal dominant
- Autosomal recessive
- X-linked dominant
- X-linked recessive
- Y-linked

If the homologous chromosomes contain both dominant genes, then the genotype is homozygous dominant and if both are recessive genes, homozygous recessive. If both dominant and recessive genes are present, then the genotype is heterozygous for that trait. This is illustrated in Punnet squares 1 and 2. Mendelian patterns of inheritance are illustrated in Punnet squares 3–12.

Punnet squares 1 and 2.

Example of homozygous and heterozygous gamete

Father has brown eyes with homozygous dominant gamete (BB) and mother has blue eyes with homozygous recessive gamete (bb).

FATHER		B	B
M O T H E R	b	Bb	Bb
	b	Bb	Bb

All offspring will have brown eyes and be heterozygous (Bb) for that trait.

If that child, when an adult, has a child with a partner who has blue eyes with homozygous recessive gamete (bb)

Child now Adult		B	b
P A R T N E R	b	Bb	bb
	b	Bb	bb

then there will be a 50% chance of the offspring having brown eyes and being heterozygous (Bb) for that trait and a 50% chance their child will have blue eyes and be homozygous recessive.

Autosomal recessive inheritance

A large proportion of genetic diseases appear to be inherited in a recessive manner. Consequently, for the gene mutation to be expressed, the offspring must be homozygous recessive for that trait. The heterozygous offspring will be carriers for that gene mutation, with the ability to transfer it to their own children. Examples of autosomal recessive disorders include cystic fibrosis, thalassaemia, sickle cell anaemia and phenylketonuria.

Test your knowledge

With autosomal recessive cystic fibrosis, if one parent has cystic fibrosis and has a child with an adult who is heterozygous for the affected mutant cystic fibrosis gene, what is the percentage chance that their offspring will:

- Be carriers of the cystic fibrosis disease?
- Have cystic fibrosis disease or that their children will be normal?

Punnet squares 3–5.

If the father is heterozygous for the mutant gene cystic fibrosis (Cc) and the mother is homozygous normal (cc)

FATHER			
M O T H E R		C	c
	c	cC	cc
	c	cC	cc

then there will be a 50% chance of the offspring having heterozygous (Cc) and being carriers for cystic fibrosis.

If the father is heterozygous for the mutant gene cystic fibrosis (Cc) and the mother is heterozygous for the mutant gene cystic fibrosis (Cc)

FATHER			
M O T H E R		C	c
	C	CC	Cc
	c	Cc	cc

then there will be a 50% chance of the offspring having heterozygous (Cc) and being carriers for cystic fibrosis, a 25% chance their child will be homozygous normal (cc) and a 25% chance that they will be have cystic fibrosis and be homozygous (CC).

FATHER			
M O T H E R		C	C
	c	cC	cC
	c	cC	cC

If a parent who has cystic fibrosis, and is therefore homozygous for the mutant affected gene, has a child with an unaffected homozygous adult their offspring will all be carriers.

For all Punnet square examples, C is the defective mutant cystic fibrosis gene.

Autosomal dominant inheritance

As illustrated by the two Punnet squares, in autosomal dominant inheritance, all affected individuals have an affected parent and there are no carriers. Diseases that have this inheritance pattern include Marfan syndrome, myotonic dystrophy, achondroplasia, neurofibromatosis and Noonan syndrome. If a parent is heterozygous affected with, for example, myotonic dystrophy, then there is a 50%

chance that their offspring will have myotonic dystrophy (Punnet 6). If both parents are heterozygous affected with the dominant mutant myotonic dystrophy then there is a 25% chance that their offspring will be normal, a 50% chance that they will have myotonic dystrophy (heterozygous expressed) and a 25% chance that they will have myotonic dystrophy (homozygous expressed), although generally the foetus is non-viable (Punnet 7).

Punnet squares 6 and 7.

EXAMPLE 6			
	FATHER		
M O T H E R		M	m
	m	mM	mm
	m	mM	mm

EXAMPLE 7			
	FATHER		
M O T H E R		M	m
	M	MM	Mm
	m	mM	mm

For both Punnet square examples, M is the defective mutant haemophilia A gene.

X-linked recessive inheritance

As illustrated by the three Punnet squares, in X-linked recessive inheritance, males are principally affected. Haemophilia A and B, and Duchenne muscular dystrophy are the more commonly known diseases that have this inheritance. If the father, for example has haemophilia A, then his sons will be normal and his daughters will be carriers of the haemophilia trait (Punnet 8). If the mother is a carrier of the recessive mutant haemophilia gene, then half the daughters will be carriers and half the boys will have haemophilia A (Punnet 9).

Test your knowledge

With sex-linked recessive haemophilia A, if the father has haemophilia A and the mother is a carrier for the defective mutant haemophilia gene, what is the percentage chance that their sons and daughters will:

- Be carriers of haemophilia A
- Have haemophilia A
- Be normal?

Punnet squares 8–10.

EXAMPLE 8			
		FATHER	
		אּ	Y
M O T H E R	X	אּ X	XY
	X	אּ X	XY

EXAMPLE 9			
		FATHER	
		X	Y
M O T H E R	אּ	אּ X	אּ Y
	X	XX	XY

EXAMPLE 10			
		FATHER	
		X	Y
M O T H E R	אּ	אּ X	אּ Y
	אּ	אּ X	אּ Y

If the mother has the disease because the mutant recessive gene is located on both the mother's X chromosome then all boys (46, XY) will express the mutation as they have no other X chromosome to challenge it.

For all three Punnet square examples אּ is the defective mutant haemophilia A gene.

X-linked dominant inheritance

As illustrated by the two Punnet squares 11 and 12, in-linked dominant inheritance, all affected individuals have an affected parent and there are no carriers. A disease that has this inheritance pattern is Fragile X syndrome. If the father is affected, for example has Fragile X syndrome, then his sons will be normal and his daughters will have Fragile X syndrome (although generally more mildly) (Punnet 11). If the mother has Fragile X syndrome then half the daughters will have Fragile X syndrome and half the boys will have Fragile X syndrome (Punnet 12).

Inherited variations

Not all diseases, however, follow the traditional patterns of inheritance. This can involve either single genes or the whole chromosome. Some diseases can express both dominant and recessive inheritance patterns, for example osteogenesis imperfecta, commonly known as brittle bone disease. Osteogenesis imperfecta is caused by an abnormality in the maturation of collagen protein, resulting in skeletal alterations such as bone fragility and low bone mass, along with connect-

Punnet squares 11 and 12.

EXAMPLE 11				EXAMPLE 12			

	FATHER		
M O T H E R		א	Y
	X	א X	XY
	X	א X	XY

	FATHER		
M O T H E R		X	Y
	א	א X	א Y
	X	XX	XY

For both Punnet square examples, א is the defective mutant Fragile X gene.

ive tissue manifestations such as hyperlaxity of ligaments and skin. Arising from both autosomal dominant and recessive forms of inheritance, or as a consequence of a spontaneous mutation, osteogenesis imperfecta has clinical features and diagnosis types ranging from mild to severe forms including perinatal lethality. The condition often leads to an increased likelihood of bone fractures, hearing impairment, loose teeth, shortness in stature and bruising. The presence of blue or grey sclera is a controversial diagnostic feature in the infant age range as it can be found in healthy individuals (Rauch & Glorieux, 2004). Table 1.1 illustrates chronic childhood conditions and their inheritance patterns.

Table 1.1   Patterns of inheritance.

Patterns of inheritance	
Autosomal dominant	**Autosomal recessive**
Achondroplasia	Cystic fibrosis
Huntington's chorea	Congenital adrenal hypoplasia
Myotonic dystrophy	Osteogenesis imperfecta
Marfan syndrome	Phenylketonuria
Neurofibromatosis	Sickle cell disease
Noonan syndrome	Thalassaemia
Ostetogenesis imperfecta	Wilson disease
Spherocytosis	
Sex-linked dominant	**Sex-linked recessive**
Fragile X syndrome	Duchenne muscular dystrophy
	Haemophilia A and B
	Hunter disease
Multi-factorial	
Neural tube defects	Cardiac defects
Cleft lip/and or palate	Renal agenesis
Pyloric stenosis	Congenital dislocation of the hip
Hypospadias	Talipes

Adapted from Wong, 1999.

Test your knowledge

(1) Using nomenclature, how would the following be described in a cytogenic report?

    (a) A normal male chromosome arrangement
    (b) A chromosomal arrangement indicative of Turner syndrome
    (c) A chromosomal arrangement of Edwards syndrome
    (d) A chromosomal arrangement where there is a microdeletion on the short arm of chromosome S

(2) Describe the change to the normal human chromosome pattern designated by the following:

    (a)   47, XY +18
    (b)   48, XXXX

(3) What are the three main areas of chromosomal anomalies?
(4) Where is the centromere positioned in acrocentric chromosomes?
(5) Name three antenatal screening techniques.
(6) Identify three important reasons why children's nurses need knowledge of genetics.

As highlighted at the beginning of this chapter, knowledge and understanding of genetics is important to children's nurses, with the Department of Health (2003) emphasising that genetic knowledge is important for health professionals at all levels. With advances in scientific findings within the field of genetics, nurses are likely to become increasingly involved in the delivery of advice and support for children, young people and their families affected by genetic deviations (Jenkins *et al.*, 2001; Skirton *et al.*, 2005). Information related to the genetic basis of a child's condition needs to be given sensitively, requiring the nurse to have the necessary knowledge, to be able to access relevant information and direct children, young people and families to appropriate sources. (See the list of websites at the end of the chapter.) This chapter will now explore the study of the causes or origins of disease or chronic conditions, defined as aetiology, of which genetics is just one aspect.

The aetiology of many chronic conditions such as cystic fibrosis (CF) or Duchenne muscular dystrophy (DMD) can be relatively simple to explain or, as in the case of type 1 diabetes or eczema, may involve complex factors that may not reflect the expression of severity of a child's condition. As previously described in this chapter, although CF results from a single gene mutation, there is multisystem involvement for the child. The aetiology of type 1 diabetes or eczema cannot be explained in such simple genetic terms. When a child has type 1 diabetes, just one cell type within the pancreas malfunctions at diagnosis or, in the case of eczema, just the skin is affected. There may be a genetic influence relating to the chronic condition, but other factors can be involved in the onset of disease. Aetiological factors can include diet, lifestyle, infection, aberrations in foetal developmental or a chronic condition being part of another syndrome. For example, epilepsy can be part of Fragile X syndrome or a metabolic disorder. (See Scottish

Inter-Collegiate Network (SIGN), 2005 guidelines for a list of conditions where epilepsy can be a feature.) A chronic condition can manifest itself at any time during childhood, from the antenatal period to 18 years of age, and into adulthood. The genetic condition, Huntington's chorea, normally manifests in adulthood and is rarely seen in childhood. Although multi-factorial conditions such as coronary heart disease are identified in adulthood, early risk factors for cardiac disease are now being identified in pre-adolescent children (Muratova *et al.*, 2002), particularly in children classed as obese. In Chapter 5, the implications of obesity in children and young people with chronic illnesses are discussed. Via various screening programmes, the identification of chronic conditions in children begins as early as the prenatal period and continues throughout childhood.

Antenatal period

Using improved antenatal screening techniques, many conditions are identified before the baby is born, leading to a chronic illness diagnosis. Problems that can be identified in the foetus include congenital heart defects (CHDs), Fragile X and osteogenesis imperfecta.

 Time out

Suggest some of the antenatal screening procedures that may be employed to identify specific chronic illnesses.

Response

- Ultrasonography to identify:
  - organ and bone structure
  - size of foetus
- Chorionic villus sampling to identify:
  - genetic or chromosomal abnormalities
- Amniocentesis to identify:
  - genetic or chromosomal abnormalities

 Case study 1.1

An ultrasound examination has identified a congenital heart defect in a foetus at 18 weeks gestation. What information could be gained from parents that may reveal the aetiology of this condition? Consider your response in relation to pre-pregnancy issues and factors during pregnancy. You may consider elements from a family history that may reveal important information leading to possible identification of aetiology for the heart condition.

Development of the heart during the foetal period is very complex and can be arrested or altered by several factors. Impairment may occur as a result of terato-genic influences such as infection or drugs taken by the mother during the first trimester of pregnancy. Drugs used in the treatment of epilepsy are known to cross the placenta (Adab *et al.*, 2005) and increase the risk of CHD in the foetus. The contraction of an infection such as rubella by the mother is known to increase the risk of CHD (Vyse *et al.*, 2002). In addition to infection, if the mother has a chronic condition, the risks increase for CHD in the child. A mother who has diabetes preconceptually has an increased risk of 3.6% for the child developing CHD compared to non-diabetic mothers (Wren *et al.*, 2003). The mechanism that leads to an alteration of foetal heart development has not yet been determined. A heart condition may not be present in isolation but be part of a broader syn-drome such as Triploidy, Trisomies 13, 18 and 21, Noonan syndrome or DiGeorge syndrome (Manning *et al.*, 2005). A family history can reveal other family mem-bers with different syndromes or heart defects and small chromosomal deletions or translocations have been implicated. Studies also reveal an increased occur-rence of CHD during foetal development where a parent has defective heart valves (Lewin *et al.*, 2004). Both autosomal recessive and dominant inheritance have been implicated.

 Case study 1.2

During an ultrasound antenatal scan, it is noted that the skeletal system of the foetus does not appear completely normal. The limbs are shorter than average and bowed. The foetus also has a degree of scoliosis. From what condition may the foetus be suffering?

There is a wide range of differential diagnoses that could be suggested (Hurst *et al.*, 2005) and the presence or absence of fractures would be significant. In the absence of fractures, it is possible that the child will have one of the dwarfing syndromes such as achondroplasia or thanatophoric dysplasia, both of autosomal dominant aetiology. If there are fractures seen on the scan, osteogenesis imper-fecta (OI) is more likely to be suggested. Again this condition, which was dis-cussed earlier, has both autosomal recessive and dominant forms.

It is not always possible to reach a diagnosis until further investigations such as genetic testing via amniocentesis or chorionic villus sample are carried out. Although the aetiology of these conditions is known to be genetic, both achon-droplasia and type 2 OI have been noted to result from new mutations in most cases (Lipson, 2005), and in some cases of OI, it has been found that a parent has cell mosaicism. If a parent is known to have a chronic skeletal condition such as OI, genetic analysis can be carried out earlier in pregnancy by chorionic villus sampling.

Time out

Using Punnet squares estimate the risk for the children in the following situations:

(1) The mother has achondroplasia and the father does not.
(2) The father is heterozygous for osteogenesis imperfecta (OI) and the mother is genetically normal for OI (does not carry the OI gene).

Response

(1) In this example the father is heterozygous for osteogenesis imperfecta and the mother does not have the condition. Because the condition is autosomal domin-ant, the risk is that 50% of the children will have the condition.

	FATHER	
M O T H E R	O	σ
σ	O σ	σ σ
σ	O σ	σ σ

(2) Again, because achondroplasia is autosomal dominant, if the mother has the condition and the father does not, 50% of the children are at risk of inheriting the condition.

	FATHER	
M O T H E R	a	a
A	A a	A a
a	a a	a a

Both amniocentesis and chorionic villus sampling can be used for other genetic and chromosomal problems

The neonatal period

During the first 28 days of life (the neonatal period), many chronic conditions can be diagnosed either following direct observation of the infant, or as a result of signs that are characteristic of certain physiological problems. When problems are suspected, further investigations need to be carried out to confirm a diagnosis. For instance, CHDs that have not been identified earlier may be suspected if the child is cyanosed and has tachypnoea. A neonate may have seizures or unexplained hypoglycaemia, which could indicate a diagnosis of a metabolic or endocrine disorder.

During the neonatal period, a range of chronic conditions can be identified by a heel prick test. This is carried out by allowing four large drops of blood to drop from the baby's heel onto a prepared absorbent paper, which is then left to dry before laboratory testing. This is sometimes called the PKU test (from phenylke-tonuria, the condition for which the test was originally devised), or the Guthrie test (from the name of the scientist who developed the test for PKU in the 1960s).

 Time out

Identify the chronic conditions that can be diagnosed by the heel prick test carried out within the first week of life. Suggest the aetiology of these.

Response

Phenylketonuria	Autosomal recessive
Duchenne muscular dystrophy	X-linked recessive
Hypothyroidism	Multifactorial
Cystic fibrosis	Autosomal recessive
Sickle cell disease	Autosomal recessive
Thalassaemia	Autosomal recessive
Galactosaemia and other metabolic disorders	Usually autosomal recessive

Identification of these conditions would not have occurred until the post-neonatal age prior to this test being carried out. Diagnosis would have been made as symptoms arose and/or the child's physical health deteriorated. There would be a deterioration of cognitive and mental health development in a child who has phenylketonuria or hypothyroidism. The aetiology of PKU is autosomal recessive inheritance whereas that of hypothyroidism has multiple origins, although genetic origins have been identified (Straight *et al.*, 2003) in about 15% of instances.

According to Hunter *et al.* (2000), 25:100 000 cases of hypothyroidism are congenital. In a comprehensive account of childhood hypothyroidism, Straight *et al.* (2003) explain the pathology that results in the condition. Agenesis, dysplasia or absence of the thyroid gland occurring as an aberration of foetal development, result in reduced or absent secretion of thyroid hormones. A lack of production of these hormones may also result from a defect of other body systems that normally would, through their release of enzymes or hormones, maintain or stimulate thyroid function. One example of this would be a defective pituitary gland that produces the thyroid stimulating hormone, an essential hormone for normal functioning of the thyroid gland. Although PKU and hypothyroidism are relatively uncommon in the UK, 1:10 000 and 1:4000 births respectively (Medical Screening Society, 1999; 2000), nurses may be involved with the family at the time of diagnosis. Due to the absence of any indication of a problem during the neonatal period, families can experience a range of emotions on being told of the diagnosis. Chapter 3 examines theories of grief and loss and models of adaptation associated with families following the diagnosis of their child with a chronic disorder.

Post-neonatal period

More commonly, conditions are diagnosed after the first month of life, even though their origins may be present earlier. A number of neuro/musculo/skeletal problems can develop such as Duchenne muscular dystrophy, which is well recognised as an X-linked recessive genetic disorder. Signs of the disorder will not be evident until the child is aged 2–4 years, when physical development milestones are not achieved and the child begins to lose motor ability. (See Chapter 7 for a more detailed discussion of a child with a neuromotor disability, the resulting physical and psychosocial effects, and the required associated care management pathway.) Other conditions identified after the first month of life include epilepsy, type 1 diabetes and juvenile arthritis.

  Time out

Identify factors that may influence the onset of epilepsy. You need to consider issues such as environmental, genetic, medical history and trauma.

Epilepsy can develop at any age, with most diagnoses being made after the neonatal period and before the age of 20 years, often causing distress for the children, young people and their families. A diagnosis of epilepsy is only made following two or more seizures and many children suffer one isolated seizure. Studies of aetiology of this condition suggest neuropathological origins. This could be an insult by an infection such as encephalitis or meningitis, or as a result of a tumour or trauma caused during delivery or an accident. However, children who exhibit the same disease process do not necessarily develop epilepsy, or, if epilepsy does develop, the same phenotypical epilepsy. It has also been noted that epilepsy can develop following complex febrile convulsions (Verity & Golding, 1991) and that febrile seizures may be a marker of a child's seizure threshold (Camfield *et al.*, 1994). As with cardiac malformations, epilepsy can be a feature of a more complex syndrome (SIGN, 2005), which would lead to the child requiring more complex care. As a single disorder, one of the features of epilepsy is the unpredictable nature of its expression. A child may have seizures infrequently and/or irregularly, and the expression of the epilepsy may be shown by a child having different types of seizure: complex and/or partial.

Other aetiological factors are known and studies have suggested a genetic influence to the development of the condition, although this is not always conclusive. A definite genetic aetiology for epilepsy, where there is no other identified pathology, accounts for at least 50% of sufferers (Johnson & Sander, 2001). Investigations into twin studies have confirmed a genetic link (Berkovic *et al.*, 1998). In dizygotic twins, the likelihood of both developing epilepsy (18%) is higher than for the general population (approximately 1% by the age of 20 years) (Hauser, 1995), and in monozygotic twins, epilepsy is expressed in 60% of twin pairs, where epilepsy is seen in one or both children. Identifying epilepsy via genetic screening would be a complex process, as mutations have been identified on several chromosomes. There are also complexities in relation to genotype and phenotype with this condition, where the same phenotype expressed in two people has been found to have different genotypes (Johnson & Sander, 2001).

 Case study 1.3

A five-year-old boy has been diagnosed with type 1 diabetes. The parents do not know of any close relatives who have the condition. What information could you give when the parents ask what has caused this?

Even greater complexity in aetiology has been highlighted for type 1 diabetes. A number of nutritional influences have been documented in studies involving children with type 1 diabetes, including failure to breast-feed or short duration of breast-feeding and the early introduction of cow's milk and soya proteins (Dahlquist, 1998). The mechanism that initiates the auto-immune process of destruction of beta cells in the pancreas and the reason why some children develop the condition and others do not, is not understood. Protective genes have been identified to prevent this process, but other gene mutations are known to influence the onset (Todd, 1999). As with epilepsy, these are not single gene mutations, but loci are found on a number of chromosomes, although a marker on chromosome 6 has been identified as a common link in some population groups (Greenberg *et al.*, 2000). Twin studies show a much lower concordance in comparison with those that investigate epilepsy prevalence, with views that genetic risk factors are stimulated by environmental influences. The levels of type 1 diabetes in children 0–16 years increased from 3.1:100 000 to levels similar to the indigenous population, 11.7:100 000, when families moved from an area where type 1 diabetes is not commonly seen to one where it is more common (Bodansky *et al.*, 1992). This may be the result of contact with resident viruses that are thought to play a role in the aetiology of type 1 diabetes, particularly in children (Hyöty & Taylor, 2002). Viruses that have been implicated as a result of infection in children and timing of onset of diabetes are enteroviruses, pertussis and rubella. A number of studies have also shown a link between maternal viral infection during pregnancy and childhood onset of type 1 diabetes (Hyöty & Taylor, 2002).

Researchers are challenged in identifying risk factors for diabetes as the incidence is increasing, which cannot be explained through genetic aetiology. Single gene, recessive or dominant conditions, or sex-linked conditions follow the same inheritance patterns over time, and the incidence remains relatively unchanged, such as with cystic fibrosis or achondroplasia. Vaccines are now used to prevent pertussis and rubella in most of the population, thus potentially decreasing the prevalence of type 1 diabetes as a result of this risk factor.

Challenges are also evident in identifying aetiology of allergic conditions affecting this age group. Again, there appear to be genetic influences, but these are not straightforward and the research is sometimes conflicting. Much of the literature discusses more than one allergic condition, including food allergies, asthma, eczema and/or allergic rhinitis (hay fever). Those affected children whose parent/s had allergic conditions were at greater risk, although this inheritance pattern was not always strong. Links between atopic disease and T helper cell function and IgE productions have been identified (Stone, 2003). Infections in childhood have been implicated in these conditions although aetiological explanations are complex, particularly for asthma and allergic rhinitis. Holt and Sly (2002) suggest there is protection against development of non-atopic asthma and allergy, but atopic asthma is triggered following respiratory infections in childhood. Exposure to older siblings has been found to reduce the risk of developing asthma, eczema and allergic rhinitis, except early onset asthma (before the age of two years) (McKeever *et al.*, 2001). Perhaps having older siblings provided an early and constant exposure to a wide variety of organisms, somehow protecting susceptible genes from being over-stimulated, leading to allergic disease. Holt and Sly (2002) speculate that a child may have genes that are susceptible to interaction with environmental triggers, with a number of triggers being recognised to exacerbate allergic chronic conditions. However, the onset of the disease process is not fully understood (Wadonda-Kabonda *et al.*, 2004). Reactions are seen in a child following ingestion of certain foods to which the child is sensitive and links have been found between food allergies and asthma (Roberts & Lack, 2003), with increasing severity of the condition when a child consumes particular foods. Unfortunately, whether the food allergy or the asthma appears first is not stated. Dietary intake can also be seen to influence atopic eczema (Fiocchi *et al.*, 2004) but it is not suggested that this is a cause of eczema.

Most cases of eczema are seen in the first three months of life, and food allergies by 12 months of age. Other factors are known to influence expression of the disease, which affects around 10% of children (McNally *et al.*, 1998). Multiple causes are suggested, including several from the environment. A class gradient is seen with a higher prevalence among social classes I and II, which may be a reflection of environmental factors such as dietary intake and pollution. This may also be related to the increased incidence among people migrating from a low prevalence area to a geographical area of higher prevalence.

Although it is well known that eczema and asthma affect children, it is not commonly recognised that chronic arthritis can affect those under the age of 18 years. Many consider that this group of chronic conditions only affect older people (Arthritis Research Campaign 2004), but there are a number of arthritic conditions that are seen in children of all ages. It is a complex group of conditions affecting the joints, causing pain, swelling and restricted movement for the child.

(L) Time out

Access the Arthritis Society website http://www.arthritis.ca/types and identify the different types of arthritis that may be seen in childhood

---

The variety, expression and types of conditions are also reflected in the range of aetiologies, which are still not fully understood (Arthritis and Musculoskeletal Alliance, 2004). Auto-immune processes are evident and infections have been implicated. Arthritis has been seen following a number of viral and bacterial infections (Lee & Hall, 2000). The rubella virus has been isolated from affected joints when neither natural infection nor vaccination has occurred. Seasonal variation of onset has been noted that may be linked with infections, which themselves may predominate at different times of the year (Murray *et al.*, 1997). In addition, there are genetic origins to juvenile chronic arthritis, with gene mutations identified on several chromosomes (Murray *et al.*, 1997).

As most children and young people will be cared for at home, children's nurses may see few children and young people admitted to hospital with arthritis. This may result in nurses having limited knowledge and understanding of juvenile arthritis, thus leading to difficulties in the nursing care of these children and families. With about 1 child per 1000 being affected (Arthritis Research Campaign, 2004), it is likely that at some time during their practice, many children's nurses will be involved in the nursing care of these children and young people, and their families. Parents may be shocked to learn of their child's diagnosis (refer to Chapter 3 for family response to recent diagnosis of their child with a chronic illness) and it is important that nurses are able to offer advice, and have an understanding of psychological and practical issues related to the care of the child. It is suggested that following initial diagnosis parents and children may need longer appointment times, in comparison with adults, to discuss some of these issues with a clinical nurse specialist (Arthritis and Musculoskeletal Alliance, 2004). Parents and children will need information, and children's nurses need to have knowledge of the problem and be able to suggest sources of information for parents and for the patient, such as the websites referenced at the end of this chapter.

Adolescent period

Some conditions, the aetiology of which have already been discussed, may begin or be first diagnosed at almost any time during childhood, such as epilepsy, type 1 diabetes, allergic conditions or arthritis. Other chronic problems are more commonly first seen during adolescence or early adulthood, although these can occasionally occur before the teenage years. One group of chronic conditions with a peak diagnostic age of 15–25 years (Parkes & Jewell, 2001) is irritable or inflammatory bowel disease (IBD), with the two most common being identified as Crohn's disease (CD) and ulcerative colitis (UC). The molecular origins of this group of conditions remain largely unknown, but significant research has identified complex factors that appear to contribute to their development. A number of research studies focus on Crohn's disease and ulcerative colitis, showing some similarities but considerable differences between aetiological elements. It is suggested by Thompson-Chagoyan et al. (2005) that an abnormality in the function of the gut barrier, when one or more of these elements is present, or increased gut permeability (Korzenik, 2005), may predispose the individual to IBD.

In a comprehensive literature review of the genetic basis of CD and UC, Parkes and Jewell (2001) identified research showing monozygotic twin concordance of 35%, and dizygotic twin concordance of 7%, for CD, with only 11% and 3% respectively for UC. They report gene mutations on a range of chromosomes for the two conditions, some of which are common to both. Another factor that may suggest a genetic link is the increased risk between certain population groups, for example among Ashkenazi Jews, and the reduced risk among the Afro-Caribbean population. This may also suggest links to lifestyle factors common to groups, which may increase the risk of developing IDB. Dietary intake has been considered as an influence in the deterioration of UC (Jowett et al., 2004; Magee et al., 2005), and thus may also trigger the onset. A high intake of meat and meat products, eggs and fat has been linked to relapses of UC (Jowett et al., 2004), and sulphur in different chemical compositions, commonly used in many processed foods, has also been shown to be detrimental to UC (Jowett et al., 2004, Magee et al., 2005). Smoking is another lifestyle factor that may reduce deterioration in UC, but certainly does cause deterioration in CD (Johnson et al., 2005). Smoking, therefore, may have some influence in the onset of CD, particularly as its onset coincides with the time when many young people begin smoking. This emphasises the importance of the role of the children's nurse in giving advice to young people on the many risks to their health of continued smoking. Alternatively, children's nurses could be challenged in their ability to give health promotion advice in relation to smoking if a young person has UC, when the condition is less severe among smokers.

In addition to these factors, infection has been implicated as contributing to IBD (Roediger & Macfarlane, 2002; Korzenik, 2005). Mycoplasms and helicobacter have been identified in patients, and measles has been implicated but not identified as being present in more patients with CD than in the general population (Ghosh et al., 2001).

Conclusion

As initially discussed at the start of this chapter, the need for children's nurses to have genetic knowledge, including the understanding of aetiology of chronic illness in children, is an important element of their practice. Several examples were given where there are opportunities for introducing strategies in care management to lead to a reduced risk of conditions occurring, or a reduction in severity for those where a condition has been identified. Examples given earlier related to advice for a young person or parents considering further pregnancies. When a known genetic cause for a chronic condition is identified such as an autosomal recessive (e.g. CF or phenylketonuria) or dominant gene mutation (e.g. osteogenesis imperfecta or achondroplasia), children's nurses can become involved in genetic advice, which can help couples come to decisions about future pregnancies. Indeed, it may be the young person who is embarking on a sexual relationship and seeks help about future children. These decisions are not easy and may be more difficult if a sporadic gene mutation is identified. Alternatively, if someone has a genetic condition and that person is considering parenthood, advice can be given regarding pregnancy and risk factors. Risk factors include the mother's health during pregnancy if she is the one with the condition.

In relation to conditions where lifestyle has an impact, nurses, health visitors and midwives can advise families, including the child who has the chronic illness, on ways to make lifestyle changes where this would be advantageous to the child or young person's well-being. Children's nurses or school nurses could implement strategies that target children and/or parents to develop healthy lifestyles. This can lead to a reduced risk of some chronic illnesses such as type 2 diabetes.

Specialist nurses are in the best position to address psychological aspects of care and provide a range of information. Following diagnosis is a time when families, including the child if he or she is old enough to understand, need information relating to the condition. Also, support is needed, which may be nursing, medical, social or psychological. This support can be more comprehensive if the nurse has a good knowledge base of the aetiology of the condition. Support for families is an important aspect of care that can influence the long-term psychological outcome for the child or young person with a chronic condition (Immelt, 2000).

With advances in genetics and the increasing impetus for the development of strategies to ameliorate or cure chronic conditions with genetic origins, it is becoming increasingly important that nurses develop competence in the area of genetics. They will need not only to give appropriate information in an understandable way to those who need the help, whatever their culture (Middleton *et al.*, 2005), but also to be aware of other multidisciplinary agencies or support networks to which young people and/or parents can be referred for counselling. Due to genetics being of high media and public interest, particularly in relation to the complexities and ethical issues surrounding cloning, the manipulation of genes through gene therapy and the uncertainties of the long-term outcomes, it is essential that nurses caring for children and young people develop their genetic knowledge and understanding. They must, along with other professionals, be able to fully participate in the relevant debates and ethical discussions that can have implications for children, young people and their families.

> **Key points**
>
> - Developing genetic knowledge and competence is essential for children's nurses and children's nursing.
> - A chronic condition can manifest itself at any time during childhood, from the antenatal period to 18 years of age, and into adulthood.

Useful websites

Antenatal screening resources
www.antenataltesting.info

Bio-News: latest genetic information
www.BioNews.org.uk

British Society for Human Genetics
www.bshg2.org.uk/

Contact a family for background information on a wide range of chronic conditions
www.cafamily.org.uk

Genetics home reference which gives basic information on genetics
http://ghr.nlm.nig.gov/ghr/page/Home

Genetic Iinterest Group: national alliance of 120 organisations that support children, families and individuals affected by genetic disorders.
www.gig.org.uk

Gene Sense, giving information on science, ethics and practice issues using case studies
www.genesense.org.uk

Human Genetics Commission
www.hgc.gov.uk

Muscular Dystrophy
www.muscular-dystrophy.org

International Society for Nurses in Genetics
www.ISONG.ORG

The Cambridge Genetics Knowledge Park
www.cgkp.org.uk

The Child Growth Foundation
www.cgf.org.uk

The Genetic Interest Group: support networks for individuals and families
www.gig.org.uk

The Turner Syndrome Support Society
www.tss.org.uk

The Wales Gene Park
www.walesgenepark.co.uk

The Wellcome Trust for information on genetics, ethics and the Human Genome Project
www.wellcome.ac.uk/en/genome/index.html

UK National Screening Committee
www.nsc.nhs.uk

http://www.arthritis.ca/types

References

Adab, N., Tudur Smith, C., Vinten, J., Williamson, P.R. & Winterbottom, J.J. (2005) Common anti-epileptic drugs in pregnancy in women with epilepsy. *The Cochrane Database of Systematic Reviews*, **4**.

Arthritis and Musculoskeletal Alliance (2004) *Standards of Care for People with Inflammatory Arthritis*. London, Arthritis and Musculoskeletal Alliance.

Arthritis Research Campaign (2004) http://www.arc.org.uk Accessed 7/12/06.

Barr, O.G. & McConkey, R. (2006) Supporting parents who have a child referred for genetic investigation: the contribution of health visitors. *Journal of Advanced Nursing*, **54** (2), 141–150.

Berkovic, S.F., Howell, R.A., Hay, D.A. & Hopper, J.L. (1998) Epilepsies in twins: genetics of the major epilepsy syndromes. *Annals of Neurology*, **16** (6), 16–20.

Bodansky, H.J., Staines, A., Stephenson, C., Haigh, D. & Cartwright, R. (1992) Evidence for an environmental effect of the aetiology of insulin dependent diabetes in a transmigratory population. *British Medical Journal*, **304** (6833), 1020–1022.

Bradley, A.N. (2005) Utility and limitations of genetic testing and information. *Nursing Standard*, **20** (5), 52–55.

Burke, S. & Kirk, M. (2006) Genetics education in the nursing profession: literature review. *Journal of Advanced Nursing*, **54** (2), 228–237.

Camfield, P., Camfield, C., Gordan, K. & Dooley, J. (1994) What types of epilepsy are preceded by febrile seizures? A population-based study of children. *Development Medicine and Child Neurology*, **36** (10), 887–892.

Dahlquist, G. (1998) The aetiology of type 1 diabetes: an epidemiological perspective. *Acta Pædiatr*, (Suppl. 425), 5–10.

Department of Health (2003) *Our Inheritance, Our Future. Realising the Potential of Genetics in the NHS*. London, The Stationery Office.

Edgar, D.A. (2004) Advances in genetics: implications for children, families and nurses. *Paediatric Nursing*, **16** (6), 26–29.

Fiocchi, A., Bouygue, G.R., Martelli, A., Terracciano, L. & Sarratud, T. (2004) Dietary treatment of childhood atopic eczema/dermatitis syndrome (AEDS). *Allergy*, **59** (Suppl. 78), 5.

Ghosh, S., Armitage, E. & Wilson, D. (2001) Detection of persistent measles virus infection in Crohn's disease: current status of experimental work. *Gut*, **48**, 748–752.

Greenberg, D.A., Durner, M., Keddache, M. *et al.* (2000) Reproducibility and complications in gene searches: linkage on chromosome 6, heterogeneity, association, and maternal inheritance in juvenile cyclonic epilepsy. *The American Journal of Human Genetics*, **66**, 508–516.

Hauser, W.A. (1995) Epidemiology of epilepsy in children. *Neurosurgical Clinics of North America*, **6** (3), 419–429.

Holt, P.G. & Sly, P.D. (2002) Interactions between respiratory tract infections and atopy in the aetiology of asthma. *European Respiratory Journal*, **19**, 538–545.

Hunter, I., Greene, S.A., MacDonald, T.M. & Morris, A.D. (2000) Prevalence and aetiology of hypothyroidism in the young. *Archives of Disease in Childhood*, **83**, 207–210.

Hurst, J.A., Firth, H.V. & Smith son, S. (2005) Skeletal dysplasia's. *Seminars in Fetal and Neonatal Medicine*, **10** (3), 233–241.

Hyöty, H. & Taylor, K.W. (2002) The role of viruses in human diabetes. *Diabetologia*, **45** (6), 531–534.

Immelt, S.C. (2000) *Correlates of Global Self-worth in Young Children with Chronic Medical Conditions*. The Johns Hopkins University, Unpublished Ph.D.

ISCN (1995) An International System for Human Cytogenetic Nomenclature. F. Mitleman (ed.). Basel, Switzerland, S. Karger.

Jenkins, J.F., Prows, C., Dimond, E., Monson, R. & Williams, J. (2001) Recommendations for educating nurses in genetics. *Journal of Professional Nursing*, **17** (6), 283–290.

Johnson, G.J., Cosnes, J. & Mansfield, J.C. (2005) Review article: smoking cessation as primary therapy to modify the course of Crohn's disease. *Alimentary Pharmacology & Therapeutics*, **21** (8), 921–931.

Johnson, M.R. & Sander, J.W. (2001) The clinical impact of epilepsy genetics. *Journal of Neurology Neurosurgical Psychiatry*, **70** (4), 428–430.

Jones, C. (2004) Genetics: overview and issues in child health. *Paediatric Nursing*, **16** (6), 37–42.

Jowett, S.L., Seal, C.J., Pearce, M.S. *et al.* (2004) Influence of dietary factors on the clinical course of ulcerative colitis: a prospective cohort study. *Gut*, **53**, 1479–1484.

Kenner, C. & Moran, M. (2005) Newborn screening and genetic testing. *Journal of Midwifery and Women's Health*, **50** (3), 219–226.

Kirk, M. (2005) Introduction to the genetics series. *Nursing Standard*, **20** (1), 48.

Kirk, M., McDonald, K., Anstey, S. & Longley, M. (2003) *Fit for Practice in the Genetics Era: A Competence-based Education Framework for Nurses, Midwives and Health Visitors*. Pontypridd, University of Glamorgan.

Korzenik, J.R. (2005) Past and current theories of aetiology of IBD: toothpaste, worms, and refrigerators. *Journal of Clinical Gastroenterology*, **39** (4), supplement 2, 59–65.

Lee, L.H. & Hall, C.B. (2000) Recognising infection-related arthritis. *Contemporary Pediatrics*. Available at: http://mediwire.sma.org/main/Default.aspx?P=Content&ArticleID=139753

Lewin, M.B., McBride, K.L., Pignatelli, R. *et al.* (2004) Echocardiographic evaluation of asymptomatic parental and sibling cardiovascular anomalies associated with congenital left ventricular outflow tract lesions. *Pediatrics*, **114**, 691–696.

Lipson, M.H. (2005) Common neonatal syndromes. *Seminars in Fetal and Neonatal Medicine*, **10** (3), 221–231.

McKeever, T.M., Lewis, S.A., Smith, C. *et al.* (2001) Siblings, multiple births, and the incidence of allergic disease: a birth cohort study using the West Midlands general practice research database. *Thorax*, 758–762.

McNally, N.J., Phillips, D.R. & Williams, H.C. (1998) The problem of atopic eczema; aetiological clues from the environment and lifestyles. *Social Science and Medicine*, **46** (6), 729–741.

Magee, E.A., Edmond, L.M., Tasker, S.M., Choon Kong, S., Curno, R. & Cummings, J.H. (2005) Associations between diet and disease activity in ulcerative colitis patients using a novel method of data analysis. *Nutrition Journal*. Available at: http://www.nutritionj.com/content/4/1/7 Accessed 7/12/06.

Manning, N., Kaufman, L. & Roberts, P. (2005) Genetics of cardiological disorders. *Seminars in Fetal and Neonatal Medicine*, **10** (3), 259–269.

Medical Screening Society (1999) *Phenylketonuria*. Available at: http://www.medicalscreeningsociety.com/screeningbriefs Accessed 7/12/06.

Medical Screening Society (2000) *Hypothyroidism*. Available at: http://www.medicalscreeningsociety.com/screeningbriefs Accessed 7/12/06.

Middleton, A., Mushtaq, A. & Levene, S. (2005) Tailoring genetic information and services to clients' culture, knowledge and language level. *Nursing Standard*, **20** (2), 52–56.

Muratova, V.N., Demerath, E.W., Spangler, E. *et al.* (2002) The relation of obesity to cardio-vascular risk factors among children: the cardiac project. *West Virginia Medical Journal*, **98** (6), 263–267.

Murray, K., Thompson, S.D. & Glass, D.N. (1997) Pathogenesis of juvenile chronic arthritis: genetic and environmental factors. *Archives of Disease in Childhood*, **77**, 530–534.

Parkes, M. & Jewell, D. (2001) *Ulcerative Colitis and Crohn's Disease: Molecular Genetics and Clinical Implications.* Expert Reviews in Molecular Medicine 3. Cambridge, Cambridge University Press. Available at: http://www.expertreviews.org/0100391Xh.htm Accessed 15/02/07.

PET/RCN (2006) *The Progress Guide to Genetics* (3rd edition) London, Progress Educational Trust (with the Royal College of Nursing).

Rauch, F. & Glorieux, F.H. (2004) Osteogenesis imperfecta (seminar). *The Lancet*, **363** (9418), 1377–1385.

Roberts, G. & Lack, G. (2003) Food allergy and asthma – what is the link? *Paediatric Respiratory Review*, **4** (3), 205–212.

Roediger, W.E.W. & Macfarlane, G.T.R. (2002) A role for intestinal mycoplasmas in the aetiology of Crohn's disease? *Journal of Applied Microbiology*, **92** (3), 377–381.

Scottish Inter-Collegiate Network (SIGN) (2005) *Diagnosis and Management of Epilepsies in Children and Young People: a National Clinical Guideline.* Edinburgh, SIGN. Available at: http://www.show.scot.nhs.uk/sign/pdf/sign81.pdf Accessed 7/12/06.

Simpson, J.L. & Elias, S. (2003) *Genetics in Obstetrics and Gynaecology* (3rd edn). Pennsylvania, Saunders.

Skirton, H. & Patch, C. (2002) *Genetics for Healthcare Professionals: a Lifestage Approach.* Oxford, Scientific Publishers Ltd.

Skirton, H., Patch, C. & Williams, J. (2005) *Applied Genetics in Healthcare.* Oxford, Taylor & Francis.

Stone, K. (2003) Atopic disease of children. *Current Opinion in Pediatrics*, **15** (5), 495–511.

Straight, A.M., Bauer, A.J. & Ferry, R.J. (2003) *Hypothyroidism.* Available at: http://www.emedicine.com/ped/topic1141.htm Accessed 21/01/06.

Thompson-Chagoyan, O.C., Maldonado, J. & Gil, A. (2005) Aetiology of inflammatory bowel disease (IBD): role of intestinal microbiota and gut-associated lymphoid tissue immune response. *Clinical Nutrition*, **24** (3), 339–352.

Thurmon, T.F. (1999) *Medical Genetics.* New York, Parthenon Publishing.

Todd, J.A. (1999) From genome to aetiology in a multi-factorial disease, type 1 diabetes. *BioEssays*, **21**, 164–174.

Verity, C.M. & Golding, J. (1991) Risk of epilepsy after febrile convulsions: a national cohort study. *British Medical Journal*, **303** (6814), 1373–1376.

Vyse, A.J., Gay, N.J., White, J.M. *et al.* (2002) Evolution of surveillance of measles, mumps, and rubella in England and Wales: providing the platform for evidence-based vaccination policy. *Epidemiologic Reviews*, **24**, 125–136.

Wadonda-Kabonda, N., Sterne, J.A.C., Golding, J., Kennedy, C.T.C., Archer, C.B. & Dunnill, M.G.S., ALSPAC Study Team (2004) Association of parental eczema, hay fever, and asthma with atopic dermatitis in infancy: birth cohort study. *Archives of Disease in Childhood*, **89**, 917–921.

Wong, D.L. (1999) *Whaley and Wong's Nursing Care of Infants and Children* (sixth edition). St Louis, Mosby.

Wren, C., Birrell, G. & Hawthorne, G. (2003) Cardiovascular malformations in infants of diabetic mothers. *Heart*, **89**, 1217–1220.

2 Context of Care and Service Delivery

Fay Valentine and Peter Mcnee

Introduction

The purpose of this chapter is to explore some of the current political, economic and social policies that are shaping the context of nursing practice and service delivery for children and young people with chronic illnesses. To analyse these external change drivers, examples of service models and nursing roles will be used, demonstrating their influence upon the shifting boundaries of clinical practice and service delivery.

The chapter intends to raise awareness of the issues and challenges that managers, practitioners and service users face as a consequence of these external influences impacting upon their service. An in-depth discussion on the complexities and contentions surrounding the multitude of, and sometimes radical, service delivery models utilised within health care is not within the scope of this chapter, although some of these and the current dialogues surrounding advancing nursing practice will be touched upon in this and subsequent chapters.

Aim of the chapter

To raise awareness and knowledge about the external political, social and economic drivers that are influencing how chronic illness services for children and young people are developing, along with the resulting implications and opportunities for children's nurses.

Intended learning outcomes

- To analyse current political, economic and social policies that are impacting upon service and practice delivery for children and young people with chronic illnesses and their families
- To examine current and future service models and the workforce required for them to be delivered in partnership with children and young people with chronic illnesses and their families
- To explore the complexities surrounding shifting health and social care workforce role boundaries, associated competencies and their impact upon service users, professionals and managers

Context of change

In relation to the provision of health care services for children and young people with chronic illnesses, several external change drivers have been influencing the development and shaping the context of nursing practice for this client group and their families. These external drivers stem from political, economic and social sources and are creating the imperative for health care leaders, managers and professional organisations to review children and young people's journeys through the health care system, reconsider the workforce required for their delivery, examine how the NHS can be more responsive to patients' needs through effective commissioning processes, and implement strategies that enhance cross-organisational boundary and multidisciplinary partnership working.

To realise a long-term vision of an NHS that is patient led, equitable, responsive and at the same time sustainable within the current and future economic and political environments, the Government has strongly influenced the introduction of some key changes. These include introducing patient choice into models of service provision, strengthening governance and accountability arrangements, relinquishing control to more local based health care services and encouraging patients to be fully 'engaged' as partners in their health care. Key political strategies to achieve this have been the development of foundation trusts, managed clinical networks, practice based primary led commissioning, payment by results and the setting of tariffs to create the right incentives to ensure overall system affordability (Wanless, 2002; Department of Health, Social Services and Public Safety Northern Ireland (DHSSPSNI), 2005; Audit Commission, 2004; Foundation Trust Network, 2005; Scottish Executive, 2005a). More recently in England, *Commissioning a Patient Led NHS*, which proposes some radical shifts in the commissioning and delivery of services, has created huge debate regarding the re-emergence of market forces within the NHS (DoH, 2005a).

Political influences

In recent years, the health care and well-being of society has been the focus of increased Governmental and public attention in the UK. This interest was partly driven by the visibility of several high profile public enquiries involving the deaths of children and young people. These reviews made transparent to the public some of the deficits of maintaining a consistently high quality and safe service within the current health care system. These safety risks and quality issues have been attributed to poor partnership working and ineffective communication networks between professional groups and agencies responsible for safeguarding and delivering services to children and young people, thereby leading to fragmentation and critical incidents. Other contributing factors include the inadequate supervision and monitoring of professional practice (Kennedy *et al.*, 2001; Laming, 2003), poor leadership, accountability and governance (Kennedy *et al.*, 2001; Redfern *et al.*, 2001; Carlile, 2002), along with a lack of involving parents in the decision making process. The outcomes from these reviews and, in light of them, mounting public pressure, have encouraged health care policies and recommendations for children and young people's services to be designed and delivered around their needs, and to safeguard them. Key policy initiatives include England's ten-year *Children's Workforce Strategy* programme (DfES, 2005) devised to implement *Every Child Matters* (DfES, 2003), and to reiterate the Government's commitment to supporting and safeguarding children. The new *Children Act* (2004) sets out how children's health, social care and education services in England and Wales will be transformed and improved, and Wales and England have produced their *National Service Framework for Children, Young People and Maternity Services* (DoH, 2004c; WAG, 2005d). Scotland and Ireland are also in the process of reviewing their children and young people's services. To implement these new policy documents and Government strategies, children and young people's services have witnessed the appointment of children's commissioners and national directors, the establishment of children's trusts, the development of managed clinical networks and integrated acute, community and school based services (DfES, 2003; WAG, 2003b; DHSSPSNI, 2005; WAG, 2004; Children and Young People's Specialised Service (CYPSS), 2005; DfES, 2005; DoI I, 2005b).

In response to the aforementioned key Government and subsequent policy documents, some founding principles for children and young people's health care services have been agreed by various professional bodies, voluntary and parent groups and children's welfare organisations. These have been incorporated into the National Service Frameworks for England and Wales (DoH, 2004c; WAG, 2005d) and numerous Royal College of Paediatrics and Child Health (RCPCH) and Royal College of Nursing (RCN) guidance and standard setting documents. These include:

- Better communication and coordination of children and young people's public services
- Child and family empowerment
- Services closer to the child's home
- Children only being admitted to hospital if medically required to do so
- The importance of considering developmental issues with the provision of age appropriate services
- Increasing emphasis upon preventative health and health promotion strategies (RCPCH, 2003a; b; RCN, 2003; 2004a; CYPSS, 2005)

This view is further supported by a recent Audit Commission document that states: 'The overriding principle of provision of services must be safe and effective services as locally as possible, not local services as safely as possible' (National Collaborating Centre for Cancer, 2005, p. 90).

Economic influences

With increasing medical technological advances, particularly in neonatal care, along with enhanced care giving practices and new medical treatments, children and young people with chronic illnesses are living longer, requiring more complex and continuing care needs to be addressed into adulthood. Meeting these needs is often dependent on interventions and equipment that in the past would have required the child or young person to be hospitalised. Today they are often provided in the local community or the child's home environment, resulting in the traditional boundaries of health care provision shifting from the acute care setting to one provided nearer to and often by the family within community and primary care settings. It is suggested that, when cared for at home, children with complex and continuing health needs have improved physical, psychosocial and development outcomes (Hewitt-Taylor, 2005), and that this service delivery mode is a more cost-effective choice for the NHS (Appiereto *et al.*, 2002). Consequently, this delivery mode is an appealing choice for the Government and health care managers who are trying to deliver quality effective services within the financial constraints of a climate of rising health care costs. It could be argued, though, that this NHS cost saving may be transferred to the family if the appropriate support services are not instigated, including financial benefits, psychosocial and educational support, or adaptations to the family home.

Social influences

To address the problems of an increasing number of children and young people with chronic illnesses and complex health care needs, Government task forces, health care managers and professional bodies have had to examine alternative service delivery models. Models advocated are those that emphasise an integrated approach between health, social care and education services and collaborative working with the voluntary and independent sector. The aim is that partnership working between these services will ensure a holistic approach, taking into account the child, young person and families' physical, developmental, social and psychological needs. The children, young people and maternity NSFs (DoH, 2004c; WAG, 2005d) both advocate this approach and recommend that appropriate family support services be put into place.

Often compounding some of the needs of children and young people with chronic illness and their families is the increasing evidence of the impact of poverty and social exclusion upon their health and welfare (DoH, 2004b; WAG, 2005a). These include the ability to access services, the financial hardship associated with parents having to give up employment to care for their child, poor public transport links, housing issues and the ability to provide adequate nutritional support. Recent Government health and social care policies have attempted to recognise service poverty, where improving public services could play a key role in breaking cycles of poverty along with influencing the development of services closer to the patient's home. Managed clinical networks for specialised services (CYPSS, 2005) and locally based commissioning arrangements in some format in the four UK countries are both being pursued in the hope that they will minimise constraints that can affect equity and access to services. Possible constraints could be geographical location, the level of local funding, or the availability of professional expertise, new medical technologies and treatments. Managed clinical networks and locally based commissioning are to be discussed in more detail in the following section.

Considering the external influences so far discussed, it is essential that health care services are sufficiently flexible to enable a responsive approach to meet the frequently complex individual needs of children and young people and consider these in relation to their level of independence, maturity, social circumstances and the features of their chronic illness process. A balance must be struck between the 'care' needs of the child or young person and their 'disease' needs (National Collaborating Centre for Cancer, 2005).

> **◁▢━◖ Key point**
>
> Figure 2.1 illustrates a summary of the political, economic and social influences for children and young people with chronic illnesses and the resulting outcomes. These outcomes will now be discussed in more detail giving practice examples of their application.

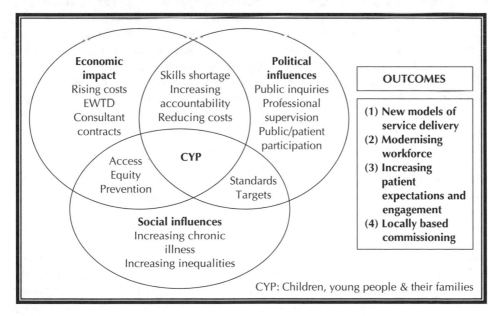

Figure 2.1 Summary of external influences and resulting outcomes health care services for children and young people with chronic illness and their families.

New models of service delivery

As previously intimated, new ways of delivering services have had to be examined in order to meet the Government's health service plans and agendas and to implement the NSFs for children, young people and maternity services (DfES, 2003; DHSSPSNI, 2005; DoH, 2004c; WAG, 2005b; d), all within an economic climate of financial constraints and rising health care costs. These service changes include where and when they are delivered and by whom.

The UK-wide review *Securing our Future Health* by Derek Wanless (2002) highlighted in particular the need for a strengthened, integrated and more streamlined model of whole system workforce redesign, which is aligned to service and able to meet future patient expectations and changing health needs. Building upon the review's findings, a subsequent Wanless *Review of Health and Social Care in Wales* again emphasised the need for a radical design and reconfiguration of services in Wales, with a need to review how best to utilise its health care resources (WAG, 2003b). This view was later further supported by the Audit Commission in Wales:

> 'Making it efficient is not just about better management or better staff or equipment. It is about the way in which services are organised with and between primary and secondary care and between health and social care services, about where and how hospital based services are delivered.' (Audit Commission in Wales, 2004, p. 4)

Service models that have been developed have tended to provide more integrated, community and ambulatory care facilities and the reconfiguration of specialised tertiary services onto one site within a locality through the establishment of managed clinical networks. These models aim to facilitate earlier discharge from hospital, prevent admissions, supporting parents as experts in the care of their child or adolescent with a chronic illness, whilst at the same time ensure safe services through centralising specialised resources. Managed clinical networks are seen by Government and professional bodies as a method of enhancing service provision through better commissioning and delivery of services for those children who require treatment and care across a range of professional groups and organisational boundaries. They have been defined as: 'Linked groups of health professionals and organisations from primary, secondary and tertiary care, and social services and other services working in a coordinated manner' (DoH, 2004c); and 'Managed local networks are fundamentally about enabling services to be formed or linked across boundaries (whether physical or financial) with the overall aim to ensure an optimal patient journey through and across services' (DoH, 2005c).

Managed clinical networks are viewed as enabling the concentration of health professionals with specialist skills and facilitating the implementation of the new consultant and general medical services contracts. They have also encouraged service leads and NHS modernisation teams to reconsider how they best use professional roles and competencies to allocate staff in the right place at the right time and with the necessary competencies to meet children, young people and families' needs within a modernised patient-led NHS.

Managed clinical networks define and support several ideal pathways of care for children and young people with particular health problems, spanning not only primary, secondary and tertiary care, but also local authority and voluntary sector based services. They provide a guide for professionals on the optimal care required for that particular problem, identifying the standards, resources and quality improvement processes. An example could be a managed clinical network for children and young people with respiratory disorders, which could support an asthma, chronic lung and cystic fibrosis pathway of care. Another example could be a managed clinical network for cancer, incorporating pathways of care for leukaemias, solid tumours, haemoglobinopathies and lymphomas. Key within these pathways is the competence of professionals and the communication networks with the child, young person and family.

Designed for Life (WAG, 2005b) advocates that over the next five years health care services in Wales would need to be explicitly based on models of managed clinical networks. In particular, it has been identified that children and young people with complex health care needs have unnecessary delays in hospital due to a lack of community provision to support them in the family home. This provision is related to service issues, such as a deficit in respite care, and also a shortage of staff with the education and training required for this important support and educative role (Hewitt-Taylor, 2005). Respite, unfortunately, is often viewed as crisis intervention rather than a method that can be included with other services to support the child or young person.

To support children and young people in the community, several service models have been developed to meet local needs. These include hospital based outreach services, community based in-reach services, the employment of specialist nurses who practise across community and acute sectors, and hospital at home or ambulatory care teams (Whiting, 2004). Innovative methods have also been applied to reduce child and parent anxiety, vulnerability and feelings of isolation, including the use of telemedicine. A project undertaken at Sheffield Children's Hospital involved the use of telemedicine to help neurologically impaired children to remain at home through having the means to speak directly to a member of the multidisciplinary neurology team. Early outcomes of the project are very positive and the plan is to evaluate the project over the next few years (Guest *et al.*, 2005).

⏱ Time out

- Consider some of the children and young people you have met with chronic illnesses whilst out on community placements.
- What type of service models did they experience?
- What were the key elements of this service?

Overall, the literature supports the existence of multi-agency working but, where this is implemented, least common is a model that delivers this through an identified contact person, except in the case of key workers for children with disabilities (Greco & Sloper, 2004). Generally, though, there are few sound evaluative studies demonstrating outcomes of multi-agency working for service users. Evidence is mainly anecdotal and focused on the process of undertaking multi-agency team working (Sloper, 2004). One exception is a multidisciplinary 24-hour diabetic home care team established over 20 years ago at Birmingham Children's Hospital, which now covers two hospitals and provides a service to 400 patients. This service has demonstrated an increase in cost savings as a consequence of a reduction in bed occupancy days.

It must be remembered, though, that one professional discipline does not have the sole responsibility of delivering the new service models. To ensure a holistic child and family focused approach, like the Birmingham example, care must be delivered throughout the child and young person's health care pathway by multidisciplinary teams including all relevant specialist staff. This requires a flexible and needs led approach rather than one based on professional boundaries. Membership and governance of these teams must be explicit and include clearly defined responsibility for clinical leadership and management. If this is done, professional tribalism and a fragility of new roles, developed as part of modernising services, should be prevented (Gibson, 2005).

Modernising workforce

Increasing globalisation has had an impact upon health care. Typical examples include the introduction of the European Working Time Directive and a shrinking, more mobile labour market for health care managers and universities to attract and recruit from (DoH, 2004a), resulting in nurses being recruited from and to overseas. This, along with the aforementioned policy agendas, financial incentives and the need to provide safe and efficient children and young people's health care services, has again forced managers and professions to look at re-defining service models, modernising pay systems and reviewing health professional roles under the umbrella term of the *Children's Workforce Strategy* (DfES, 2005). Integral to workforce and service delivery transformations is to ensure their synergy with pay modernisation programmes incorporating *Agenda for Change* (DoH, 2002), the *NHS Knowledge and Skills Framework* (DoH, 2003) and career pathways (WAG, 2005c). This approach should ensure long-term recruitment and retention of a larger NHS workforce, including those with highly specialised skills (DoH, 2004b; WAG, 2004; Scottish Executive, 2005b).

The implementation in April 2004 of the new General Medical Services (GMS) Contract for England and Wales introduced the option for GPs to opt out of providing out-of-hours provision, creating some potential difficulties for children and young people's health care services, for example an increasing use of accident and emergency departments. However, this withdrawal of service could provide opportunities for health care professionals to examine and develop new roles and ways of delivering services that are more child and family focused, for example delivering a greater range and enhanced quality of nurse led community based services. Similarly, *Agenda for Change* could present the potential for children and young people's health care practitioners to expand their roles and examine the scope of working flexibly across professional groups within an agreed skill and competency framework.

To achieve real change for children and young people, it will be a necessary to focus on staff groups such as nursing or health care support workers and develop an overall workforce strategy that considers cross-professional and service sector roles (WAG, 2005c). This will require a collective will to change, partnership working, shared accountability and major workforce changes between health care settings, social care and education sectors. Applying these issues to children and young people with chronic illnesses, such a cross-sector role could be an adolescent transitional care practitioner who would work across adult and children's health care services and in partnership with health, social care and educational sectors. This role could facilitate a coordinated and planned transition programme for young people from child to adult services and enable their physical, psychosocial and educational or employment needs to be incorporated within this plan.

(🕐) Time out

- Can you think of any other potential roles that could be developed that would facilitate more effective services to be delivered for children and young people with chronic illnesses across organisations and different health care sectors?
- Compare your thoughts to some potential roles identified at the end of this chapter.

Over the last few years, children and young people's health care services have witnessed an increasing number of condition specific specialist/advanced practitioner/consultant nurse positions. These roles, however, differ from one region to another in terms of job titles, role descriptors, areas of accountability, qualifications, competencies required to fulfil the role and pay and employment conditions (NMC, 2005). Frequently, these positions incorporate extended roles that have traditionally been those of junior medical doctors. This could include nurse led outpatient clinics, baseline assessments, reviewing treatment programmes, prescribing medicines, providing valuable health education, family support services, undertaking research, influencing policy agendas and delivering specialist staff education and training programmes. The RCN Children and Young People's Forum have produced useful guidance and a role framework for preparing children and young people's nurses for future roles, incorporating a useful example of the role descriptors and role elements for a children's diabetes specialist nurse, an advanced nurse practitioner and a nurse at consultant level practice (RCN, 2004b). However, professional nursing bodies have expressed caution regarding the professional regulation of these advanced roles

(DHSSPSNI, 2005; NMC, 2005). A key concern is the need to ensure that these roles are redesigned based upon quality improvement strategies and meeting the child, young person and families' needs rather than just taking on an area of responsibility or practice that is no longer deemed an important aspect of another profession's role. To safeguard children and young people and professionals, these advanced roles need to be supported by protocols, clear guidelines, agreed accountability structures and supervision networks.

A useful illustration of a consultant nurse role is a children and young person's consultant oncology nurse, whose role and responsibilities will include elements of delivering expert clinical practice, professional leadership, developing education programmes and support systems, scholarly activity and consultancy work across professional and organisational boundaries. Extended advanced elements of the role could include the ordering and interpreting of appropriate screening, laboratory and other diagnostic tests, and administering timely supportive treatment regimes according to agreed protocols. However, when new roles are planned, often challenging traditional working patterns and role boundaries, a strategic approach is required. This strategy would need to be based upon robust systems and frameworks that support enhanced quality and effectiveness of services so that professionals, children, young people and their families can clearly identify the longer term advantages.

Increasing patient expectations and engagement

So far, this chapter has illustrated that an intricate range of services is required for children and young people with chronic and complex illnesses. The underpinning rationale for this is sustained continued care provision, which often involves many disciplines and professional staff crossing organisational and institutional boundaries. Integrated pathways incorporating processes for referral, assessment, service delivery and review, which also give young people and families a central role in planning services, are essential.

Emphasised in policies and guidance (DoH, 2005a; b; WAG, 2005a) is the importance of involving users in their health care practices, and evaluating and considering existing and new service developments. As children and young people's views about their own needs may not be the same as those of their parents or adult proxies, increasing interest has evolved regarding how they can be consulted (Cavet & Sloper, 2004), including the provision of children's advocacy services to enable children and young people to complain and give suggestions for service improvement (WAG, 2003a).

A study by Lightfoot and Sloper (2003), investigating the views of young patients who have taken part in NHS service development projects, identified several issues that need to be considered when involving young patients to ensure positive results. These include the need for a lead member of staff, support and reassurance for the young participants, and the development of a 'listening culture'. More research needs to be undertaken with larger sample groups and the inclusion of younger children and children from different ethnic backgrounds to provide further information to guide participation work.

Parents, whose child or teenager requires ongoing medical or technological interventions within the community or family home environment, often have to deliver some care practices that traditionally would have been carried out by children's nurses or health care support workers. Supporting parents to perform these care practices, cope with the demands of administering treatments, provide 24-hour care, and deal with general aspects of parenting and family life can be challenging. Alternative models of health care delivery services that strengthen community provision, and a review of the type of staff required and the associated role competencies are required. Methods of actively engaging children and young people and their families in services and treatment options requires highly tuned communication skills and an understanding that these parents often have increased knowledge and skills (Kirk & Glendinning, 2002).

Parents of children and young people with chronic conditions and complex health needs are often very knowledgeable about their child's condition and the practicalities of managing their child's symptoms, care and treatment choices. These 'expert parents' can be assertive and may challenge professional views regarding treatment options and care strategies (Shaw & Barker, 2004). Health care professionals must work in partnership with children, young people and parents to negotiate new roles and responsibilities to take on supportive and educative roles (Hewitt-Taylor, 2005). These new roles in the community and family home require specific competencies to be developed. The nature of the relationship has changed regarding the power equation in the familiarity of the environment and also the knowledge base in relation to some rarer chronic medical conditions (Glendinning & Kirk, 2000; Hewitt-Taylor, 2005). Parental role transfer and the implications for nursing skill development will be expanded upon later in the chapter.

⏱ Time out

- Reflecting on the parents of children and young people with chronic illnesses that you have met in practice, what skills:
  - Did these parents undertake what normally would have been done by a nurse?
  - Did the nurses need to support these parents?
- Compare your thoughts with the section on parental roles later on in this chapter.

Locally based commissioning

Planning, commissioning and funding all aspects of care for children and young people across the whole health care system should be coordinated to ensure that there is an appropriate balance of service provision and allocation of resources to address local social, economic and environmental factors that affect people's health and well-being (DHSSPSNI, 2005; WAG, 2005a; b).

There have been changes to the mechanisms for funding and commissioning health care services to encourage more integrated local needs based commissioning and increasing accountability and governance of health care expenditure (DoH, 2005a; b). New commissioning organisations and processes, which vary across the four countries in the UK, all have elements that strengthen the governance and accountability arrangements of clinicians and managers over budgets, achieving national and local health performance targets, such as equity, efficiency and cost containment, alongside facilitating meaningful engagement of children, young people and their families to ensure responsiveness to their needs. These drivers have produced an opportunity to reconfigure services to develop sustainable models of provision, with integrated approaches to care delivery that are often community based alternatives to hospital care.

Challenges for the commissioning bodies include delivering the right commissioning models within an overall context of community engagement and partnership working. They need to address health inequalities, meet national priorities and performance targets, determine clinical service models and ensure patient choice. Consider for instance, a children's diabetes service that has to meet the needs of a local population that geographically encapsulates both a densely populated city and a rural community. Effective access and equity of services for all children and young people with diabetes would require the development of services within the city and locally in the rural areas. Delivery of care closer to home can result, for example, in reduced travelling costs, less disruption to family life, reduced school absences, sibling social and family participation and less employment time loss. Furthermore, there could be the added advantage of children, young people and families developing increased confidence in local services. Unfortunately, the costs incurred by increasing the provision of local services and the provision of appropriate support to families and carers closer to home have not been addressed, for example the continuing development of children's community nursing teams.

The remainder of this chapter will consider some of the implications of the political, social and economic drivers upon service from a practice context. It will particularly highlight the impact on the roles of parents and nurses, and service challenges that need to be addressed to support these changes.

Staffing implications

As intimated earlier, due to advances in treatment and innovative life promoting technologies, children whose conditions would have been deemed incompatible with life are now surviving and are able to be cared for at home (Hewitt-Taylor, 2005). This shift towards the provision of home care raises a number of issues for those tasked with providing that care. One of the key debates for home care concerns who should deliver it. A number of reports have identified the need for wider service provision that crosses traditional organisational boundaries (DoH, 1998; 2004c). Children with chronic illness and complex health needs often require skilled intervention, and it has often fallen on parents to provide home care with little or no preparation or training (Glendinning & Kirk, 2000).

Staff education and competence

Key to providing the appropriate care to meet and support children and young people's needs in both home and hospital environments is the effective education and training of staff involved in the delivery of this provision. Children who require advanced technological support, including those requiring long-term ventilation, often experience difficulty in having those needs met (Noyes, 2002). This group of children with chronic illness can often have protracted periods of hospitalisation due to a lack of collaboration between the acute and community settings. This requires services to be established and presents nurses with the opportunity to develop roles that can facilitate well planned, coordinated transitional programmes from hospital to home environments.

Margolan *et al.* (2004) found four consistent causes for delayed discharge: the provision of health authority funding, the need to employ community carers, adaptation of the child's home and the purchase of equipment and consumables in order to provide and establish a safe home care environment. It was also clear from this study that parents often felt excluded from the discharge process and confused by the input from a variety of health and social care organisations.

To facilitate a seamless transition from hospital to home, there is a need for a coordinated approach across organisational boundaries, with perhaps an identified named nurse commissioning the whole process. With such a current ad hoc approach to discharge planning, it would be appropriate for nursing staff to develop guidelines and protocols concerning the purchase of equipment and consumables and the maintenance of ordering systems. Management plans should also be in place, which identify the various components of the commissioning process from home adaptation to the recruitment and training of carers. Margolan *et al.* (2004) highlight the need for children to be nursed in an appropriate environment, including high dependency units and transitional care beds, to avoid the stress of children's intensive care units. Whilst barriers exist across organisational boundaries, the commissioning process of services for children requiring long-term ventilation will remain unwieldy, failing to meet the most basic and essential needs of the child.

Glendinning & Kirk (2000) found a number of issues regarding the organisation and the commissioning of care that impacted heavily on parents. The study involved interviewing 24 parents whose children had chronic health needs, and identified that parents often assumed primary responsibility for their child's care to ensure a more rapid discharge from the hospital setting. This can be seen to exploit the parental role if adequate service provision is not available. It is estimated that there are up to 6000 technology dependent children living in the UK, and the cost of equipment and, in some cases, ventilatory support, is approximately £130 000 per annum per child (Glendinning & Kirk, 2000). Their study also identified that parents increasingly found their homes loaded with technology, with the focus on technical proficiency rather than the psychological aspects of undertaking often distressing procedures on their own children. In this area, where ongoing care is required over a 24-hour period, parents are expected to perform what would be traditionally understood as nursing interventions, including suctioning, tracheostomy care and the setting up of intravenous infusions.

To try to meet these needs, a number of roles have been developed, including the key worker role, which will be discussed later on in the chapter. Nurses undertaking coordinating roles need to assist in the establishment of multidisciplinary care management pathways, which identify professional roles and responsibilities within the process and provision of appropriate resources to individual children and young people.

Hewitt-Taylor (2005) undertook a pilot study to ascertain the training needs of staff involved in the care of children and young people with chronic illness. A wide range of educational and training needs were identified as important, including the knowledge and skills related to invasive therapies such as assisted ventilation and tracheostomy care. To be effective, planned education and training needs have to be targeted to ensure that they meet the needs of both qualified and unqualified nurses, as they are the professionals delivering care outside the hospital environment (Robinson & Jackson, 1999). Much of the input is focused on the acquisition of clinical knowledge and skills but it is equally important to ensure that there is equivalent attention paid to the psychological and developmental needs of the children. This would suggest that there is a role for shared education between children's nurses, mental health nurses and professionals working within child psychology teams. It must be ensured that care is delivered holistically so that all the health and social care needs of the family are met (Hewitt-Taylor, 2005).

Reflection

Reflecting on the parents of children and young people with chronic illnesses that you have met in practice what:

- Impact did their child's chronic illness have upon them?
- Strategies were used by professionals to minimise these impacts?
- Roles and services could be provided to help support children and young people in their homes?

Meeting parental needs

The diagnosis of a chronic illness is a life-changing event for the family concerned. Meleski (2002) described parents as experiencing a period of disequilibrium, where identified roles and family routine were adversely affected by the adaptation process. This is especially apparent during the transition phase when parents are coming to terms with having a child with a chronic condition (Meleski, 2002). Parents often experience a significant change in their role because they have to become primary care givers in order to meet their child's needs. They often become dependent on the provision of home carers to meet the ongoing needs of their children. Margolan *et al.* (2004) found wide variations between the recruitment and ongoing training of carers, with some organisations having no specific training programmes available. Only one service was identified that provided ongoing training of home carers, where families' needs were regularly reviewed with input increased or decreased as the needs of the child and family changed. This type of responsive service provision ought to be the norm not the exception, with other service providers and commissioning bodies taking note of best practice to further develop their own services. The process of transition and adaptation can cause an inordinate amount of stress on the whole family, which requires health care professionals to be aware of the individual and holistic needs of all members of the family group. It is essential that children's nurses are educationally prepared to deliver this kind of responsive service through post-registration education and supervision by management teams.

Effective communication is essential if service provision is to meet the holistic needs of families coping with a child with an ongoing chronic illness (Fawcett et al., 2005). Various authors have identified parental needs as the desire for normality and certainty, particularly around the diagnosis and ongoing management of disease processes, the need for information and the need for a sense of partnership with members of the multidisciplinary team involved in the provision of services and care delivery (Fisher, 2001). This partnership approach has to be established across a range of health care and social settings including the educational environment. Perhaps one reason why service provision is fragmented, and at times uncoordinated, is a lack of recognition of the role of children's community nurses. The work undertaken by community teams is often hidden as it is not high on the political agenda in comparison to the provision of acute services. Byrne (2003) recognises that this issue impacts on the role and development of services within the home care environment. Much of the work undertaken by community workers is not wholly transparent. Byrne (2003) found that a variety of nursing strategies are employed to meet the needs of children and young people with complex needs but much of this work was not evidenced in documentation, such as assessment charts, as it focused on psychological and social care, an area that is often undervalued and immeasurable. A clear gap emerges between documentation and the scope of nursing within the home environment. Nurses have developed and combined a range of skills that focus on empowerment, physical assessment and care, teaching and providing effective guidance and support to families (Byrne, 2003). To provide community care, families will require a broad range of nursing input from both qualified nurses and unqualified carers.

Reflection

Reflect upon the children and young people with chronic and complex illness within the community. What differing skills and knowledge do you require to meet their needs in this environment, as opposed to providing care for them in the acute setting? Consider the following to guide your thoughts:

- Professional responsibility and accountability
- Parents as experts in the care of their own child
- Resource issues
- The environment of care

It is important to establish the correct skill mix and division of labour to ensure that care needs are fully met. To achieve this, community teams need to collaborate and ensure that all team members have access to ongoing training and development to fulfil the required roles. When establishing community teams, educational programmes need to be developed to ensure that a broad range of knowledge and skills are taught to the participants. With the varied skill mix in some community teams, the topics taught have to meet the needs of both trained and untrained nurses (Hewitt-Taylor, 2005). The delivery of nursing care to children in their own homes requires a comprehensive level of knowledge and skill acquisition. The ability to meet care needs through a combination of nursing and parentally delivered care will remain problematic whilst commissioning and funding deficits remain. The skills and knowledge required for effective delivery of care to children and young people in the community setting should include:

- Sound interpersonal skills in order to develop good working relationships with families and professionals
- Knowledge of ethics and the law to advocate on behalf of children, young people and their families
- A thorough knowledge of both statutory and voluntary provision
- The ability to provide holistic care, including meeting the physical, social, emotional and psychological needs of those in their care.

It is of paramount importance that nurses establish an evidence base for the effectiveness of community-based care, for the needs of children and young people with chronic illness to be met. Home nursing care delivery needs to be both identifiable and measurable for the development of best practice, clear and consistent discharge planning and the commissioning of services.

Innovative practices – new roles

A variety of strategies and schemes have been developed to support children and young people and their families in their home, including telemedicine, which will be discussed later in the chapter. A range of professionals will be involved in care delivery. It is envisaged that there will be a growth in the development of roles such as consultant nurses, key workers and the further development and enhancement of children's community nursing teams to meet the needs of children, young people and their families (DoH, 2004c; WAG, 2005b; d). What is required to take these services forward is nurse leadership in the development and provision of care packages. The recognition and development of the role of the children's nurse, not only in delivering but commissioning services, has been clearly recognised (WAG, 2004). Increasing integration and commissioning of services is being seen as a way of ensuring quality of care and reducing duplication in the assessment and sometimes delivery of services. The role of the consultant nurse in the community setting is intended to ensure clear lines of care provision and communication. Caerphilly Local Health Board (LHB) in Wales has established the role of the children's community nurse consultant in delivering coordinated care to children and young people with ongoing and complex needs. This follows on from the 2005 partnership strategy for health, social care and well-being (Caerphilly LHB, 2005), which sought to plan, administer and deliver a range of services across the health and social care arena. This approach to coordination across traditional boundaries is intended to provide targeted and cost-effective services to children, young people and their families in a range of settings and circumstances.

 Time out

Consider the role of the nurse in the provision of care to children and young people with a chronic illness in the community setting:

- How do health and social care influences affect the provision of care?
- How could new nursing roles such as a consultant nurse improve this situation?

Telemedicine

Telemedicine has been seen as an opportunity for parents to opt for more care to be provided for children and young people in their own homes. Telemedicine has been defined as: 'The use of information and communication technology to deliver health or social care in new ways on a person-to-person basis, where those people are physically apart' (TEIS UK, 2004).

In the past, this has served to combat issues around geographical distance and the high cost of bringing children and young people to regional centres for consultation. Guest et al. (2005) highlighted the benefits of telemedicine for a specific group of neurologically impaired children, but potentially this has far-reaching implications for a range of children with chronic illness and severe disability. Clear benefits arise from this technology, including a reduction in time consuming home visits and instant help and advice via a real time video link. This appears to have real benefits for families living in rural communities or in locations that are not well served by specialist services. This approach to care delivery could have a much broader application particularly when providing care for technology dependent children. This group of children often experience delays in the discharge process while services are configured to meet their needs (Wang & Barnard, 2004). For children requiring long-term ventilation, telemedicine offers the possibility of real time support, which is important for both parents and carers (Edwards et al., 2004). The benefits of such technology are clear, but it is important that clear policies are developed to ensure appropriate children and young people access this provision. Guidelines also need to be developed for practitioners to ensure safe practice and accountability, alongside appropriate education and skills development.

Key worker role

Fragmented service provision and a lack of coordination between professional disciplines, agencies and health care settings has often been raised as an issue for the parents of children and young people living with a chronic illness (National Collaborating Centre for Cancer, 2005). Within the NHS, over recent years, a number of nursing roles have been established, which are often disease orientated, For example clinical nurse specialists in oncology, cystic fibrosis and diabetes. A number of outreach and specialist services have made some impact on providing services that are across organisational boundaries, particularly from tertiary centres, but this type of service has been hampered at times by organisational culture and economic factors. However, there is some evidence of success in this approach (Brewis, 2004). It has become increasingly apparent that a key worker role is essential if service delivery is to be targeted at the needs of children and young people with chronic illness.

 Time out

What type of roles and responsibilities do you think a key worker might have to undertake to ensure the delivery of a coordinated package of care?

Various reports outline the role of a key worker, particularly regarding services for children and young people with complex health care needs or oncological conditions where there may be shared health care between tertiary and secondary organisations, often in different health authorities. This role includes the coordinated provision of information, the provision of care and treatment plans and communication with members of the wider multidisciplinary team to ensure effective and timely interventions appropriate to the care of the child or young person concerned (National Collaborating Centre for Cancer, 2005). It has been found that a number of titles are used to describe the key worker role, including care coordinator, family support worker and link worker (Greco & Sloper, 2004), which has led to some confusion in attempting to identify the prerequisites of the role and its potential boundaries.

As far back as the Warnock committee report (Department of Education and Science, 1978), it was recognised that there was a need for an identified professional to whom parents could turn for advice and support in accessing services. Glendinning and Kirk (2000) identified the benefits of the key worker role for families as: the reduction of multiple visits by numerous professionals, an improvement in communication between the hospital and community settings and less confusion about the role boundaries of the multitude of professionals involved in the care of a single child and family. Difficulties in advancing the key worker role are often related to a lack of detailed action plans, a lack of commitment and the existence of territorialism by a number of agencies, poor communication and a lack of access to a designated budget (Mukherjee *et al.*, 1999). However, the *Health Act* (1999) allowed for pooled budgets between health and social care, leading to a slow emergence of the key worker role. Many care coordination schemes are established on short-term funding, and joint funding by statutory agencies remains uncommon (Greco & Sloper, 2004). What is not clear is how widespread key worker roles and care coordination services are within the UK. The key worker role affords the child and family the opportunity for some continuity of care and integration of the primary, secondary and tertiary roles. This role encompasses health, social care and education (National Collaborating Centre for Cancer, 2005).

Both the DoH (2001) and National Assembly for Wales (2001) have recognised the importance of this expansive role. To be successful, key workers need to be able to span all agencies involved in the care and treatment of children and young people living with a chronic illness. This role, from a nursing perspective, involves the care and support of the individual family concerned and may involve teaching new clinical skills, case management between clinical settings and the coordination of future treatment and care. The key worker needs to be accessible to both the families and other professionals (National Collaborating Centre for Cancer, 2005). Greco and Sloper (2004) found evidence of good practice within care coordination schemes, which was partly due to most schemes having all three statutory agencies of health, social care and education involved in establishing schemes. There was also good evidence of parental involvement. However, this was not extended to children and young people, whose views are continually overlooked in the commissioning and development of services. The challenge facing key workers has been found to be a lack of training (Greco & Sloper, 2004). To develop and fulfil the role, it is important to be clear about what services will be provided for the family, the areas of responsibility and to whom the key worker is accountable. A coordinated approach to training across the UK needs to be developed to ensure consistency and best practice in service delivery.

Role diversification is becoming more prevalent within a range of clinical settings; traditional nursing roles are evolving, leading to opportunities for both qualified and unqualified nurses. The development of the role of the registered nurse has led to an expansion in the role of the health care support worker, who will continue to provide basic nursing care (Scottish Executive, 2005b), and perhaps more complex procedures in both acute and community settings. Within nursing, as previously discussed, there are huge opportunities for nurses to take lead roles in assessing, delivering, coordinating and evaluating packages of care and their effectiveness. Nurses now face the challenge of taking the key worker role forward in order to meet the complex health needs of children and young people with chronic illness.

Mental health issues

Children and young people living with a chronic illness will, over time, experience a range of physical, psychological and emotional issues that may impact on their sense of worth and mental well-being. Although medical advances have increased survivability, the challenges of living with a chronic illness through adolescence and into adulthood remain. Mental health has been defined as the ability to develop psychologically, emotionally, intellectually and spiritually (DfES, 2001). Children and young people with chronic illness experience a range of issues that impact on the development and maintenance of this health dimension. To attempt to meet these needs, it is important that, as children's nurses, we recognise the limitations of our skills and knowledge and refer on, when necessary, to specialist services. A possible solution in attempting to meet the holistic needs of children, young people and families is to increase interprofessional collaboration. It is important that children's nurses share their knowledge and skills and, where deficits are identified, appropriate professional involvement should be encouraged.

In attempting to meet the mental health needs of children and young people, it would be appropriate for children's nurse managers to employ mental health nurses within community nursing teams. This is by no means a unique situation as we have seen mental health nurses employed on adolescent units and children's nurses employed in child and adolescent mental health settings. LeBovidge et al. (2005) examined adjustment to chronic illness in 75 children and young people aged 8–18 years with chronic arthritis. The data were collected using a questionnaire which examined attitudes towards illness, depressive symptoms and anxiety. A range of psychosocial stressors was experienced, which impacted on day-to-day living and the individual mental health of the children concerned. Parents of the children also completed a measure of psychosocial adjustment. From this study, it became clear that health care professionals and others involved in the care, support and treatment of this specific group of children needed to develop interventions in order to assist children and young people to come to terms with their illness and develop coping mechanisms. Only with the appointment of nurses with the appropriate skills, or by establishing multidisciplinary teams, will these needs be met.

Multi-agency working

The impact of chronic illness upon children and young people in relation to their physical, social and psychological well-being emphasises the importance of children's nurses being able to work in partnership with other members of the multidisciplinary team. This would help ensure that all aspects of children and young people's needs are met to minimise the risk of complications occurring, such as behavioural problems, depression, non-compliance or poor educational attainment. King et al. (2006) highlight the use of a multidisciplinary approach in attempting to meet the educational needs of children with sickle cell anaemia and cerebral infarcts. In this study, the multidisciplinary team included a nurse practitioner, social worker, neurologist and neuropsychologist, amongst others. Their role was aimed at reducing absenteeism and lost education by providing home tutoring and ensuring that educational environments were geared for children's needs when they were in school. The role of the nurse was to provide ongoing care in both the acute and ambulatory setting. What is important is that this type of coordinated approach to care delivery is being established and used across a wide range of settings so that children and young people have full access to education, health and social care.

Multidisciplinary team (MDT) working

Kenny (2002) highlights how knowledge and skills have changed over recent years and the importance of interprofessional collaboration. This may entail developing close working relationships with groups of professionals whose working methods are relatively unknown to nurses. In terms of mental health, joint appointments and commissioning of posts appears to be the most effective way forward. For service provision to be holistic, children's community nursing teams must have a varied skill mix, with nurses able to meet the wide range of complex health needs, not just physical needs but also mental health and educational needs.

A number of high profile reports and recommendations have recognised gaps in service delivery and fragmentation of services. This has contributed to a lack of workforce planning and poor integration of services (DoH, 2004c). Danvers *et al.* (2003) found a number of issues that impact on the role and function of the MDT. These included a lack of standardised documentation, tension between services providing input to the same child and family and a lack of coordinated shared education and training. The establishment of Diana children's community teams has provided nurse led services aimed at establishing high quality seamless services focusing on supporting children with life-threatening or life-limiting illnesses, which in turn has led to an increase in multi-professional collaboration and partnership across agencies (Danvers *et al.*, 2003). Problems around effective inter-professional working have been identified since the NHS was introduced (Atwal & Caldwell, 2005).

MDT working is a key aspect of effective health care delivery, with teams varying in composition, leadership styles and culture. This variation can have a profound impact upon the clinical effectiveness of service delivery and ultimately on the management of care for the individual child and family. Gaps and omissions in services and the fragmented approach to care delivery is a Government priority that is clearly identified throughout the various NSFs. Caldwell and Atwal (2003) identified clear advantages of the MDT approach. These included improved planning, clinical effectiveness, avoidance of duplication and fragmentation of services and a more patient centred responsive approach to care. An effective MDT approach can lead to the eradication of dysfunctional professional barriers, which have impacted on the service provision and ultimately the quality of care delivered (Royal College of Physicians, 2004). Danvers *et al.* (2003) identify various positive examples within multi-professional collaborative approaches, including the development of joint visiting and a palliative care pathway. The value of developing a pathway that can be used by the wider team has clear benefits to the care and treatment of children and young people with a range of life-limiting or threatening conditions, particularly in ensuring that the holistic needs of the individual service user are met by the wider agencies involved in care provision.

Time out

Reflecting on the parents of children and young people with chronic illnesses that you have met in practice, can you:

- Identify key members of the MDT and their roles within the acute or community setting?
- Identify barriers that may have impacted on effective MDT working?

Nursing implications, challenges and opportunities in MDT working

Some barriers that have been identified in relation to effective multidisciplinary working include individual team members placing their own achievements above those of the team, professionals' lack of self-confidence (Eilertsen *et al.*, 2004), and a lack of clear aims and poor communication networks (Reder & Duncan, 2003). However, within this collaborative approach there are clear opportunities for the children's nurse to develop shared policies and standards, thereby avoiding duplication and confusion around referral processes and appropriate access to professional care. Danvers *et al.* (2003) recognise the need to evaluate the multi-agency approach to children's community services, with audit and validation enabling the implementation of further service development. To establish the cost effectiveness and validity of a multi-agency approach, different service delivery models and partnership approaches need to be evaluated. This would appear to be a good opportunity to establish and justify the role of a children's community nurse consultant, presenting the evidence base for this approach to the delivery of care to those with the most complex health care needs. Within this MDT approach, opportunities will present themselves for the integration of inter-professional research and education and also the potential for children's nurses to expand their roles and skills.

Conclusion

This chapter has considered the political, social and economic influences on service provision. To meet the future physical and psychosocial health care needs of children and young people with chronic illnesses and their families, it is apparent that policy makers, commissioners and deliverers of children and young people's health, social and education services must work together to remove some of the real and potential barriers of dysfunctional professional boundaries, organisational infrastructures, unresponsive commissioning processes and outdated routine practices. There is a need to ensure integration and coordination of care within primary, secondary and tertiary care settings and between the voluntary sector, health, social care and educational organisations.

This requires coordinated planning, commissioning and funding arrangements. However, this breaking down of barriers and the building of effective partnership working arrangements will require children, young people and their families to be truly 'engaged' in shaping new services and working practices. This chapter has also examined some of the implications for children's nurses of increasing integration of services, changing role boundaries and practice settings along with an increasing engagement with children, young people and their families.

Useful websites

www.auditcommission.gov.uk
www.dhsspsni.gov.uk
www.dfes.gov.uk
www.foundationtrustnetwork.org
www.kingsfund.org.uk
www.nice.org.uk
www.rcn.org.uk
www.rcpch.org.uk
www.wales.gov.uk

References

Appiereto, L., Cori, M., Binnchi, R. *et al.* (2002) Home care for chronic respiratory failure in children: 15 years experience. *Paediatric Anaesthesia,* **12** (4), 345–350.

Atwal, A. & Caldwell, K. (2005) Do all health and social care professionals interact equally: a study of interactions in multidisciplinary teams in the United Kingdom. *Scandinavian Journal of Caring Science,* **19**, 268–273.

Audit Commission (2004) *Payment by Results: Key Risks and Questions to Consider for Trust and PCT Managers and Non-executives.* London, Audit Commission.

Audit Commission in Wales (2004) *Transforming Health and Social Care in Wales: Aligning the Levers of Change.* London, Audit Commission for LAs and NHS in England and Wales.

Brewis, E. (2004) Oncology outreach: history in the making. *Paediatric Nursing,* **16** (9), 24–27.

Byrne, M.W. (2003) Culture-derived strategies of a paediatric home-care nursing speciality team. *International Nursing Review,* **50**, 34–43.

Caerphilly Local Health Board (2005) *A Partnership Strategy for Health, Social Care and Well-being in Caerphilly County Borough.* Caerphilly, Caerphilly Local Health Board.

Caldwell, K. & Atwal, A. (2003) The problems of inter-professional health care practice in the hospital setting. *British Journal of Nursing,* **12**, 1212–1218.

Carlile, A. (2002) *Too Serious a Thing: the Review of Safeguards for Children and Young People Treated and Cared for by the NHS in Wales.* Cardiff, National Assembly for Wales.

Cavet, J. & Sloper, P. (2004) Participation of disabled children in individual decisions about their lives in public decisions about service development. *Children and Society,* **18**, 278–290.

Children Act (2004) London, The Stationery Office.

Children and Young People's Specialised Service Project (CYPSS) (2005) *All Wales Universal Standards for Children and Young People's Specialised Health Care Services: Consultation Document.* Cardiff, Welsh Assembly Government.

Danvers, L., Freshwater, D., Cheater, F. & Wilson, A. (2003) Providing a seamless service for children with life-limiting illness: experiences and recommendations of professional staff at the Diana Princess of Wales Children's Community Service. *Journal of Clinical Nursing*, **12**, 351–359.

Department of Education and Science (1978) *Special Educational Needs: Report of the Committee of Enquiry into the Education of Handicapped Children and Young People*. The Warnock Report. London, HMSO.

Department for Education and Skills (2001) *Promoting Children's Mental Health within Early Years and School Settings*. London, Department for Education and Skills.

Department for Education and Skills (2003) *Every Child Matters*. London, Department for Education and Skills.

Department for Education and Skills (2005) *Children's Workforce Strategy: a Strategy to Build a World-class Workforce for Children and Young People: Every Child Matters: Change for Children*. London, Department for Education and Skills.

Department of Health (1998) *Paediatric Intensive Care Framework: Future Targets and Milestones*. London, Department of Health.

Department of Health (2001) *The NHS Cancer Plan*. London, Department of Health.

Department of Health (2002) *Agenda for Change: a Modernised NHS Pay System*. London, Department of Health.

Department of Health (2003) *The NHS Knowledge and Skills Framework (NHS KSF) and Developing Review Guidance*. London, Department of Health.

Department of Health (2004a) *A Compendium of Solutions to Implementing the Working Time Directive for Doctors in Training from August 2004*. London, Department of Health.

Department of Health (2004b) *The Chief Nursing Officer's Review of the Nursing, Midwifery and Health Visiting Contribution to Vulnerable Children and Young People*. London, Department of Health.

Department of Health (2004c) *National Service Framework for Children, Young People and Maternity Services: Standard 8. Disabled Children and Young People and those with Complex Health Needs*. London, The Stationery Office.

Department of Health (2005a) *Commissioning a Patient Led NHS*. London, Department of Health.

Department of Health (2005b) *Practice Based Commissioning: Promoting Clinical Engagement*. London, Department of Health.

Department of Health (2005c) *A Guide to Promote a Shared Understanding of the Benefits of Local Managed Networks*. London, Department of Health.

Department of Health, Social Services and Public Safety Northern Ireland (2005) *A Healthier Future: A Twenty-year Vision for Health and Well-being in Northern Ireland*. Belfast, Department of Health, Social Services and Public Safety Northern Ireland.

Edwards, E.A., O'Toole, M. & Wallis, C. (2004) Sending children home on tracheostomy dependent ventilation: pitfalls and outcomes. *Archives of Disease in Childhood*, **89**, 251–255.

Eilertsen, M.E.B., Reinfjell, T. & Vik, T. (2004) Value of collaboration in the care of children with cancer and their families. *European Journal of Cancer Care*, **13**, 349–355.

Fawcett, T.N., Bagley, S.E., Wu, C., Whyte, D.A. & Martinson, I.M. (2005) Parental responses to health care services for children with chronic conditions and their families: a comparison between Hong Kong and Scotland. *Journal of Child Health Care*, **9** (1), 8–19.

Fisher, H.R. (2001) The needs of parents with chronically sick children: a literature review. *Journal of Advanced Nursing*, **36** (4), 600–607.

Foundation Trust Network (2005) *Foundation Trusts: Future Thinking, Challenges and Change*. London, The NHS Confederation Publications.

Gibson, F. (2005) Advancing nursing practice – nurse practitioners: the door to the future in paediatric oncology (editorial). *Journal of Pediatric Oncology Nursing*, **22** (5), 249.

Glendinning, C. & Kirk, S. (2000) High tech care: high skilled parents. *Paediatric Nursing*, **12** (6), 25–27.

Greco, V. & Sloper, P. (2004) Care coordination and key worker schemes for disabled children: results of a UK wide survey. *Child, Care, Health and Development*, **30**, 13–20.

Guest, A., Rittey, C. & O'Brien, K. (2005) Telemedicine: helping neurologically impaired children to stay at home. *Paediatrc Nursing*, **17** (2), 20–22.

Health Act (1999) London, The Stationery Office.

Hewitt-Taylor, J. (2005) Caring for children with complex needs: staff education and training. *Journal of Child Health Care*, **9** (1), 72–86.

Kennedy, I., Howard, R., Jarman, B. & Maclean, M. (2001) *Learning from Bristol: the Report of the Public Inquiry into Children's Heart Surgery at the Bristol Royal Infirmary 1984–1995*. Norwich, The Stationery Office.

Kenny, G. (2002) Children's nursing and inter-professional collaboration: challenges and opportunities. *Journal of Clinical Nursing*, **11**, 306–313.

King, A., Herron, S., Mckinstry, R. *et al.* (2006) A multidisciplinary health care team's efforts to improve educational attainment in children with sickle cell anaemia and cerebral infarcts. *Journal of School Health*, **76**, 33–37.

Kirk, S. & Glendinning, C. (2002) Supporting 'expert' parents – professional support and families caring for a child with complex health care needs in the community. *International Journal of Nursing Studies*, **39** (6), 625–635.

Laming, W.H. (2003) *The Victoria Climbie Inquiry – Report of an Inquiry by Lord Laming Presented to Parliament by the Secretary of State for Health and the Secretary of State for the Home Department by Command of Her Majesty*. Norwich, The Stationery Office.

LeBovidge, J.S., Lavigne, J.V. & Miller, M.L. (2005) Adjustment to chronic arthritis of childhood: the roles of illness related stress and attitude towards illness. *Journal of Pediatric Psychology*, **30** (3), 273–286.

Lightfoot, J. & Sloper, P. (2003) Having a say in health: involving young people with a chronic illness or physical disability in local health service development. *Children and Society*, **17**, 277–290.

Margolan, H., Fraser, J. & Lenton, S. (2004) Parental experiences of services when their child requires long-term ventilation. Implications for commissioning and providing services. *Child: Care, Health and Development*, **30** (3), 257–264.

Meleski, D.D. (2002) Families with chronically ill children. *American Journal of Nursing*, **102** (5), 47–54.

Mukherjee, S., Beresford, B. & Sloper, P. (1999) *Unlocking Key Working*. Bristol, Policy Press.

National Assembly for Wales (2001) *Improving Health in Wales: a Plan for the NHS and its Partners*. Cardiff, National Assembly for Wales.

National Collaborating Centre for Cancer (2005) *Improving Outcomes in Children and Young People with Cancer: the Manual*. London, National Institute for Health and Clinical Excellence.

Noyes, J. (2002) Barriers that delay children and young people who are dependent on mechanical ventilators from being discharged from hospital. *Journal of Clinical Nursing*, **11** (1), 2–11.

Nursing and Midwifery Council (2005) *Consultation on a Framework for the Standard for Post-registration Nursing*. London, Nursing and Midwifery Council.

Reder, P. & Duncan, S. (2003) Understanding communication in child protection networks. *Child Abuse Review*, **12**, 82–100.

Redfern, M., Keeling, J.W. & Powell, E. (2001) *The Royal Liverpool Children's Inquiry*. London, House of Commons.

Robinson, C. & Jackson, P. (1999) *Children's Hospices: a Lifeline for Families?* London, National Children's Bureau.

Royal College of Nursing (2003) *Children and Young People's Nursing: a Philosophy of Care. Guidance for Nursing*. London, RCN Publications.

Royal College of Nursing (2004a) *Adolescent Transition Care: Guidance for Nursing Staff*. London, RCN Publications.

Royal College of Nursing (2004b) *Services for Children and Young People: Preparing Nurses for Future Roles: RCN Guidance*. London, RCN Publications.

Royal College of Paediatrics and Child Health (2003a) *Health Care for Adolescents*. London, Royal College of Paediatrics and Child Health.

Royal College of Paediatrics and Child Health (2003b) *Specialist Health Services for Children and Young People: a Guide for Primary Care*. London, Royal College of Paediatrics and Child Health.

Royal College of Physicians (2004) *Clinicians, Services and Commissioning in Chronic Disease Management in the NHS: the Need for Coordinated Management Programmes*. London, Royal College of Physicians.

Scottish Executive (2005a) *Building a Health Service Fit for the Future*. Edinburgh, Scottish Executive.

Scottish Executive (2005b) *Framework for Developing Nurses' Roles*. Edinburgh, Scottish Executive.

Shaw, J. & Barker, M. (2004) 'Expert patient' dream or nightmare. *British Medical Journal*, **32** (7442), 723–724.

Sloper, P. (2004) Facilitators and barriers for coordinated multi-agency services. *Child, Care, Health and Development*, **30** (6), 571–580.

TEIS UK *Telemedicine and E-Health Information Service* (2004) Available at: www.teis.nhs.uk Accessed 16/5/06.

Wang, K. & Barnard, A. (2004) Technology – dependent children and their families: a review. *Journal of Advanced Nursing*, **45** (1), 36–46.

Wanless, D. (2002) *Securing our Future Health: Taking a Long Term View. Final Report*. London, HM Treasury.

Welsh Assembly Government (2003a) *National Standards for the Provision of Children's Advocacy Services*. Cardiff, Welsh Assembly Government.

Welsh Assembly Government (2003b) *The Review of Health and Social Care in Wales*. Cardiff, Welsh Assembly Government.

Welsh Assembly Government (2004) *Nurturing the Future: a Framework for Realising the Potential of Children's Nurses in Wales*. Cardiff, Welsh Assembly Government.

Welsh Assembly Government (2005a) *A Fair Future for Our Children: the Strategy of the Welsh Government for Tackling Child Poverty*. Cardiff, Welsh Assembly Government.

Welsh Assembly Government (2005b) *Designed for Life: Creating World Class Health and Social Care for Wales in the 21st Century*. Cardiff, Welsh Assembly Government.

Welsh Assembly Government (2005c) *Making the Connections: Connecting the Workforce: The Workforce Challenge for Health. (Consultation Document)* Cardiff, Welsh Assembly Government.

Welsh Assembly Government (2005d) *National Service Framework for Children, Young People and Maternity Service in Wales*. Cardiff, Welsh Assembly Government.

Whiting, M. (2004) The future of community children's nursing. *Archives of Disease in Childhood*, **89**, 987–988.

3 Impact upon the Child and Family

Lesley Lowes

Introduction

The whole family are likely to experience a number of losses when a child is diagnosed with a chronic condition, a situation that may represent a life-changing event for parents and their child. As changes need to be introduced to accommodate the needs of the child with chronic illness, the whole family are presented with many challenges that may upset the equilibrium of their everyday life. However, a diagnosis of chronic childhood illness does not impact upon the family solely during the peri-diagnostic period but can have considerable impact upon their life and lifestyle over many years following diagnosis.

Aim of the chapter

The purpose of this chapter is to critically examine the impact of the diagnosis on the child/young person with chronic illness and family, and to identify factors that may contribute to family stress and disruption during the peri-diagnostic period. Issues will be explored from the perspectives of the affected child, siblings and parents and will be considered at different stages of growth and development, from infancy to adolescence, and up to twelve months after diagnosis.

This chapter does not intend to be all inclusive concerning the possible impact of childhood chronic illness on the child and family but to engender an awareness of the topic and the associated theories to stimulate further learning. Issues will be explored within a theoretical framework of grief, loss, change, adjustment and adaptation, which will allow the impact of chronic illness to be considered from various standpoints, including cultural influences. Also examined will be the impact of chronic illness on finances, employment, socialising and relationships within the family. Type 1 diabetes in childhood is used as a case study to introduce, examine and apply some of the theories and social and practical issues that may confront families of children with chronic illness.

Intended learning outcomes

- To analyse the models and theories of grief, loss, change, adjustment and adaptation, and how they apply to children with chronic conditions and their families
- To examine how childhood chronic conditions can impact emotionally, socially and practically on the child and family, taking cultural influences into account
- To explore the effect of childhood chronic illness on the family as a unit, the factors that may contribute to family stress and conflict, and consider these issues in the context of family-centred care
- To explore the role of the children's nurse in helping families cope with, and adapt and adjust to, a diagnosis of chronic illness in childhood

Theories of grief, loss and change

The period immediately following a diagnosis of childhood chronic illness is often an anxious and distressing time for the whole family. Parents, in particular, may find it difficult to come to terms with the diagnosis, which they may view as the end of 'normal' health and a familiar lifestyle. The profound impact of the diagnosis on family life often engenders feelings of grief arising from the losses imposed by the chronic condition (Lowes *et al.*, 2004; 2005; Webb, 2005). Grief experienced in the context of childhood chronic illness may not have an endpoint and needs to be considered well beyond the time of diagnosis. Some theories of grief, loss and change are introduced here to provide a framework for the ensuing discussion throughout this chapter.

Reflection

Before reading the next section, take a few minutes to reflect on your own knowledge and experiences, and identify key points that arise from your understanding of loss and grief.

Much of the work that has been undertaken on grief as a response to loss has focused on the bereaved or care of the dying. However, it is well recognised that a diagnosis of chronic illness can trigger a similar grief response in affected individuals and their families and this is discussed later in the chapter. As you read the following section, you may find it helpful to try to relate the theories of grief, loss and change to the grief response that may arise from losses incurred by a diagnosis of childhood chronic illness.

A classic *stage theory* developed by Kubler-Ross (1970) has played a major role in increasing understanding about the grieving process. Kubler-Ross describes five stages of emotional reaction to death and dying: denial, anger, bargaining, depression and acceptance. The belief that the experience of loss can be divided into stages is common to a number of grief theories, some of which suggest there is a sequential progression through stages of grief, which vary in definition according to different theoretical perspectives (Kamm, 1985; Clubb, 1991; Worden, 1995). Traditional *stage* or *time-bound theories* about grief have usually been developed through work undertaken with the bereaved, and describe similar end stages such as acceptance (Kubler-Ross, 1970) and resolution (Engel, 1962). However, the experience of grief is unique to each individual and influenced by many factors such as the type of loss, circumstances leading up to the loss, and personal, cultural and social values and beliefs (Worden, 1995). Thus, different stages of grieving vary in their intensity for individuals and may not be experienced in their entirety by everybody, with no predetermined order or pattern to the grieving process (Cook & Phillips, 1989; Clubb, 1991; Taylor, 1995; Worden, 1995; Coles, 1996).

The idea of grief being experienced in stages or phases, while appropriate to the concept of grieving as a process, implies a kind of passivity – something mourners must pass through (Worden, 1995). Worden discusses *adaptation to loss* in the context of four basic grief tasks: to accept the reality of the loss, to work through the pain of grief, to adjust to the environment of the loss, and to emotionally relocate the deceased (the loss) and move on with life. Worden believes tasks offer mourners hope through purposeful activity, which can help overcome feelings of helplessness, but suggests that incomplete mourning can result if all these tasks are not accomplished.

Thus, traditional theories propose that the grieving process normally results in acceptance or resolution, with failure to reach this stage seen as an abnormal response (Teel, 1991). However, some authors who have studied chronic illness believe it may be very difficult to reach this stage and suggest that failure to achieve acceptance or resolution is not 'abnormal' (Dashiff, 1993; Murgatroyd & Woolfe, 1993; Hainsworth *et al.*, 1994; Tinlin, 1996; Lowes *et al.*, 2005). Grief may be perpetual, with periods of remission and periods of intensification of grief symptoms (Clubb, 1991; Murgatroyd & Woolfe, 1993; Tinlin, 1996). The perception of grief as a recurring state may have implications for parental adaptation to the diagnosis of childhood chronic illness because, as Clubb (1991) suggests, parents of children with chronic illness may never reach the acceptance or closure stages of time-bound theories. This is because the affected child serves as a constant reminder of the loss, which consequently inhibits resolution of the grief response (Teel, 1991). For example, parents of a child with type 1 diabetes are constantly reminded about the loss of their 'healthy child' when insulin has to be administered at least twice a day to keep their child alive. Even if the treatment becomes 'part of their daily lives' (Lowes *et al.*, 2004), their grief may resurface under certain circumstances, such as their child moving to a new school or being restricted in employment choices. Thus, when exploring grief in chronic illness, theories that analyse grief in the context of bereavement may have limited applicability (Teel, 1991; Hainsworth *et al.*, 1994; Tinlin, 1996).

Chronic sorrow is an approach that views the parental reaction to childhood chronic illness as one of functional adaptation to, but not acceptance of, the child's condition (Clubb, 1991). Chronic sorrow does not resolve over time, and is defined as a recurring sadness, interwoven with periods of neutrality, satisfaction and happiness (Teel, 1991). Olshansky (1962) introduced the theory of chronic sorrow to explain the response of lifelong episodic sadness in parents of children with impaired cognitive abilities. He proposed that parents never fully recover from the impact stage and, although they adjust and adapt to the situation, their efforts do not represent acceptance. Thus, Olshansky disputes that parents of children with chronic illness ever reach the closure stage of time-bound models and defines chronic sorrow as a normal response to ongoing loss. On the other hand, Solnit and Stark (1961) view chronic sorrow as a disruption of the traditional time-bound grief theories understood in the light of psychoanalytical theory. This reflects a critical difference between Solnit and Stark (1961) and Olshansky (1962) in their perception of chronic sorrow. Whereas Olshansky believes chronic sorrow to be a natural response to ongoing loss, Solnit and Stark view it as an abnormal grief reaction – a disruption of the time-bound grieving process (Teel, 1991). The theory of chronic sorrow has been elaborated by workers such as Copley and Bodensteiner (1987) who identified two phases of reaction to loss when working with parents of children with disability. The first phase is impact, denial and grief, experienced as a cycle of emotional peaks and troughs. This leads to the second phase, during which parents employ appropriate coping measures to systematically resolve crises, and begin to adapt to their changed life situation. Emotional turmoil continues, but is less intense in the second phase. While sorrow fades with time, it never ends. Copley and Bodensteiner suggest parents of some children with disability never progress to phase two due to the ongoing nature of their loss, remaining in the phase of emotional turbulence.

Most of the work on chronic sorrow has involved parents of children with severe disability, and the relationship between the profundity of the child's condition and the presence of chronic sorrow is not yet clear. Phillips (1991) suggests that chronic sorrow is elicited when there is hopelessness regarding progress, cure or normalcy, as in the case of the parents of children with severe disability in Olshansky's original work, who face the reality of their situation everyday. It could, however, be argued that ongoing losses are also experienced by parents of children whose condition is chronic but without severe disability or cognitive impairment. These parents may also experience events or situations that periodically bring their child's condition to the forefront, reawakening feelings of sadness and guilt or reinforcing a sense of disparity, for example absence of menstruation due to infertility in certain genetic conditions. More recently, Eakes *et al.* (1998) have emphasised the role of 'disparity' in creating chronic sorrow as a normal response to ongoing loss or the loss occasioned by bereavement. Disparity is described as the difference between an individual's current reality and idealised reality that, periodically, is brought into focus by trigger events or milestones, such as an anniversary or a difference in developmental milestones. When working with families of children with chronic illness, children's nurses need to accept that chronic sorrow exists and use strategies to reduce its impact (Langridge, 2002).

Key points

- A diagnosis of chronic illness in childhood can trigger a grief response in the child and family.
- Traditional stage or time-bound theories of grief suggest there is a sequential progression through stages of grief culminating in an endpoint such as acceptance.
- In chronic sorrow, grief is believed to be perpetual with no endpoint such as resolution, and is characterised by periods of remission and periods of intensification of grief symptoms.
- An understanding of the grief experienced by children with chronic illness and their families can assist children's nurses to help them as they try to adapt and adjust their lives to incorporate the demands of disease management.

Time out

What key physical and social developmental events may trigger a reminder in parents of children/young people with chronic illness?

A diagnosis of childhood chronic illness represents many losses or consequences for families and these will reflect the different stages of their child's physical and social development. Key milestones that may be adversely affected in the presence of chronic illness include those associated with communication, social skills, toilet training, play patterns, motor skills and maturation. For example, in younger children, developmental events such as walking and talking may be delayed, or not reached at all. In older children, maturation may be problematic, for example some diseases, such as Turner syndrome, delay maturation and development, while others, such as spina bifida, cerebral palsy and some endocrine conditions, may cause premature development (Boas *et al.*, 1995). Young people may also experience problems with events related to increasing independence, such as maintaining steady employment or leaving home.

Recent work suggests that the grief experienced by parents of a child with newly diagnosed diabetes arises from an awareness of a discrepancy between a world 'that should be' and a world 'that is' (Lowes *et al.*, 2005). Data exploring parents' experience of having a child diagnosed with type 1 diabetes (Lowes *et al.*, 2004) was examined within the framework of the *Theory of Psychosocial Transition* (Parkes, 1993; 1996). Parkes proposes that when faced with a life-changing event or 'psychosocial transition', such as a diagnosis of childhood diabetes, individuals are required to review and modify assumptions about the world that they have built up over many years. A familiar world suddenly becomes unfamiliar, causing feelings of anxiety and fear. For parents of children with newly diagnosed diabetes, the world 'that should be' is their world as they knew it before diagnosis. The world 'that is' is their world after diagnosis that needs to incorporate the demands and challenges of having a child with diabetes.

Reflection

Reflect on how the above theories might apply to children and young people with chronic conditions.

Much of the work on grief and loss in relation to childhood chronic illness has focused on parents, predominantly mothers, as the main carers, and very little work has been undertaken with children with chronic conditions. Contemporary research ethics and governance frameworks make research with children and young people a complex undertaking, but quite rightly so, because children's rights and well-being must take paramount importance over the need for research. Research that aims to elicit an understanding of people's experiences of loss and grief is usually qualitative in design, with in-depth interviewing the main data collection method. Some adult respondents have found being interviewed about emotive topics a helpful, even 'therapeutic', activity (Lowes & Gill, 2006) but in-depth interviewing can bring to full consciousness feelings and emotions hitherto unacknowledged and it is not known how this outcome may affect children and young people. Selecting a research sample from this population may also be problematic due to the different stages of cognitive, emotional and physical development potentially affecting how children and young people experience loss and grief.

It is difficult to estimate the impact of a diagnosis of chronic illness on a child's life because this will be determined by a number of influencing factors, including age at diagnosis, stage of development, gender, personality, temperament and coping styles (Cooper, 1999). The impact will be influenced by the characteristics of the chronic condition, including nature of onset, disease trajectory, effects on appearance, effects on daily functioning, effects on behaviour and ability to relate to others and the care required. It is probable, too, that the impact on the child will be influenced by parental response and coping. For example, children whose social activities are severely restricted due to parental over-concern about safety might experience a greater loss of freedom.

It is easy to see how children with chronic illness may grieve the 'normal' life they enjoyed before diagnosis and experience a number of losses caused by the diagnosis. Those losses could include a loss of freedom (this could be freedom from worry, freedom from having to think about managing their condition or freedom in the context of being restricted in social activities), a loss of the good health they previously enjoyed, a loss of self-esteem and a loss of confidence.

However, perhaps surprisingly, most studies have shown that children with chronic illnesses are as emotionally healthy as their peers and, in some cases, even surpass their peers in confidence and optimism (Deaton, 2006). Deaton suggests that this is because children with chronic illness have faced challenges that most children have not faced and have successfully overcome the hurdles.

Initial impact

 Case study 3.1

Background information

Taleisha is an 11-year-old girl who developed type 1 diabetes two weeks ago. Her father (42 years of age) is Caribbean, has lived in England for twenty years and is employed as a store manager for a large national computer company. Her mother (39 years of age) is white British and a part-time hairdresser at a local salon. Taleisha was born in England and has a 13-year-old brother and a 4-year-old sister. The family are social class 2 (based on the National Statistics Socio-Economic Classification (NS-SEC)) and live in a cul-de-sac of four bed-roomed modern detached houses in a semi-rural village. Taleisha has been attending the local primary school for the past five years but will be transferring to the local comprehensive school in four months time. Her widowed paternal grandmother lives in Antigua, and her maternal grandparents live a hundred miles away in Leeds and work full time in a family run hardware store. No other family members are known to have diabetes.

Test your knowledge

- What are the classic sequential symptoms that indicate a diagnosis of type 1 diabetes?
- What are the essential elements of type 1 diabetes management?
- Why is it important to obtain and sustain optimal glycaemic control?

Type 1 diabetes

Type 1 diabetes, one of the most common lifelong childhood disorders, is occurring with increasing frequency. A lack or relative insufficiency of insulin results in hyperglycaemia, polyuria, polydipsia, lethargy and weight loss. If untreated, severe fluid, electrolyte and acid–base disturbances will lead to vomiting, dehydration, coma and death (Brink, 1995). The management of childhood diabetes is relentless and invasive, involving two or more insulin injections a day, blood glucose monitoring up to four times a day, a healthy diet and regular exercise. In addition to the short-term complications of diabetic ketoacidosis and hypoglycaemia, poor glycaemic control increases the risk of life-threatening microvascular and neurological complications in later life (Diabetes Control and Complications Trial (DCCT) Research Group, 1993).

For more information on type 1 diabetes and its management, readers are referred to the suggested reading list and websites at the end of this chapter.

Impact on parents

Taking the case study as an example, parents of a child with newly diagnosed diabetes have been found to experience a grief response similar to that normally associated with bereavement (Almeida, 1995; Hatton *et al.*, 1995; Lowes *et al.*, 2004; 2005), and a diagnosis of childhood diabetes may represent multiple losses to Taleisha's parents.

  Time out

Consider what losses you think may be experienced by parents of a child with newly diagnosed childhood diabetes.

Feelings of loss will vary from family to family depending upon, for example, their view of the world, their past experience, the extent to which their life needs to change and their expectations of the future. Losses that Taleisha's parents may experience include the loss of the healthy child they thought they had, loss of a certain lifestyle, loss of freedom, loss of former support systems, loss of social acceptance, potential loss of their child's life, and a loss of confidence in their ability to protect their child from danger (Lowes *et al.*, 2004; 2005).

Following the diagnosis, Taleisha's parents are likely to experience a range of emotions such as disbelief, anger, sadness, guilt, anxiety, fear and confusion. For some time after diagnosis, diabetes will be the first thing Taleisha's parents think about in the morning and the last thing they think about at night. They have received a lot of information about diabetes and its management in addition to having to learn the practical skills of insulin administration and blood glucose monitoring. Taleisha's father works long hours as a store manager and it will fall to Taleisha's mother to take responsibility for the day-to-day management of her daughter's condition. This includes thinking about the timing and content of meals, and how this is all going to fit in with her part-time job as a hairdresser. Findings from a recent study suggest that mothers of children with diabetes might even experience post-traumatic stress disorder (Horsch *et al.*, 2006), which may interfere with their ability to manage their child's diabetes.

Indeed, parents may find that having a child with a chronic illness impinges on almost all aspects of their life, including finances, employment, childcare, parenting, marital relationships and roles, sibling relationships and socialising (Goble, 2004). One or both parents must devote extra time and attention to help their child cope with the demands of the condition. This can create problems, for example, with conflict about disciplining the affected child, sibling rivalry and attention seeking behaviour, and disagreement about approaches to parenting or management of the chronic condition. Childcare becomes difficult, either because parents are worried about handing over the care of their child to untrained or inexperienced carers, or because carers are concerned about taking responsibility for routine medication or managing potential emergency situations (Miller, 2005). This can affect the parents', particularly the mother's (who are usually the main care givers) ability to work outside the family home, which in turn may reduce the family income. Childcare difficulties may also severely curtail the social activities of children with chronic illness and their parents (Hatton *et al.*, 1995).

🔑 Key points

- A diagnosis of chronic illness can represent a number of losses for affected children/young people, their parents and families.
- The presence of chronic illness in childhood can impinge on almost all aspects of family life.

It is important to remember, however, that some parents of young people with chronic illness may identify positive aspects of the parenting experience, including recognising family strengths and adopting a healthier lifestyle (Mellin *et al.*, 2004).

🕐 Time out

Consider how a diagnosis of chronic illness might impact on children and young people at different developmental stages, for example preschool, school-age and adolescent.

Impact on the child/young person with chronic illness

A diagnosis of chronic illness will also have a profound effect on the affected child. Children with chronic diseases are confronted with a specific interpersonal situation – they have to cope with the fact that their condition is not only affecting their own lives but also that of their parents and siblings (Eiser & Berrenberg, 1995; Eiser, 1996; Varni & Wallander, 1998; Seiffge-Krenke, 1998; Schmidt *et al.*, 2002). They also face the challenge of coping with the unique demands of their chronic condition, while coping at the same time with the developmental tasks associated with their particular age group (Meuleners *et al.*, 2002).

   Children's stage of development will affect their response to the diagnosis. Although infants (0–2 years of age) will clearly not realise the implications of having a chronic condition, the process of bonding between the parents and infant may be affected. Management of the condition and extended periods of illness or hospitalisation can interfere with 'normal' interaction between the infant and parents and create difficulties with attachment (Cooper, 1999). Having a chronic condition is stressful for toddlers and preschool children. Their drive for autonomy and self-control may be hindered due to the restrictions and effects of chronic illness, and if parents are overprotective, they may lose independence and the opportunity to meet developmental tasks. They will be unable to understand the rationale for, sometimes painful, treatment and their developing self-concept may be strongly influenced by the condition and discomfort experienced (Ball & Bindler, 2006). Preschool children with a chronic illness are at an emotionally vulnerable age and their condition and treatment may adversely affect their feelings of security, their self-esteem and perception of their body image (Cooper, 1999). Preschool children often have a 'literal' grasp of language, which has implications both for them and for health care providers. For example, a four-year-old child who is told that he/she has diabetes might well understand this as meaning he/she is going to 'die of the betes', a frightening misinterpretation, particularly if they feel unable to voice their fears. It is important, therefore, that children's understanding of a situation is assessed and any misunderstandings corrected. Primary school-age children enter the stage of concrete operational thought (Piaget, 1962) at about seven years of age, when they have an increased ability to understand their condition but in the present timeframe (O'Conner-Von, 2002). School-age children (6–11 years of age) develop their sense of identity, belonging and self-esteem through involvement and acceptance by their peer group (Cooper, 1999), and this process can be affected in the presence of chronic illness. In adolescence, peer relationships take on even greater importance, often to the detriment of family relationships, as young people face the major developmental task of establishing independence from parents. Limitations imposed by a chronic condition can complicate this struggle for autonomy as young people try to integrate management of the condition into their lives (Garwick & Millar, 1996). (Chronic illness in adolescence is discussed in Chapters 9 and 10.)

At 11 years of age, Taleisha is coming to a stage in her life when she is beginning to strive for a degree of independence from her parents, maybe going to friends' houses for sleepovers or to the local shops with friends at weekends. These activities are made more difficult in the presence of diabetes because she now has to consider issues such as insulin injections, blood glucose monitoring and eating regular carbohydrate containing foods. She has to try to avoid and, when necessary, recognise and treat hypoglycaemic episodes. Her increasing shift towards independence may be hindered due to parental concerns about new safety issues and she may start to feel different to her friends who do not have these restrictions in their lives. Feeling 'different' is often a major problem for school-age children with a chronic condition.

Children with chronic illness are presented with unique problems in school, where they may encounter a range of academic, social and emotional difficulties (Shiu, 2004). Depending upon the age of the child and the demands of the chronic condition, they and their parents may rely heavily upon support from school staff to help the child cope with their disease management away from the home setting. Children with chronic conditions such as diabetes, epilepsy, asthma and cystic fibrosis may require some form of intervention during the schoolday. Notaras *et al.* (2002) found that parents felt that teachers lacked adequate knowledge to provide care related to their child's condition in school. This finding was supported by Clay *et al.* (2004) in a survey of 480 US schoolteachers, 59% of whom reported no professional training and 64% no in-house training for dealing with issues of chronic illness, a lack of knowledge that can adversely impact on the family's quest for a 'normal' life. Variable attendance and isolation from peers may impact upon the possible level of educational attainment (Shiu, 2004). To help children cope with chronic illness in school, a multidisciplinary and inter-agency approach (see Chapter 2) is essential.

Key points

- It is important that children who are chronically ill are facilitated to integrate the management of their condition into school life, participating in sports/activities and achieving their full academic potential.
- To achieve this, there needs to be effective communication between the child and family, school staff and health professionals, including the school nurse and the primary and secondary health care teams.

Before Taleisha returned to school following her diagnosis, it was important that the children's diabetes specialist nurse educated school staff about diabetes and the extra care and support that Taleisha would need (RCN, 2005), particularly in relation to hypoglycaemic episodes. This was relatively straightforward in Taleisha's primary school setting, where her class teacher assumed primary responsibility for her care, but will be more difficult when Taleisha moves to the larger comprehensive school, where she will transfer to various classrooms with different teachers, to be taught specific subjects. Although the ideal solution is to regularly educate all school staff about diabetes at an inset day, this is sometimes not possible due to increasingly full agendas at inset sessions, and responsibility for the care of children with chronic illness often falls to the staff member qualified in first aid and the head of year.

Time out

Think of four factors that may influence how successfully Taleisha copes with diabetes management in school.

You may have thought about:

- The level of teachers' knowledge and understanding of diabetes
- The understanding and support of her peer group and immediate circle of friends

- The provision of somewhere private to go to undertake blood glucose monitoring
- Taleisha's confidence to deal with situations such as hypoglycaemic episodes
- Whether she is subjected to teasing or bullying for being 'different'
- Is she included unconditionally on school trips or do the school insist that a family member accompanies her?
- Has she received support from the school nurse?

School nurses play a major part in helping children and young people with chronic illnesses integrate the management of their condition into school life. They have a pivotal role in ensuring effective communication between children with chronic illness and their parents, teachers, health care teams in primary and secondary care and other professionals. They also have a remit, alongside specialist health care professionals, to educate school staff about specific chronic conditions and their implications for school life.

Continuing care

 Case study 3.2

Four months after diagnosis

Taleisha has made a successful transition to the comprehensive school. However, problems are emerging in relation to Taleisha feeling that she is being treated differently to her siblings who, in turn, are jealous of the attention being given to Taleisha. Uncharacteristically, her 13-year-old brother has begun teasing her unkindly, particularly when she gets upset about having to do injections or blood glucose monitoring. He is also refusing to carry out his normal household tasks. Her 4-year-old sister is continually vying for their mother's attention, crying and trying to sit on her lap when she is assisting Taleisha with her diabetes care. Although Taleisha's parents are trying to ensure that all the children receive attention, the situation is causing a lot of conflict within the family, which is exacerbating the tiredness experienced by her parents due to the continuous demands of diabetes management. Fortunately, Taleisha has good glycaemic control (blood glucose levels mainly 4–9mmol/l, HbA1c 7.2%) as she is still in the honeymoon phase.

Impact on siblings

Sibling relationships are important throughout life, and can influence how individuals develop and the type of people they become. Siblings often spend a lot of time together, particularly in early or middle childhood, and a diagnosis of chronic illness in a brother or sister can have a considerable impact on the unaffected siblings. However, few studies have investigated this topic. A meta-analysis of the literature found that siblings of children who are chronically ill were more at risk for negative psychological effects (i.e. depression and anxiety) than those without, and that chronic illnesses requiring daily treatment regimens were more likely to affect siblings than those that did not (Sharpe & Rossiter, 2002). Sharpe and Rossiter concluded, though, that more methodologically sound studies need to be undertaken in this area.

 Time out

How do you think Taleisha's brother and sister might be affected by her diagnosis of diabetes?

The effect of childhood chronic illness on siblings will vary from family to family, and will depend greatly upon parenting styles, family structure (e.g. where the affected child sits within the family), previous and present sibling relationships, age differences, past experience, individual characteristics and the nature/demands of the chronic condition. However, Taleisha's siblings might experience:

- Jealousy – everything revolves around her
- Restrictions – we are unable to eat sweets in front of her, nothing nice to eat is kept in the house anymore
- Anger at the illness itself – this should not have happened
- Sadness – this is a dreadful thing to have happened to her, and there's nothing we can do to make it better
- Distress – it is awful that she has to give injections and do blood glucose monitoring and that mum and dad are upset all the time
- Worry – that she might die, or that we might also develop diabetes; can we catch it?
- Confusion – we do not know enough about diabetes, why did this happen?
- Protectiveness – we need/want to look after her
- Responsibility – we need to make sure she's safe

A recent Swedish study by Wennick and Hallstrom (2006) found that siblings of a brother/sister with newly diagnosed type 1 diabetes sensed that they received less parental attention than the affected child, and experienced anxiety and restricted independence. However, the presence of childhood chronic illness also allows siblings to view life from a different perspective, which can result in positive outcomes. These might include strengthening family relationships, achieving more personal independence, gaining satisfaction from seeing improvement in their brother/sister's condition (Derouin & Jessee, 1996), becoming more altruistic, and being more accepting of those who are unable to lead a 'normal' life.

A study by Williams (2000) found that young people managed chronic illness (asthma and diabetes) in gendered ways. Most girls showed greater adaptation than boys, incorporating their condition and associated treatment regimens into their social and personal identities. Taleisha's positive transition to comprehensive schooling suggests that she has successfully integrated diabetes into her life outside the home environment. At a clinic visit, though, it transpired that there was conflict between Taleisha and her mother concerning her mother's reluctance to allow Taleisha the freedom she enjoyed pre-diagnosis. Research has shown that parents, especially mothers, are often afraid to 'let go' following a diagnosis of childhood diabetes (Lowes *et al.*, 2004). Problems with 'letting go' arise mainly from a parental fear that their child might have a severe hypoglycaemic episode when out on their own or with friends and no one will know how to treat it. Parents need to feel in control of the diabetes management. This is a difficult problem to resolve because it is important that Taleisha socialises with her peer group, but equally important that her mother's concerns are addressed. Taleisha's father suggested that he buy her a mobile phone, thus allowing easy contact between Taleisha and her mother, a solution that pleased Taleisha and offered some reassurance to her mother.

Povlsen *et al.* (2005) found that younger people with type 1 diabetes from ethnic minorities living in Denmark had significantly poorer metabolic control. This was related to limited educational backgrounds, insufficient language skills and marginalised social positions. Taleisha's mixed race parentage does not seem to have been problematic in relation to her family's adaptation to the diagnosis. The family are highly respected in the community. Her father has lived in the UK for many years, speaks very good English and holds a well paid and influential position in a large national company. The family diet is healthy and varied. Although Taleisha's mother sometimes cooks African-Caribbean meals, she now avoids typical sweet dishes and concentrates on starchy foods (e.g. yam, sweet potato, rice, hard dough bread), fruit and vegetables (e.g. banana, mango, melon, okra, pepper), meat, fish and other protein alternatives (e.g. kidney beans, black-eye beans, lentils).

⏲ Time out

Can you identify characteristics of specific cultures and religions that may impact on a family's ability to adapt and adjust to a diagnosis of chronic illness in childhood?

Religion and culturally different beliefs about health and illness can influence coping, adaptation and adjustment to a diagnosis of chronic illness. For example, in Vietnamese culture, it is disrespectful to ask a doctor a question (Shanahan & Bradshaw, 1995), which has implications for successful, patient-centred chronic disease management. In some cultures (e.g. India, China and Japan), parents of a child with a chronic illness such as type 1 diabetes or epilepsy will fear social stigmatisation, which may result in families being burdened with a sense of shame and lead to secrecy about the condition (Koizumi, 1992; Coclami & Bor, 1993; Pal *et al.*, 2002; Mu, 2005). Dietary management of certain conditions, such as diabetes, may be affected by religious beliefs. Moslem families, for example, may wish to observe Ramadan, which requires fasting from sunrise to sunset, although diabetes is one condition that exempts affected individuals from keeping this rule. Some religious beliefs can result in more serious outcomes. For example, Jehovah's Witnesses believe that blood represents life itself and may consequently refuse blood transfusions even in life-threatening situations, and members of the Church of the First Born believe in prayer rather than medicines to treat the sick. Tragically, since the mid-1970s, in Colorado 11 children whose parents were members of the Church of the First Born have died or been stillborn after medical treatment was withheld. The last, in 2001, was a 13-year-old girl who died of complications from untreated diabetes (Lofholm, 2001). Chapter 4 also discusses psychosocial issues in relation to culture and spirituality in the context of childhood chronic illness.

Key points

- A diagnosis of chronic illness in a brother or sister can have a considerable impact on unaffected siblings.
- Children's nurses need to be aware of the potential impact on siblings and include them in discussions and, if appropriate, involve them in the care of their affected brother or sister.

Coping, adaptation and change

It is generally accepted that a diagnosis of childhood diabetes represents a major stressor event for parents (Lowes & Lyne, 1999; 2000). Influenced by a variety of interpersonal and environmental factors, parents may approach the process of coping in different ways. Over the four months since diagnosis, Taleisha's parents will have used various strategies to help them cope with the changes to their lifestyle necessitated by the diagnosis. Some theories of coping, adaptation and change, two of which are classical theories underpinning much of the work of contemporary theorists in this area, are introduced below. Coping strategies that may be used by parents of children with chronic conditions are also discussed.

Reflection

Think about the last time you experienced stress. Reflect on how you coped with this and the strategies you use to resolve or minimise the stress.

Theories of stress and coping

Coping, or the responses of an individual to a stressor event, is an important component of stress management (Powell & Enright, 1990). Historically, stress has been defined as either the physiological and/or psychological responses to a threatening or demanding situation (response-based model) or as the event or set of circumstances which threatens a person's well-being and gives rise to a stress reaction (stimulus-based model). However, both these models fail to take into account the meaning of events to those experiencing them (Clark, 1990). Families cope with change in many ways, and a wide range of theories about coping has been developed. In this chapter, two classical theories relating to stress, coping, adaptation and change are introduced: the *family adaptation model* (McCubbin & Patterson, 1983) and *cognitive appraisal and coping* (Lazarus & Folkman, 1984), both of which recognise the many factors that may influence individual responses to the same stress experience.

The family adaptation model

This model by McCubbin and Patterson (1983) is based on four assumptions drawn from family research and crisis theory. It describes the family as responding to a stressor event through the two phases of adjustment and adaptation. In the *adjustment phase* the family's vulnerability to a crisis is believed to be dependent upon the actual stressor event and prior strains, the family's existing resources and the family's subjective perceptions of the seriousness of the stressor event. Adjustment to the stressor event, therefore, varies with individual families. Some families absorb the change into routine family functioning, whereas for other families, more adjustment is necessary and can develop into a crisis. In the *adaptation phase*, the family attempts to adapt and achieve a new sense of balance in the family system, with the level of adaptation dependent upon the accumulation of demands on the family, the family's strengths and resources and the family's perception of the crisis. For example, if other stressful events happen at the same time as the diagnosis, less energy may be available for coping with the chronic condition. Adaptation is also influenced by the family's use of general coping processes in acquiring and allocating resources.

Cognitive appraisal and coping

According to a theory of stress and coping developed by Lazarus and colleagues (Lazarus & Folkman, 1984; Folkman *et al.*, 1986), coping is the person's constantly changing cognitive and behavioural efforts to manage specific external and/or internal demands that are appraised as taxing or exceeding the person's resources. The stress experience is moderated by two basic cognitive appraisals, through which people assess the level of threat and their own resources for dealing with it. These appraisals will be influenced by the personal characteristics of individuals, such as patterns of motivation (values, commitments or personal goals), beliefs about themselves and the world, and personal recognition of resources for coping (social skills, problem solving skills or finances). Appraisal processes are also influenced by environmental variables such as the nature of the danger, whether it is imminent, whether it is ongoing or short term and whether it is an ambiguous type of threat or not, as well as the existence and quality of social support (Banyard & Hayes, 1994). Other potential influences on individuals' ability to cope with stressful situations include their previous experiences, existing coping strategies, health status and cognitive ability.

Thus, stress is the product of the interaction between a person and their environment. An event is only stressful if it is perceived as such by the individual. Stress is believed to arise when there is an imbalance between the perceived demand and the perceived capability to cope with that demand (Bailey & Clarke, 1989; Sutherland & Cooper, 1990). In a chronic illness such as diabetes, the process of coping entails different challenges, tasks and responses at various points in time (Kovacs *et al.*, 1985a; b).

Coping strategies

When a stressor event occurs, people use coping strategies to try to change or alleviate the situation and manage the demands imposed upon them. As the process of coping is influenced by a number of factors, the coping strategies used to manage any particular stress event will vary considerably between individuals (Lazarus & Folkman, 1984). Lazarus and Folkman identify two different approaches to coping:

- Problem-focused coping (a direct approach where the problem is evaluated and action is taken to change or avoid the situation)
- Emotion-focused coping (a more indirect approach with the focus on reducing anxiety rather than dealing with the problem causing the anxiety)

Coping strategies are sometimes described as 'adaptive' or 'maladaptive' (Lu & Chen, 1996). *Adaptive strategies* are believed to alleviate stress and re-establish equilibrium, enabling the individual to adjust appropriately while gaining from the experience. Adaptive coping might include understanding what is going on, recognising demands and resources and taking action to reduce demands. *Maladaptive strategies* are defined as those that exacerbate existing demands, fail to stabilise the situation and do not allow the individual to adjust, resulting in misery and unhappiness. Maladaptive coping might include failing to recognise and understand what is happening, denial, avoiding situations which produce anxiety and withdrawal from social support (Powell & Enright, 1990; Roger & Nash, 1995).

 Time out

Can you think of some coping strategies that Taleisha's parents might use?

A variety of coping strategies used by parents of children with chronic illness can be elicited from the literature (Lowes & Lyne, 1999). These are presented in Table 3.1,

Table 3.1   Coping strategies.

Emotion-focused coping strategies

- Not focusing on the diabetes
- Unburdening themselves/expressing the stress
- Maintaining the image of a healthy child
- Gaining confidence to manage family life
- Resignation (diabetes is better than some illnesses)
- Putting the implications of the disease into perspective
- Holding out (I have to treat this child)
- Thinking positively about life with diabetes
- Belief in religion
- Clinging to hope for an early cure
- Accepting a lack of support from fearful friends and relatives
- Reminiscing about the time of diagnosis
- Realising that the complex regimen must be continued for their child to live
- Trusting others
- Taking charge of the situation/being in control
- Staying calm/taking one day at a time
- Normalisation
- Seeing their child happy
- Looking for a cause

Problem-focused coping strategies

- Dealing with their children's needs
- Allowing their child a certain amount of responsibility
- Being assertive and advocating for their child
- Acquiring cooperation from other family members
- Maintaining family integrity
- Developing a social support network
- Talking to other parents
- Becoming technically competent
- Strict adherence to the treatment regimen
- Liasing/working with professionals
- Educating others about diabetes
- Getting knowledge about/understanding of the condition
- Parental sharing of responsibilities
- Taking charge of the situation
- Normalisation
- Looking for a cause

Sources   Benoliel, 1975; Anderson, 1981; Gallo, 1990; Koizumi, 1992; Hatton *et al.*, 1995; Faulkner, 1996; Seppanen *et al.*, 1999; Lowes *et al.*, 2004; 2005; Mu, 2005; Van Hooren *et al.*, 2005; Webb, 2005.

classified as either emotion-focused or problem-focused strategies, although the categorisation of some of the strategies may be contentious depending upon subjective interpretation. A major coping strategy used by parents of children with chronic illness is normalisation.

Normalisation

The aims of normalisation are to reduce feelings of being different and enable children and their families to have a sense of control over their lives (Krulik, 1980).

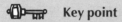 **Key point**

Parents of children with chronic illness face difficulties not experienced by other parents (Purssell, 1994).

The experience of having a child with chronic illness in the family is extremely demanding, with adjustment and adaptation by the family requiring recurrent modification in response to environmental, social and cognitive pressures (Muller *et al.*, 1994). Parents use normalising tactics to minimise the effects of, and thereby reduce the impact of, chronic illness (Krulik, 1980; Muller *et al.*, 1994). Parents define normalisation as: 'constant process of actively accommodating the changing physical and emotional needs of the child or adolescent, with the goal of integrating the child into the family rather than making him or her a "special nucleus"' (Deatrick *et al.*, 1988, p. 17).

Normalisation involves parents in promoting normal experiences for their child with chronic illness, while constantly assessing, and adapting to, potential problems or limitations resulting from their child's condition. This involves effort beyond that of the usual parenting role (Bossert *et al.*, 1990), and may encompass neighbourhoods, schools and other agencies involved in issues relating to the child's needs. Knafl and Deatrick (1986) undertook an analysis of the concept of normalisation based on ways in which families manage chronic conditions. The child's age and the nature and severity of the condition were found to influence families' abilities to normalise their situation, with normalisation during childhood easier than during either preschool or adolescent years.

 Time out

Can you think of some coping strategies that Taleisha might use?

Coping strategies used by children and young people with chronic illness will depend upon their personal characteristics, which include level of confidence, self-esteem, usual coping style, view of the world, past experiences, developmental stage, cognitive ability, family structure and dynamics, and how parents, family and friends perceive, and cope with, the condition. Taleisha has reached a developmental stage where friends are important. She is beginning to want to socialise independently of her parents and siblings. Therefore, Taleisha might:

- Seek information to become expert about her condition
- Develop a supportive relationship with her health care team
- Actively participate in decisions about her care
- Learn self-care skills to minimise the daily effects of her condition and enhance her self-esteem and autonomy
- Pursue interests and hobbies
- Explain the condition, its treatment and the restrictions it imposes to supportive friends
- Normalise diabetes in the context of her life and lifestyle

 Case study 3.1

A year after diagnosis

Taleisha's glycaemic control is deteriorating. She is attending clinic with very few blood glucose readings and her HbA1c (12.3%) indicates that she is probably not administering all of her insulin, the dosage of which has been gradually increased as her body is now producing little or no endogenous insulin. The school nurse has contacted the diabetes team due to a concern about Taleisha's attendance rate at school. Taleisha's mother broke down at their last attendance at clinic and appears to be depressed, partly because coping with Taleisha's diabetes management is causing major conflict within the family unit. A multidisciplinary, inter-agency meeting is to be convened at the school to include Taleisha and her parents.

Psychosocial problems are not unusual in children and young people with chronic illness, or their parents (Streisand *et al.*, 2005), and may occur for any number of reasons. The *National Service Framework for Diabetes in Wales* (WAG, 2003) recognises that diabetes is often more difficult to control during puberty and adolescence. Children and young people with type 1 diabetes may experience psychological disturbances such as anxiety, behavioural and conduct disorders and family conflict, and it is recommended that they and their families should receive timely and ongoing access to mental health professionals (NICE, 2004; Diabetes UK, 2005). This is reinforced by the *National Service Framework for Children, Young People and Maternity Services* (DoH, 2004; NHS Wales, 2005), which recommends that targeted and specialist services should be available to ensure that parents receive appropriate support, when required, at any time during their child's journey to adulthood. However, the reality is that there are too few mental health professionals working in this field, which, along with cost implications, means that many paediatric diabetes services do not have access to appropriate services (Hartnett, 2005). Having worked as a paediatric diabetes specialist nurse for the last eleven years, the author estimates that 50% of her workload involves working with parents and children and teenagers with type 1 diabetes with psychosocial issues. Psychosocial distress in young people with chronic conditions often results in poor adherence to treatment, poor behaviour, acting out, and non-adaptive and risk-taking behaviours (Rosina *et al.*, 2003). The target HbA1c (glycosylated haemoglobin) for children and young people with type 1 diabetes is 7.5% or below (NICE, 2004). Thus, Taleisha's high HbA1c result is cause for concern, and it is clear that, for whatever reason, she is not having enough insulin.

 Time out

Can you identify why Taleisha may not be receiving enough insulin?

It may be that Taleisha is omitting or inappropriately reducing some of her insulin doses, or that she has come out of the honeymoon period (i.e. her pancreatic beta cells are no longer producing insulin) and, because she is doing little or no blood glucose monitoring, she is unaware of her resulting high blood glucose levels. She could be omitting some of her insulin doses to lose weight, which is a common reason, for girls particularly, not to adhere to or comply with, the insulin regimen (Barber & Lowes, 1998). Although Taleisha is not overweight, she may have an altered perception of her body image. She may be testing the boundaries or simply be 'fed up' with the inconvenience of insulin injections and blood glucose monitoring. She may not want to feel 'different' from her non-diabetic peers and be ignoring her diabetes management to fit in with their relatively unrestricted lifestyle, particularly if she is trying to avoid hypoglycaemic episodes. It is possible that she is rebelling against her parents' strict adherence to diabetes care. She might be experiencing bullying at school, feel that no one appreciates what she has to 'suffer' on a daily basis, or resent her invasive diabetes care becoming an accepted part of her life, whereas immediately after diagnosis she was treated as 'special'. Due to her stage of development, Taleisha may have a growing awareness of the perpetuity of her condition, be frightened about the future or have an increased sense of her own mortality.

These are just a few scenarios that may have been the catalyst for the deterioration in Taleisha's glycaemic control. What is clear is that psychosocial issues often impact on glycaemic control and, due to an increased risk of diabetes-related complications in later life (Diabetes Control and Complications Trial Research Group, 1993), there is a need to try and resolve the underlying problem. It is sometimes difficult for health professionals to understand why children and young people endure high blood glucose levels for extended periods of time because they will undoubtedly experience polyuria, nocturnal enuresis, polydipsia and lethargy, have mood swings and feel generally below par. Children and young people with poor glycaemic control may have frequent readmissions to hospital with diabetic ketoacidosis (DKA), a life-threatening acute complication of type 1 diabetes. Furthermore, it is not unheard of for children and young people with type 1 diabetes to engineer admissions to hospital to escape a threatening situation, such as sexual abuse.

> **⟨Key⟩ Key point**
>
> Children's nurses in the ward environment are in a unique position to develop a trusting relationship with children and young people with chronic illness who suffer repeated readmissions, and work with them and other health professionals to uncover the underlying cause.

Taleisha's mother is concerned and upset about the HbA1c result, which is an average blood glucose measurement over 6–8 weeks. Parents often view the HbA1c as an 'exam' they have to pass at their child's clinic visit (Lowes *et al.*, 2004) and feel guilty or inadequate if it deteriorates, even if they believe they have done all they can to try and achieve good glycaemic control. This is, perhaps, when the concept of chronic sorrow could be applied. Other parents do not have to worry about these sorts of issues. Repeatedly over time, parents are forced to realise that their child or young person with chronic illness is 'different' under certain circumstances (Lowes & Lyne, 1999).

NICE (2004) recommends that children with chronic illness and their parents should be offered structural behavioural intervention strategies for reducing diabetes related family conflict. Morrison *et al.* (2003) discuss the benefits of a therapeutic model to support parents of children with chronic illness. The therapeutic model assumes that childhood chronic illness and disability can represent a trauma that impacts on day-to-day activities for the whole family, as discussed in the first section of this chapter. The study by Morrison *et al.* identified that families needed ongoing supportive interventions and counselling, referred to as 'psychological first aid', from diagnosis and at subsequent times of crisis.

The multidisciplinary paediatric diabetes team worked with Taleisha and her parents to try to resolve the problem. The approach included ongoing diabetes education, which was age appropriate and commensurate with Taleisha's stage of growth and cognitive development (International Society for Pediatric and Adolescent Diabetes, 2000; NICE; 2003; Diabetes UK, 2005). The paediatric diabetes specialist nurse consulted with Taleisha on her own because it was felt that she might have had issues she needed to discuss that she felt unable to talk about in the presence of her parents. However, taking Taleisha's age into account, if there were problems that were detrimental to her well-being, confidentiality might have had to be broken (legal and ethical issues are discussed in Chapter 6). Taleisha's parents also found it beneficial to discuss their problems and emotional responses to the diagnosis with an experienced member of the paediatric diabetes team. Although not necessary for Taleisha and her parents, children with chronic illness and their parents may require referral to a skilled mental health professional with expertise in this area of care.

The multidisciplinary, inter-agency meeting at the school, which was attended by Taleisha and her parents, was convened to address her poor school attendance rate of 42%. It transpired that Taleisha was finding it difficult to fit her diabetes management into school life and felt alienated from her peer group because she perceived herself as 'different', a belief compounded by her mixed race parentage in a school attended by predominantly white Caucasian children. Another problem concerned her friends' parents' reluctance to invite her to sleepovers or birthday outings because they were concerned about taking responsibility for her diabetes management. It was agreed that a 'buddy' system would be put in place, where a close friend would be educated about diabetes, be allowed to accompany her to do her pre-lunch blood glucose monitoring and attend the outpatient clinic with her during the school holidays. During the meeting, it was also identified that Taleisha's parents would allow her to stay at home if her blood glucose level was more than 15 mmol/l, because they worried about her becoming unwell at school. They were reassured regarding the unlikelihood of this happening and were offered further education about managing hyperglycaemia. Arrangements were also made for school staff to receive further diabetes education at the next inset day to reassure Taleisha and her parents about her safety while at school.

These interventions resolved the family conflict, and Taleisha subsequently improved her diabetes control and school attendance. However, life in the presence of childhood and adolescent diabetes is rarely that simple. In the author's experience, children and young people who present with problems relatively soon after diagnosis often continue to experience difficulty with diabetes management. Problems change in nature as the young person moves through different developmental stages, presenting children, young people, parents and the paediatric diabetes team with different challenges.

 Time out

Considering the content of this chapter, what is the role of children's nurses caring for families with a new diagnosis of childhood chronic illness?

Children's nurses should not underestimate the impact that a diagnosis of chronic illness may have on the lives of children, young people and their parents. As the father of a two-year-old boy diagnosed with type 1 diabetes said: 'There's a sense of loss in a way because we can't do it exactly like we used to do it . . . there's a change in routine, a change in the way you do things . . . it's made me think of the life that used to be and the life that is now' (Lowes *et al.*, 2004).

Thus, children's nurses need an in-depth knowledge of the theories of grief, loss, adaptation and change, and need to be able to understand and apply the underlying theoretical principles in the context of the care they provide to children with chronic illness and their families. They need to maintain an acute awareness of the intense grief that may be experienced by children and their families, and how this may affect their ability to adapt and adjust to the diagnosis. Insensitivity by children's nurses to the grieving process has the potential to inhibit expression of feelings, make affected children and their parents feel that they should be coping better and result in lowered self-esteem. Children's nurses also need knowledge of child development to be able to recognise maladaption or regression and put preventative or remedial strategies into place.

Children's nurses should be non-judgemental. It is important that they accept that different families cope in different ways and adapt the care they provide in response to individual need. For example, although some parents of a child with newly diagnosed diabetes may be prepared to inject their child with insulin on the day of diagnosis, others may find this extremely distressing. It is essential that children's nurses also take cultural and religious influences into account when addressing the care of a child with a chronic condition. Is there a need to adapt the dietary management? What are the implications of a diagnosis of chronic illness in relation to stigma or perceived suitability for marriage, particularly if infertility is a characteristic of the condition?

Children's nurses need to tailor education about a chronic condition to the needs of individual families. Complex regimens may be difficult to understand, depending upon cognitive ability, and the shock experienced at diagnosis may affect the capability to retain information. Language barriers may need to be crossed through the use of trained interpreters or pictorial information. Children's nurses should be able to direct families to voluntary organisations specific to particular conditions that have information in a variety of languages, or be able to download such information via the Internet for families.

Children's nurses are often best placed to work with children with chronic illness admitted to hospital. By developing close relationships with these children and their families during periods of hospitalisation, children's nurses may be privy to information that could ultimately affect the care they receive. They need to liaise closely with specialist teams and share information to ensure that children and their families receive optimal care during hospitalisation and after discharge home.

Conclusion

Children and young people with chronic illness, their parents and families are faced with coping with the demands of chronic conditions on a daily basis. They live with a lifestyle that changes, and different problems that arise, as the child passes through developmental stages to adulthood. Grief experienced at diagnosis will subside, but may resurface at particular times in the lives of children and young people with chronic illness and their parents. Different coping strategies will be used by children and parents to minimise the impact of the diagnosis and normalise the illness within the context of their lives, but their lives will always be different and more complicated than those of families who do not have to contend with the demands of a chronic condition.

Despite the challenges, however, many children and young people with chronic illnesses and their families, cope extremely well with the demands this places on them. The scenario provided in this chapter was designed to illustrate how a diagnosis of chronic illness may impact upon the family as a whole and give readers an opportunity to reflect upon and examine their understanding and knowledge of the topic.

Acknowledgement

The author would like to thank the editors of the *Journal of Advanced Nursing* and the *British Journal of Nursing* for their kind permission to reproduce two previously published papers in part (Lowes & Lyne, 1999; 2000).

Useful websites

Children's National Service Framework
www.doh.gov.uk/nsf/children/index.htm

Diabetes UK
www.diabetes.org.uk

International Society for Pediatric and Adolescent Diabetes
www.ispad.org

Juvenile Diabetes Research Foundation
www.jdrf.org.uk

National Institute for Clinical Excellence
www.nice.org.uk

National Service Framework for Diabetes
www.doh.gov.uk/nsf/diabetes/index.htm

RCN Paediatric and Adolescent Diabetes Forum
www.rcn.org.uk/cyp

 Recommended reading

Cooper, C. (1999) *Continuing Care of Sick Children. Examining the Impact of Chronic Illness.* Wiltshire, Mark Allen Publishing Ltd.

Lowes, L., Gregory, J.W. & Lyne, P. (2005) Newly diagnosed childhood diabetes: a psychosocial transition for parents? *Journal of Advanced Nursing*, **50** (3), 253–261.

References

Almeida, C.M. (1995) Grief among parents of children with diabetes. *The Diabetes Educator*, **21** (6), 530–532.

Anderson, J.M. (1981) The social construction of illness experience: families with a chronically-ill child. *Journal of Advanced Nursing*, 6, 427–434.

Bailey, R. & Clarke, M. (1989) *Stress and Coping in Nursing*. London, Chapman and Hall.

Ball, J.W. & Bindler, R.C. (2006) *Child Health Nursing. Partnering with Children and Families.* New Jersey, Pearson Education Inc.

Banyard, P. & Hayes, N. (1994) *Psychology. Theory and Application*. London, Chapman & Hall.

Barber, C.J. & Lowes, L. (1998) Eating disorders and adolescent diabetes: is there a link? *British Journal of Nursing*, **7** (7), 398–402.

Benoliel, J.Q. (1975) Childhood diabetes: the commonplace in living becomes uncommon. In: *Chronic Illness and the Quality of Life* (ed. A.L. Strauss), pp. 89–98. C.V. Mosby, St Louis.

Boas, S.R., Falsetti, D., Murphy, T.D. & Orenstein, D.M. (1995) Validity of self-assessment of sexual maturation in adolescent male patients with cystic fibrosis. *Journal of Adolescent Health*, **17**, 42–45.

Bossert, E., Holaday, B., Harkins, A. & Turner-Henson, A. (1990) Strategies of normalisation used by parents of chronically ill school-age children. *Journal of Child and Adolescent Psychiatric and Mental Health Nursing*, **3** (2), 57–61.

Brink, S.J. (1995) Presentation and ketoacidosis. In: *Childhood and Adolescent Diabetes* (ed. C.J.H. Kelnar), pp. 213–240. London, Chapman and Hall Medical.

Clark, E. (1990) Stress. In: *Knowledge for Practice* (eds S. Hinchliff, E. Clark & K.M. Robinson). London, Distance Learning Centre, South Bank Polytechnic.

Clay, D.L., Cortina, S., Harper, D.C., Cocco, K.M. & Drotar, D. (2004) Schoolteachers experiences with childhood chronic illness. *Children's Health Care*, **33** (3), 227–239.

Clubb, R.L. (1991) Chronic sorrow: adaptation patterns of parents with chronically ill children. *Pediatric Nursing*, **17** (5), 461–465.

Coclami, T. & Bor, R. (1993) Family relationships in Greek insulin-dependent diabetics. *Counselling Psychology Quarterly*, **6**, 267–279.

Coles, C. (1996) Psychology in diabetes care. *Practical Diabetes International*, **13** (2), 55–57.

Cook, B. & Phillips, S.G. (1989) *Loss and Bereavement*. London, Austin Cornish Publishers Limited in association with the Lisa Sainsbury Foundation.

Cooper, C. (1999) *Continuing Care of Sick Children. Examining the Impact of Chronic Illness*. Wiltshire, Mark Allen Publishing Ltd.

Copley, M.F. & Bodensteiner, J.B. (1987) Chronic sorrow in families of disabled children. *Journal of Child Neurology*, **2**, 67–70.

Dashiff, C.J. (1993) Parents' perceptions of diabetes in adolescent daughters and its impact on the family. *Journal of Pediatric Nursing*, **8** (6), 361–369.

Deaton, A.V. (2006) *Chronic Illness*. Richmond VA, Children's Hospital. Available at: http://childrenshosp-richmond.org/families/health/chronic_ill.htm

Deatrick, J.A., Knafl, K.A. & Walsh, M. (1988) The process of parenting a child with a disability: normalisation through accommodations. *Journal of Advanced Nursing*, **13**, 15–21.

Department of Health (2004) *National Service Framework for Children, Young People and Maternity Services*. London, Department of Health. Available at: www.dh.gov.uk Accessed 20/11/06.

Derouin, D. & Jessee, P.O. (1996) Impact of a chronic illness in childhood: siblings' perceptions. *Issues in Comprehensive Pediatric Nursing*, **19** (2), 135–147.

Diabetes Control and Complications Trial Research Group (1993) The effect of intensive treatment of diabetes on the development and progression of long-term complications in insulin dependent diabetes mellitus. *The New England Journal of Medicine*, **329** (14), 977–986.

Diabetes UK (2005) *Resources to Support the Delivery of Care for Children and Young People with Diabetes*. London, Diabetes UK.

Eakes, G.G., Burke, M.L. & Hainsworth, M.A. (1998) Middle-range theory of chronic sorrow. *Image: Journal of Nursing Scholarship*, **30** (2), 179–184.

Eiser, C. (1996) Helping the child with chronic disease: themes and directions. *Clinical Child Psychology and Psychiatry*, **1**, 551–561.

Eiser, C. & Berrenberg, J.L. (1995) Assessing the impact of chronic disease on the relationship between parents and their adolescents. *Journal of Psychosomatic Research*, **39**, 109–114.

Engel, G. (1962) *Psychological Development in Health and Disease*. Philadelphia, W.B. Saunders.

Faulkner, M.S. (1996) Family responses to children with diabetes and their influence on self-care. *Journal of Pediatric Nursing*, **11** (2), 82–93.

Folkman, S., Lazarus, R.S., Dunkel-Schetter, C., DeLongis, A. & Gruen, R.J. (1986) Dynamics of a stressful encounter: cognitive appraisal, coping and encounter outcomes. *Journal of Personality and Social Psychology*, **50** (5), 992–1003.

Gallo, A.M. (1990) Family management style in juvenile diabetes: a case illustration. *Journal of Pediatric Nursing*, **5** (1), 23–32.

Garwick, A. & Millar, H. (1996) *Promoting Resilience in Youth with Chronic Conditions and Their Families*. Washington, DC, Maternal and Child Health Bureau, Health Resources and Services Administration, US Public Health Service.

Goble, L.A. (2004) The impact of a child's chronic illness on fathers. *Issues in Comprehensive Pediatric Nursing*, **27**, 153–162.

Hainsworth, M.A., Eakes, G.G. & Burke, M.L. (1994) Coping with chronic sorrow. *Issues in Mental Health Nursing*, **15**, 59–66.

Hartnett, B. (2005) Room for improvement. *Diabetes Update. Diabetes UK*, Winter.

Hatton, D.L., Canam, C., Thorne, S. & Hughes, A.M. (1995) Parents' perceptions of caring for an infant or toddler with diabetes. *Journal of Advanced Nursing*, **22**, 569–577.

Horsch, A., McManus, F., Kennedy, P. & Edge, J. (2006) Can having a child with diabetes cause post-traumatic stress disorder in mothers and interfere with diabetes management. *Archives of Disease in Childhood. Royal College of Paediatrics and Child Health. Proceedings of the 10th Spring Meeting*, **91** (Suppl. 1), A20–A22.

International Society for Pediatric and Adolescent Diabetes (2000) *Consensus Guidelines 2000*. Netherlands, Medical Forum International. Available at: www.ispad.org Accessed 20/11/06.

Kamm, J.A. (1985) Grief and therapy: two processes in interaction. In: *Psychotherapy and the Grieving Patient* (ed. M. Stern), pp. 59–64. New York, Harrington Park Press.

Knafl, K.A. & Deatrick, J.A. (1986) How families manage chronic conditions: an analysis of the concept of normalisation. *Research in Nursing and Health*, **9**, 215–222.

Koizumi, S. (1992) Japanese mothers' responses to the diagnosis of childhood diabetes. *International Pediatric Nursing*, **7** (2), 154–160.

Kovacs, M., Feinberg, T.L., Paulauskas, S., Finkelstein, R., Pollock, M., Crouse-Novak, M. (1985a) Initial coping responses and psychosocial characteristics of children with insulin-dependent diabetes mellitus. *The Journal of Pediatrics*, **106** (5), 827–834.

Kovacs, M., Finkelstein, R., Feinberg, T.L., Crouse-Novak, M., Paulauskas, S. & Pollock, M. (1985b) Initial psychological responses of parents to the diagnosis of insulin dependent diabetes mellitus in their children. *Diabetes Care*, **8** (6), 568–575.

Krulik, T. (1980) Successful 'normalising' tactics of parents of chronically-ill children. *Journal of Advanced Nursing*, **5**, 573–578.

Kubler-Ross, E. (1970) *On Death and Dying*. London, Tavistock.

Langridge, P. (2002) Reduction of chronic sorrow: a health promotion role for children's community nurses. *Journal of Child Health Care*, **6** (3), 157–170.

Lazarus, R.S. & Folkman, S. (1984) *Stress, Appraisal and Coping*. New York, Springer.

Lofholm, N. (2001) Prayed-over girl died of untreated diabetes. *Denver Post Western Slope Bureau*. Available at: http://www.rickross.com/reference/firstborn8.html Accessed 22/02/06.

Lowes, L. & Lyne, P. (1999) A normal lifestyle: parental stress and coping in childhood diabetes. *British Journal of Nursing*, **8** (3), 133–139.

Lowes, L. & Lyne, P. (2000) Chronic sorrow in parents of children with newly diagnosed diabetes: a review of the literature and discussion of the implications for nursing practice. *Journal of Advanced Nursing*, **32** (1), 41–48.

Lowes, L. & Gill, P. (2006) Participants' experiences of being interviewed about an emotive topic. *Journal of Advanced Nursing*, **55** (5), 587–595.

Lowes, L., Lyne, P. & Gregory, J.W. (2004) Childhood diabetes: parents' experience of home management and the first year following diagnosis. *Diabetic Medicine*, **21**, 531–538.

Lowes, L., Gregory, J.W. & Lyne, P. (2005) Newly diagnosed childhood diabetes: a psychosocial transition for parents? *Journal of Advanced Nursing*, **50** (3), 253–261.

Lu, L. & Chen, C.S. (1996) Correlates of coping behaviours: internal and external resources. *Counselling Psychology Quarterly*, **9** (3), 297–307.

McCubbin, H.I. & Patterson, J.M. (1983) Family transitions: adaptations to stress. In: *Stress and the Family: Coping with Normative Transitions, 1* (eds H.I. McCubbin & C.R. Figley) pp. 5–25. New York, Brunner/Mazel.

Mellin, A.E., Neumark-Sztainer, D. & Patterson, J.M. (2004) Parenting adolescent girls with type 1 diabetes: parents' perspectives. *Journal of Pediatric Psychology*, **29** (3), 221–230.

Meuleners, L.B., Binns, C.W., Lee, A.H. & Lower, A. (2002) Perceptions of the quality of life for the adolescent with chronic illness by teachers, parents and health professionals: a Delphi study. *Child: Care, Health and Development*, **28** (5), 341–349.

Miller, M. (2005) *Impact of Chronic Illness on Families*. Denver, National Jewish Medical and Research Center. Available at: http://nationaljewish.org/disease-info/diseases/psych-soc/families.aspx Accessed 20/07/05.

Morrison, J.E., Bromfield, L.M. & Cameron, H.J. (2003) A therapeutic model for supporting families of children with a chronic illness or disability. *Child and Adolescent Mental Health*, **8** (3), 125–130.

Mu, P.-F. (2005) Paternal reactions to a child with epilepsy: uncertainty, coping strategies, and depression. *Journal of Advanced Nursing*, **49** (4), 367–376.

Muller, D.J., Harris, P.J., Wattley, L. & Taylor, J.D. (1994) *Nursing Children. Psychology, Research and Practice* (second edition). London, Chapman and Hall.

Murgatroyd, S. & Woolfe, R. (1993) *Coping with Crisis. Understanding and Helping People in Need*. Milton Keynes, Open University Press.

National Institute for Clinical Excellence (2003) *Guidance on the Use of Patient Education Models for Diabetes: Technology Appraisal 60*. London, NICE. Available at: www.nice.org.uk Accessed 20/11/06.

National Institute for Clinical Excellence (2004) *Type 1 Diabetes: Diagnosis and Management of Type 1 Diabetes in Children and Young People*. London, NICE. Available at: www.nice.org.uk Accessed 20/11/06.

NHS Wales (2005) *Children's National Service Framework*. Cardiff, NHS Wales. Available at: www.wales.nhs.uk Accessed 20/11/06.

Notaras, E., Keatinge, D., Smith, J., Cordwell, J., Cotterrell, D. & Nunn, E. (2002) Parents' perspectives of health care delivery to their chronically ill children during school. *International Journal of Nursing Practice*, **8**, 297–304.

O'Conner-Von, S. (2002) Growth and development of the school-aged child. In: *Pediatric Nursing. Caring for Children and Their Families*. (eds N.L. Potts & B.L. Mandleco), pp. 283–304. New York, Thomson Learning Inc.

Olshansky, S. (1962) Chronic sorrow: a response to having a mentally defective child. *Social Casework*, **43**, 190–193.

Pal, D.K., Chaudhury, G., Das, T. & Sengupta, S. (2002) Predictors of parental adjustment to children's epilepsy in rural India. *Child: Care, Health and Development*, **28** (4), 295–300.

Parkes, C.M. (1993) Bereavement as a psychosocial transition: processes of adaptation to change. In: *Handbook of Bereavement. Theory, Research and Intervention*. (eds M.S. Stroebe, W. Stroebe & R.O. Hansson), pp. 91–101. Cambridge, Cambridge University Press.

Parkes, C.M. (1996) *Bereavement. Studies of Grief in Adult Life* (third edition). London, Routledge.

Phillips, M. (1991) Chronic sorrow in mothers of chronically ill and disabled children. *Issues in Comprehensive Pediatric Nursing*, **14** (2), 111–120.

Piaget, J. (1962) *Play, Dreams and Imitation in Childhood*. New York, Norton.

Povlsen, L., Olsen, B. & Ladelund, S. (2005) Diabetes in children and adolescents from ethnic minorities: barriers to education, treatment and good metabolic control. *Journal of Advanced Nursing*, **50** (6), 576–582.

Powell, T.J. & Enright, S.J. (1990) *Anxiety and Stress Management*. London, Routledge.

Purssell, E. (1994) The process of normalisation in children with chronic illness. *Paediatric Nursing*, **6** (10), 26–28.

Roger, D. & Nash, P. (1995) Coping. *Nursing Times*, **91** (29), 42–43.

Rosina, R., Crisp, J. & Steinbeck, K. (2003) Treatment adherence of youth and young adults with and without a chronic illness. *Nursing and Health Sciences*, **5**, 139–147.

Royal College of Nursing (2005) *Specialist Nursing Services for Children and Young People with Diabetes. An RCN Guidance*. London, RCN. Available at: www.rcn.org.uk Accessed 20/11/06.

Schmidt, S., Petersen, C. & Bullinger, M. (2002) Coping with chronic disease from the perspective of children and adolescents – a conceptual framework and its implications for participation. *Child: Care, Health and Development*, **29** (1), 63–75.

Seiffge-Krenke, I. (1998) The highly structured climate in families of adolescents with diabetes: functional or dysfunctional for metabolic control. *Journal of Pediatric Psychology*, **23**, 313–322.

Seppanen, S.M., Kyngas, H.A. & Nikkone, M.J. (1999) Coping and social support of parents with a diabetic child. *Nursing and Health Sciences*, **1**, 63–70.

Shanahan, M. & Bradshaw, D.L. (1995) Are nurses aware of the differing health care needs of Vietnamese patients? *Journal of Advanced Nursing*, **22**, 456–464.

Sharpe, D. & Rossiter, L. (2002) Siblings of children with a chronic illness. *Journal of Pediatric Psychology*, **27** (8), 699–710.

Shiu, S. (2004) Positive interventions for children with chronic illness: Parents' and teachers' concerns and recommendations. *Australian Journal of Education*, **48** (3), 239–252.

Solnit, A.J. & Stark, M.H. (1961) Mourning and the birth of a defective child. *The Psychoanalytic Study of the Child*, **16**, 523–537.

Streisand, R., Swift, E., Wickmark, T., Chen, R. & Holmes, C.S. (2005) Pediatric parenting stress among parents of children with type 1 diabetes: the role of self-efficacy, responsibility and fear. *Journal of Pediatric Psychology*, **30** (6), 513–521.

Sutherland, V.J. & Cooper, C.L. (1990) *Understanding Stress. A Psychological Perspective for Health Professionals*. London, Chapman and Hall.

Taylor, S.E. (1995) *Health Psychology* (third edition). New York, McGraw-Hill, Inc.

Teel, C.S. (1991) Chronic sorrow: analysis of the concept. *Journal of Advanced Nursing*, **16** (11), 1311–1319.

Tinlin, J. (1996) A time to mourn. *Practical Diabetes International*, **13** (3), 86–87.

Van Hooren, R.H., Widdershoven, G.A.M., van der Bruggen, H., van den Borne, H.W. & Curfs, L.M.G. (2005) Values in the care for young persons with Prader-Willi syndrome: creating a meaningful life together. *Child: Care, Health and Development*, **31** (3), 309–319.

Varni, J.W. & Wallander, J.L. (1998) Effects of pediatric chronic physical disorders on child and family adjustment. *Journal of Child Psychology and Psychiatry*, **39**, 29–46.

Webb, C.L. (2005) Parents' perspectives on coping with Duchenne muscular dystrophy. *Child: Care, Health and Development*, **31** (4), 385–396.

Welsh Assembly Government (2003) *National Service Framework for Diabetes in Wales. Delivery Strategy*. Cardiff, Welsh Assembly Government. Available at: www.wales.nhs.uk

Wennick, A. & Hallstrom, I. (2006) Swedish families' lived experience when a child is first diagnosed as having insulin-dependent diabetes mellitus. An ongoing learning process. *Journal of Family Nursing*, **12** (4), 368–389.

Williams, C. (2000) Doing health, doing gender: teenagers, diabetes and asthma. *Social Science and Medicine*, **50**, 387–396.

Worden, J.W. (1995) *Grief Counselling and Grief Therapy. A Handbook for the Mental Health Practitioner* (second edition). London, Routledge.

A Holistic Approach to Meeting Physical, Social and Psychological Needs

Beverly Hodges and Julia Tod

Introduction

The physical needs of children and young people with chronic illness can often impact on their psychological well-being and social development. As highlighted in the previous chapter, families can become consumed by the care requirements of their child with chronic illness, to the detriment of other aspects of their life such as education, socialisation and promotion of independence. Therefore, assessment that encompasses all aspects of life for these children and young people and their families is an essential skill in contemporary nursing.

Whilst nurses should have an ability to negotiate and manage resources within the arena of multi-agency and inter-disciplinary teamworking, partnership and negotiation with children, young people and their families needs to be inherent in the relationship.

Aim of the chapter

Using the case study of a child with eczema, learners will be able to explore a number of social and psychological factors that are relevant to families who have a child with a chronic health need and, through reflection, also explore their own responses to some of the psychosocial factors described. Particular physical needs of the child with eczema will be considered and particular reference made to the continuing needs of the child, and the implications for nursing practice.

This chapter aims to provide an overview of some elements of physical, psychological and social issues that can affect the well-being of children, young people with chronic illness and their families. A detailed critique of social and psychological theory will not be undertaken. Before reading this chapter, therefore, learners will need to have an understanding of the physiology and function of the skin, allergic response mechanisms, theories of pain and developmental child psychology.

Intended learning outcomes

- To explore the physical, psychological and social implications for the child/young person and family living with chronic illness
- To discuss how physical symptoms can impact on social and psychological factors
- To examine the relationship between development theories and management interventions for children/young people with eczema
- To critically evaluate how children's nurses can support children/young people and their families to enable them to achieve 'a good quality of life'

Prevalence of eczema

The child in the case study below will be referred to as Isabella, one of many suffering from atopic eczema, a common skin problem in childhood. Over the last 30 years, the prevalence of atopic eczema has risen throughout the Western world, affecting as many as one in five children in the UK alone (National Eczema Society, 2003). Environmental factors such as being 'too clean', with a reduction in exposure to micro-organisms that help develop natural immunity in early life, and being exposed to pollution have been suggested as reasons for the increase in prevalence (Lui & Murphy, 2003; British Association of Dermatologists, 2004). There is, however, a genetic element to the condition that cannot be ignored, with studies demonstrating the link between parental atopic skin problems and childhood atopic eczema. Fathers are as likely as mothers to pass on the eczema predisposition (Wadonda-Kabonda *et al.*, 2004). There is also a strong association between eczema and other atopic diseases such as asthma and hay fever. These are important considerations when establishing a patient's history. Isabella's family background and current presentation of her skin is explored below.

 Case study 4.1

Background information

Isabella is a five-year-old Eastern European child who lives with her parents in an affluent suburban area in the UK. The family migrated to the UK six months ago after Goran, Isabella's father, gained promotion in a steel company. His wife, Merelee, has not worked since the move. She had worked as a personal assistant in the steel company in their home country before Isabella's birth. Both parents are in their early thirties and Isabella is an only child.

Isabella was diagnosed with atopic eczema at the age of six months; both her parents have a history of mild atopy. Due to her diagnosis, emollients are Isabella's current mainstay of treatment, but recently her skin has become difficult to manage as she is suffering from an acute exacerbation of eczema. There has been an escalation of the inflammation, swelling and irritation of her skin, which has led to an uncontrollable 'itch scratch cycle'. Isabella is not sleeping and is upset, irritable and in pain. Merelee is extremely tired, as she is sleeping with Isabella to avoid disturbing Goran, is homesick and is distressed about her daughter's condition. Goran is supportive and plays with Isabella but is not involved with her ongoing care needs. Merelee has rudimentary English and is finding it difficult to 'settle' as she misses her extended family and the community she has left.

Isabella has recently started school and, a lone child, is finding this challenging because she has not previously attended nursery. The headmistress has contacted the school nurse with a number of concerns about Isabella's care needs and her relationship with other children. There are currently no 'specialists' involved in her care as there has been a delay in her referral to the local children's hospital. Due to the concerns raised, her health visitor and general practitioner have been informed and a clinical appointment has been arranged to review all aspects of her care.

 Time out

Having read the case study what do you consider are the main nursing implications?

Nursing considerations

It is hoped that you will have recognised from the case study that Isabella needs to be assessed. This next section of the chapter will focus on considerations for children's nurses in the following areas:

- Recognising the signs of eczema and the importance of assessing the skin of children/young people with eczema
- The treatment of eczema with emollients
- The impact of the itch scratch cycle
- Family coping mechanisms

These issues will be discussed in relation to the role of the children's nurse throughout the text. The presentation of eczema will be discussed in the first instance.

Presentation of eczema

Key points

- One of the key roles of the children's nurse is to assess the current status of the skin of the child/young person with eczema, as it is an inflammatory skin condition that can present with the following physiological problems:

  — Patches of dry skin
  — Redness and inflammation of the epidermis
  — Scaly and itchy skin

- The skin can deteriorate if not assessed regularly and there is ineffective management, which can potentially lead to:

  — Blistering
  — Weeping
  — Infection
  — Lichenification (thickening and hardening of the skin)
  — Scarring

The problems associated with eczema are multi-factorial, and some of the above symptoms are synonymous with the acute exacerbation of Isabella's condition. In Chapter 1, the term 'multi-factorial' and some environmental and dietary influences on eczema were briefly discussed. It is not surprising that Isabella is feeling miserable, as she is caught up in an itch scratch cycle, is in pain and unable to sleep, a situation that is exacerbating her inability to integrate properly into her new school.

Key point

Having established the skin status of the child/young person, the children's nurse can begin to assess the effectiveness of the current treatment regimen. Thorough assessment will enable changes to be made concerning the choice of skin preparations to be used.

Isabella's assessment will take place at the clinical appointment referred to in the second part of the case study.

Treatment of eczema with emollients

Isabella's current eczema treatment regimen comprises emollients that are applied to the skin. Emollients are necessary to treat eczema due to an associated reduction in the lipid barrier function of the skin. Daily use of emollients promotes the barrier function of the skin, helping to maintain skin health. Bath additives, soap substitutes and topical emollients are recommended.

Topical emollients

Topical emollients are moisturisers, in the form of lotions, creams and ointments, which are used to recreate the moisture barrier of the skin, as they trap water in or allow water to be drawn from the dermis to the epidermis. They can be applied after bathing. Table 4.1 outlines the use of non-soap products and topical emollients. Daily application of emollients creates an additional burden for the family, due to the time taken to apply the product, gaining the child's cooperation and additional laundering of bedding and stained clothes. Further

Table 4.1   The use of non-soap products and topical emollients.

Non-soap products Aqueous cream	Topical emollients Lotions
Can be used as soap, applied on to the skin via a cloth or using hands. When rinsed off there should be minimal irritation from it. Aqueous cream is less greasy than emulsifying ointment. It should be avoided if there is a known sensitivity to it.	Lotions can be helpful for application during the day as they are not very greasy and are quite light in consistency. They are absorbed quickly and require frequent application. Due to their lack of oil content, lotions are not as effective as other emollients, even though they are often preferred due to the unobtrusive nature of the product.
Emulsifying ointment	**Creams**
A greasy product that can be used by whisking the ointment in very hot water to dissolve it and then adding it to a bath.	Children usually accept creams for use because even though they have an increased oil consistency, they do tend to sink into the skin quite easily. Creams are useful for the daytime.
Bath oils	**Ointments**
These help wash the skin and trap moisture into it as it leaves an oily film over the surface of the skin.	Ointments are very greasy products and are often not favoured by children because they leave skin looking shiny and the product does not absorb quickly. Due to the greasy nature of ointments, staining of clothing can occur. Ointments are the most effective type of emollient for a child with extremely dry, fissured skin. Ointments are often applied before a child goes to bed. Some children will need to avoid the use of ointments if they develop sensitivity.

Sources   Gould, 2001; Lawton, 2004; Burr & Penzer, 2005.

pressure can occur due to mothers wanting to keep their house clean and free from dust or anything that might cause greater irritation to their child's skin (Hawkins, 2005).

 Key point

The treatment regimen of children with chronic illness can impact on all aspects of family life.

 Time out

Outline the advantages and disadvantages of the various eczema treatments discussed.

Effects of the itch scratch cycle

As identified in the case study, a child with atopic eczema is often caught in an itch scratch cycle, which can be one of the most distressing experiences for the child, and equally distressing for the onlooking adult, who feels helpless. The distress and discomfort caused by the itch scratch cycle can cause significant disturbance to the night-time routine of the child and family, as it is often difficult for the child to settle, and sleep is often disrupted (Hawkins, 2005). Children may scratch their skin so much that it becomes red, inflamed and breaks down, causing infection, pain and discomfort as a weakness in the skin barrier occurs. Erythema can appear as a result of neuropeptide induced vasodilation that raises the temperature of the skin (Beltrani, 1999).

Sleep deprivation leads to children and their families being tired, irritable and unable to concentrate in school/work. It can have a huge impact on children/ young people in relation to their ability to make friends, schooling and educational achievement, and physically in relation to their height and pubertal development, as sleep is necessary for growth and repair to take place. Children and young people who are not developing at the same rate as their peers can often feel embarrassed and may become withdrawn as they try and cope with their emotions. In the longer term, this can lead to more acute mental health problems such as self-harm (Karstadt & Woods, 1999). The external appearance of the skin can have a huge influence on how a person feels and how others react and treat a person. It can influence socialisation as it affects society's perceptions of accepting or rejecting a person (Burr & Penzer, 2005). Merelee is very aware of this in relation to her daughter, which adds to her maternal anxiety and is affecting her ability to cope. It can also impact on parents' ability to work effectively, which can influence their economic contribution to their family and society. Parents, fearful of leaving their sick children to go to work, may choose to stay at home, thus limiting their own social contact with others. Working parents, kept awake all night by their sick children, may find their ability to be productive in work during the day affected, which can potentially impact on their ability to maintain employment. As a consequence, the confidence and self-esteem of children with a chronic condition such as eczema and their families is often diminished, which, as discussed in Chapter 3, can lead to chronic sorrow (Gould, 2001; Melnyk *et al.*, 2001).

   Key point

The itch scratch cycle can be extremely distressing for the child and equally disruptive to family life as a whole. Children's nurses must incorporate this consideration into their assessment to ensure appropriate strategies are put in place for the child and family.

Family stress and coping

The stress of caring for a child with chronic illness extends beyond the initial diagnosis. This is demonstrated in the care burden highlighted in the case study. This, together with the move from a supportive community to a new country, has altered Merelee's response to Isabella's condition. Chen (1999) suggests that some people may benefit from the care giver experience and see it as an opportunity for growth, while others may perceive it as burdensome and unpleasant. Research findings suggest that most (47–80%) care givers are women, and that men may focus more on task accomplishment and experience less stress (Chou, 2000). Care givers' sense of responsibility may also discourage them from taking part in and enjoying social activities. The burden associated with care giving tasks may be reduced by delegation and sharing responsibilities (Chen, 1999). However, social support is not always caring, and as Cuijpers (1999) found, visits by others were perceived as intrusive rather than helpful.

Following the diagnosis of a chronic condition, families often seek to define family life as essentially normal (Knafl & Deatrick, 1986), acknowledging the existence of impairment while engaging in behaviour that demonstrates their normality. The effort of managing their child's illness, whilst presenting family life as 'typical', results in a constant struggle. Periods of transition such as initial diagnosis, moving to a new setting and an increase of symptoms can have an impact on the family's equilibrium, affecting emotions and increasing stress, and the family's need to use effective coping strategies to adapt to the changed situation. See Chapter 3 for further discussion. It is important that nurses recognise that stress is an inevitable part of the lives of families with a child with a chronic condition.

(L) **Time out**

- Think of a family that you have nursed. What strategies were used to help alleviate stress?
- Were these strategies effective?

Strategies have been identified that help individuals cope with stress and avoid stress-related illness. How many did you identify?

- A sensible pattern of diet, sleep and physical activity is a simple coping strategy. The cycle of sleep deprivation may lead to a lack of enthusiasm for exercise. Encouraging Merelee to attend group exercise would allow her to be active and establish friendships.
- Social support has a significant effect on coping skills (Melnyk *et al.*, 2001). It cannot always be presumed that family will provide support; they may in fact be an additional source of stress. Children's nurses should be able to assess the family member's ability to express their needs, evaluate existing support systems (neighbours, religious groups, work colleagues) and act as a liaison between support services. Support groups such as the Eczema Society can provide local group meetings and meeting other parents in similar situations may provide an extended network.
- An adaptive response to stress is to create positive feelings. Positive events such as celebrations or improving environmental factors (pleasant music, fragrances) can enhance mood. Encouraging Merelee to avoid dwelling on negative feelings and encouraging her to engage in things that she finds enjoyable will enable her to reassess her response to Isabella's condition.
- Effective coping strategies vary for individuals and some techniques may need to be taught (e.g. deep breathing techniques); some families may benefit from a stress and coping course. (Royal College of Nursing, 2001)

The transition to school for a child with chronic illness is often stressful and may represent one of the times that force parents to recognise their child's physical cognitive or social differences (Melnyk *et al.*, 2001). Relinquishing the daily care management to teachers and other professionals can also be a source of concern. Children may face teasing and difficulties with friendship, and Isabella's skin condition may result in rejection by her peers. A loss of self-esteem can result in unruly behaviour that may lead to negative attention from teachers and ostracism by school-friends (Hardwick & Bigg, 1997). Loss of school-time due to hospitalisation can also affect performance in class, cognitive development and long-term success. Clearly, the educational and socialising experience of school is important, and good liaison between the care and education teams can ameliorate some of these difficulties.

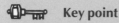   **Key point**

Children's nurses can encourage families to use various strategies to help them cope with caring for a child or young person with chronic illness.

   Case study 4.2

A thorough assessment at the clinic appointment by the consultant paediatrician and paediatric dermatology nurse established that Isabella's treatment was ineffective and needed to be reviewed and adjusted. The health visitor, who attended the appointment, explained that Merelee had no support network, was isolated and, as a result, was unable to manage Isabella's condition. The sleepless nights were unacceptable for all the family. Alleviation of Isabella's pain and the itch scratch cycle was seen as a priority. At this clinic appointment, Isabella told the nurse specialist, 'No one will play with me! I get called names in school, please make my skin better'. Isabella was asked where it hurt and she was able to point to the inflamed areas of her skin. Merelee is worried that Isabella is being bullied and is losing confidence. The health care team discussed the treatments currently being used on Isabella's skin and the frequency of application. Merelee explained that she was applying the lotion to Isabella's skin every day, in the morning and before bedtime. However, she did not think the treatment was helping, so she had been using alternative therapies including homeopathy. A short admission to hospital for immediate intervention was arranged and a multidisciplinary team meeting was organised in order to develop an action plan.

  Time out

From the case study, what do you think you would need to consider in your assessment and care plan?

Assessment and immediate intervention

Part two of the case study has highlighted the need for assessment and intervention to help improve Isabella's skin condition and meet the needs of the family in relation to her skin status. Priorities for care and immediate management will focus on the following key areas:

- The effectiveness of Isabella's treatment regimen, adherence and application technique
- Isabella's level of pain as a result of the itch scratch cycle
- The effects of the exacerbation of eczema on Isabella's psychological and social well-being, particularly as she may be a target for bullying and finding it hard to integrate into her new school

- The physical, psychological and social effects of Isabella's condition, on Merelee and Goran
- Current family support mechanisms

> ⌑━🔑 **Key point**
>
> Isabella needs to be admitted to hospital to assess her pain and stabilise her condition. Treating her physiological symptoms and promoting comfort will help ease the psychological and social burden that has been highlighted in this chapter.

Current care management plan

Due to the inflammation, swelling and irritation of Isabella's skin, it is evident that her overall treatment regimen is ineffective. This is potentially due to a number of reasons:

- Unsuitable skin care products being used to manage Isabella's eczema
- Not applying the skin care treatments correctly
- Changes in the home circumstances/environment
- Non-adherence with treatment, for example infrequent application of treatments

Wet wraps

Children with eczema who are caught up in an itch scratch cycle can often be helped by using wet wraps to treat the skin. Gould (2001) describes the process of wet wrapping, which involves the application of warm semi occlusive bandages over an emollient and if necessary a topical steroid. Wet wraps can be applied to any area of skin that is affected by eczema. They have the advantage of cooling and rehydrating the skin, which alleviates the itching, reduces pain due to the soothing effect of the treatment and promotes skin healing. Wet wraps are usually used when other forms of treatment such as bath oils, emollients, lotions, creams and mild steroids have become ineffective.

Wet wrapping is not recommended when eczema has become infected, as highlighted by Gould (2001), who recommends that skin should be clean and the eczema dry. Increased moisture introduced by wet wraps can cause an increase in formation of bacteria if an area of skin is already infected. Potent steroids are not recommended with wet wraps due to the increased permeability of the skin.

Although Isabella's skin was red and inflamed, it was not infected or oozing any exudates, so this form of treatment was an appropriate part of her management for the first 24 hours. Subsequent wet wrap treatments were carried out at night-time only for the next few days. Wet wrapping should not be used on a continuous basis as it is meant for short-term use in acute exacerbations. Prolonged use can increase the chances of skin infection, and would be a very time consuming process for parents to manage (Hindley *et al.*, 2006).

Topical steroids

Children with eczema sometimes require treatment with topical steroids if emollients are ineffective. Topical steroids help to reduce inflammation of the skin, and are available in different strengths, with the level of potency chosen dependent upon the severity of the skin condition. Topical corticosteroids are recommended for application to the affected areas of the skin no more than twice a day (NICE, 2004). An additional burden can be placed on the child and family if treatment is not properly explained.

> **Key point**
>
> A key role of the nurse is to inform children, young people and parents about the side effects of topical steroids and their rate of absorbency (Gould, 2001).

Pain assessment

Due to inflammation and swelling of her skin, Isabella is experiencing pain. When skin becomes inflamed, a chemical reaction occurs, which stimulates the nerve endings. The perception of pain occurs as a result of a message being transmitted to the brain via the dorsal horn of the spinal cord (Carr & Mann, 2000).

Pain is a complex experience that can vary between each child and young person. According to Springhouse (2003), pain can be influenced by a variety of factors, including cultural background, previous experience and cognitive and emotional responses. Children with a chronic illness such as atopic eczema are in a vulnerable position, and assessment of pain status should always be a priority to ensure appropriate control and management of the condition.

Untreated pain can be overwhelming and traumatic for children and young people (Savins, 2002). Table 4.2 outlines a philosophy of care relating to pain management put forward by the Royal College of Nursing (2002). This philosophy of care needs to be considered when assessing any child/young person in pain. A widely recognised model of care that is synonymous with this philosophy

Table 4.2   Pain management philosophy of care.

Pain management philosophy of care
(1)   Children are listened to and believed
(2)   Children and their families are viewed as partners in care
(3)   Care is individualised and holistic
(4)   Care is family centred
(5)   A collaborative, multi-professional approach is provided by knowledgeable professionals
(6)   Attention is paid to the organisational issues and systems that enable effective management to take place

is **QUESTT**, which involves **Q**uestioning the child, **U**sing a pain rating scale, **E**valuating behaviour and physiological changes, **S**ecuring parental involvement, **T**aking the cause of pain into account and **T**aking action in evaluating results (Baker & Wong, 1987). The RCN (2002) also provides clear recommendations and guidance for the recognition and assessment of pain in children.

After questioning Isabella about her pain, she was able to point to the inflamed areas of her skin and where she was hurting. It is an important role of the children's nurse to obtain a pain history from the child and parent and learn the words that a child uses to describe their pain (e.g. baddie, hurt), as this can help reduce a child's anxiety (RCN, 2002). Cultural factors, which may influence pain and its management, also need to be identified and therefore nurses require key knowledge and skills in this area. When in pain, some children are very stoical and prefer to be left alone, while others prefer to have company. Response to pain may be dependent on family and societal influences, personality, religion, values and beliefs (Twycross *et al.*, 1998).

On assessment, Isabella's behavioural and physiological response to her atopic eczema is one of distress, irritability and inability to sleep. Through assessment of this response, questioning and using an age appropriate pain rating scale, Isabella's level of pain was recognised, enabling the appropriate intervention to promote her comfort.

 Key point

Pain management of the child with eczema is multi-dimensional and needs to focus on several aspects of care.

To provide holistic care, pain relief such as the use of wet wraps, antihistamines, play and distraction should be used. These methods of pain relief act on the sensation fibres of the skin, known as the 'A beta fibres', preventing the transmission of pain. This closes the 'gate' to pain. (See indicative reading to learn more about 'gate control theory'.)

Time out

Considering cultural factors, what signs may indicate that Isabella is in pain?

Antihistamines

Due to Isabella's physiological and behavioural responses of being irritable, not sleeping and continuously scratching, which is increasing her level of pain, the introduction of an antihistamine was found to help. Although an antihistamine is not a usual method of pain relief, it can be useful in an acute episode of eczema due to its sedative effects, which can help re-establish a sleeping pattern and control itching and discomfort. As this treatment is meant for short-term use only, Isabella had antihistamines for three nights.

Play and distraction

Play is an essential element of care when looking after a child with chronic illness, who is in pain. Children like Isabella can be suffering from high levels of anxiety because they do not really understand their illness or the reason for particular health care interventions. Introducing play that is appropriate to children's age and stage of development can allow them to express their feelings, and help them to re-enact events that have occurred to gain a greater understanding of their situation (Gariepy & Howe, 2003). Play is a way of helping children to gain emotional stability and control that can help them cope with their illness, as well as enabling them to communicate with others. Gariepy and Howe (2003) discuss the importance of children's choice of toys, suggesting that the toys and type of play selected can be symbolic in helping the child to express specific fears, anxieties and guilt. Children's nurses, alongside hospital play specialists, can assist in facilitating play with the child and family through an awareness of cultural beliefs, attitudes towards health, illness and play, understanding family dynamics and having a good knowledge of the child's condition and prior experience (Webster, 2000). This can enhance the child's rate of recovery and return to normalisation.

  Time out

Reflect on a clinical situation that you have encountered with a child that required distraction techniques to be used. What distraction techniques were used? Were they beneficial?

Distraction techniques provide a focus to divert the child's attention by interacting with the child and family using developmentally appropriate play techniques that can improve coping mechanisms as well as relieve stress (Webster, 2000). Distraction techniques are useful when carrying out procedures, and work best in partnership with preparation. For example, before Isabella has wet wraps applied, she could observe or be involved in wet wrapping a doll. Examples of play, distraction and coping strategies are outlined in Table 4.3.

Bullying

Isabella is being bullied in school; no one will play with her and children are calling her names. Patterson (2005) suggests that bullying occurs among many

Table 4.3 Examples of play, distraction and coping strategies.

Coping strategy	Examples
Breathing techniques	Blowing bubbles and balloons
Relaxation techniques	Guided imagery
Books, games and puzzles	Where's Wally? I spy
Imagery and make believe	Puppets, dolls
Music and television	Singing, videos
Sensory experiences	Play-dough, fibre optics
Positive reinforcement	Stickers, certificates

Reproduced with permission from Gaskell, 2005, © RCN Publishing Co. Ltd.

primary schoolchildren and defines bullying as a person purposely harming someone else. Olweus (1994) examines the power relationship between the victim and the bully and agrees that bullying involves 'intentional harm'. Bullying can be categorised as physical or verbal. Physical harm may include pushing or hitting, whereas verbal bullying may include being isolated by others, teased and being called names, like Isabella in the case study. Such bullying and victimisation can lead to psychological harm such as depression, withdrawal, lack of confidence and low self-esteem (Karstadt & Woods, 1999). If bullying is not resolved, it can lead to continued psychological problems as the child grows into adulthood. Bullies themselves may also have a low self-concept and develop a depressive state of mind, as they often have problems occurring in their own lives (Karstadt & Woods, 1999), such as problems at home, or they may be frightened themselves of being 'picked on' by others.

When children are being bullied, they may be too frightened to tell anyone and may make excuses not to go to school, for example they may develop symptoms of illness such as headaches and abdominal pain. Fortunately, Isabella has informed the nurse that she is being called names, giving her physical appearance as the reason she is being bullied. Often, children do not accept other children that they perceive to be 'different' from themselves and their peer group.

School nurses are in a prime position to help children caught up in a bullying cycle, as it is their role to safeguard children in their care. This includes 'promoting good emotional health and well-being' (Patterson, 2005). According to Townley (2002), schoolchildren feel they are able to confide in the school nurse and discuss the issue of bullying, which allows the school nurse to make assessments of general mental health and enables liaison and support between the school and families. The school nurse, the nurse in attendance at the assessment visit and the schoolteachers can all work together with the family to help Isabella to feel confident and happy to return to school. The school may have a policy to deal with the issue of bullying. The school nurse may speak to small groups of children within the school to help the situation. The family should be supported and may be advised to log any further bullying so that it can be dealt with in an appropriate and sensitive manner.

Case study 4.3

Isabella has been in hospital for five days, her skin has improved and she no longer has inflammation, following wet wrap treatment. Play specialist intervention and meeting other children with the same condition has enabled Isabella to make friends and become less self-conscious.

While Isabella was in hospital, Merelee chose not to stay overnight with her, to gain some respite, and is no longer feeling as tired. Isabella's grandmother, who has come to stay for a month to help and support Merelee as Goran has been unable to take time off work, has said that alternative therapies are part of the family's tradition and spiritual belief and that she wishes this to continue to be part of Isabella's treatment alongside medical intervention.

Isabella has gained some weight and the paediatric dietician has been in contact with the family. The dermatology nurse has discussed the new treatment plan with Isabella and her family, and has taught them the application techniques. Liaison with the school nurse and health visitor has been arranged to ensure there is appropriate support on discharge.

The headmistress has contacted Merelee and asked if she would like to help in the school at lunchtime. Merelee has agreed, recognising that this would be a way to meet new people and support Isabella in school. A clinic appointment in a month's time has been made, and contact numbers for the hospital and information regarding support groups for children and young people with eczema have been given to the family.

It is evident within the case study that Isabella's condition has now stabilised. Merelee is feeling more settled as she has received support from her mother. Ongoing spirituality needs have been considered when planning care.

 Time out

What key elements need to be considered by the children's nurse when discharging Isabella?

Research highlights that the following key elements will need to be considered for discharge:

- Providing information about support groups
- Health promotion and education of the child/young person and family concerning the current treatment regime
- Providing education appropriate to age and stage of development
- Involvement of the child and family in decision making and planning care
- Liaison with the multidisciplinary team
- Appropriate liaison with the child's school

- Ensure appropriate follow-up appointment is made
- Consider ongoing spiritual needs when planning care
- Gaining an understanding of alternative therapies (particularly those used in Isabella's care) (Gould, 2001; Narayanasamy, 2001; Thorne *et al.*, 2002; WAG, 2005)

Case study 4.3 identifies the family's need to maintain traditional spiritual beliefs. It is the role of the children's nurse to uphold families' beliefs and values. This section will consider some of these issues in detail.

 Time out

- Reflect upon your own understanding of spirituality.
- How does this influence your nursing practice?

Spirituality

Contemporary nursing subscribes to the concept of holistic care provision for children and families. However, if nurses caring for children and young people are to embody the concept of holism, this must include an equal emphasis on spiritual needs. *The Patient's Charter* (DoH, 1992) suggests that NHS staff will be sensitive to, and respect, an individual's religious, spiritual and cultural needs at all times. For both staff and patients, spirituality is synonymous with religion. However, in present times, it is recognised that there are different forms and expressions of spirituality. Bash (2004) suggests that there are three ways to define spirituality:

- Secular approach (material world), which is often related to concepts of belonging, meaning and value
- The theistic approach (belief in a god or gods), which is related to a force or being
- The media approach, which uses secular terms but relates them to matters, typically the concern of religion, the search for truth and a reverence for the mysteries of life

Narayanasamy (2001) suggests that differences in definition relate to the variety of belief systems and values of the authors that describe them. This lack of clarity concerning a definition of spirituality may be due to its deeply personal nature, but this can result in difficulties for nurses when seeking to support the spiritual needs of families. Govier (2000) proposes five areas that may provide a foundation for assessing spiritual needs (see Table 4.4), but emphasises that nurses performing this kind of assessment must consider their professional ability to deal with the consequences.

McSherry (2000) warns against mechanistic tick box style spiritual assessment. Nursing assessment and the subsequent provision of spiritual care should arise

Table 4.4   Assessing spirituality.

Reason and reflection	A desire to search for, or find meaning and purpose in one's life
Religion	A means of expressing spirituality through a framework of values and beliefs
Relationships	A longing to relate to oneself, others and a deity/higher being
Restoration	The ability of the spiritual dimension to positively influence the physical aspects of care

Source   Govier, 2000.

out of recognition of its importance and impact on the child, young person and family, and should avoid becoming a 'paper exercise'. Spiritual meaning for Isabella's family relates to some specific New Age beliefs relating to responsibility for, and interconnectedness with, the environment. This form of spirituality that emphasises the 'mystical', and in which the individual's feelings and experience are paramount, will affect the family's response to chronic illness and some forms of treatment. It will also influence Isabella's beliefs, as children's spiritual development does not occur in isolation from their family's beliefs. Cognitive development will also have direct impact on how she provides meaning to experiences. Fowler's theory of 'stages of faith' (Fowler, 1981, cited in Robinson *et al.*, 2003) is based on Erikson's (1963) development cycle, which described critical periods of psychosocial development through the life cycle. Fowler's stages offer an explanation of the characteristics of faith development but, as with any stage theory, should not be taken too rigorously. Table 4.5 illustrates his description of the period from infancy to late adolescence. Isabella is at a stage where children are influenced by powerful images, and rituals. Her grandmother's visit reaffirms the importance of the ritual of the family's faith and may have as great an influence on Isabella as it does on the rest of the family. Aldridge (2000) considers it significant that discussion of spirituality is now legitimate in health care delivery.

⌿⎯ᴑᴑ   Key points

- Spirituality can be vital as a coping mechanism for children, young people and families experiencing chronic illness.
- Where spirituality is an important component of home routine, a lack of assessment may lead to disruption of normal routine and a lack of respect for the family's beliefs.

🕐   Time out

- What has been your experience of complementary medicine?
- Has your experience affected your attitudes, behaviour and belief in relation to alternative treatments and therapies? If so, how?

Table 4.5   Fowler's stages of faith.

Fowlers stages of faith (1996)	Age	
Undifferentiated or primal faith	Infancy	A pre-linguistic, pre-conceptual stage in which the infant is gradually recognising distinction between environment and self. Self-worth is based on unconditional or conditional grounds.
Intuitive projective – faith	2–6	This stage builds on development of language and the imagination. With no cognitive operations that could test perceptions and thus reverse beliefs, children grasp experience in and through powerful images. The child is attentive to ritual and gesture.
Mythic – literal faith	7–12	There is a reliance on stories and narrative that is implied in the family faith experience. Belief is valued in a concrete sense; it can involve testing of meaning.
Synthetic – conventional faith	12–21	Development of life meaning is built on the original faith system and compiled of conventional elements it is accompanied by a need to keep the faith group together.

Source   adapted from Robinson *et al.*, 2003.

Complementary and alternative medicine

Complementary and/or alternative medicine (CAM) is an area where conventional biomedical ideas are changing. CAM can be defined as therapies that originate from traditions distinct from Western biomedical science (NIH Panel on Definition and Description, 1997), and can range from Chinese traditional medicine, aromatherapy and homeopathy to Shamanic healing. Individuals may use CAM for comfort and symptom management, or may consider them to be curative. In their research, Thorne *et al.* (2002) describe how adult sufferers of chronic illness found it helpful if health care professionals were reasonably supportive of CAM options. Conflicting or hostile attitudes did not discourage exploration of alternatives but forced participants in the study to become involved in covert behaviour and no longer discuss their therapies with health professionals. Through an awareness of these factors, nurses can help families discuss their fears and concerns, allowing informed choice. If health care systems set CAM in opposition to conventional medicine, a barrier to the practice of self-care management may be created. Although this research relates to adult chronic illness sufferers, this information is transferable to the care of children, young people and their families. Fisher (2004) suggests that children with eczema often do very well with homeopathic treatment; the holistic and individualised nature of the treatment allows variability of the condition to be taken into consideration. Mantle (2001) discusses hypnosis as an effective technique, particularly in children aged 7–12 years, to help manage symptoms and reduce the itch scratch cycle previously described.

It is clear from the literature that people have found the use of CAM therapies helpful, but there has only been limited scientific evidence relating to some therapies. The issue of regulation of complementary medicine has led to ongoing debate. The existence of three pan-professional bodies, the Institute of Complementary Medicine, the Council for Complementary and Alternative Medicine and the British Complementary Medicine Association, and variability in standards of training may cause confusion for the families seeking a CAM therapist. Many families may consider that 'natural' equals safe but this is not always the case if other forms of 'conventional' treatment are also used or if treatment (e.g. steroids) are stopped suddenly. Encouraging open discussion of CAM between the child, the family, the multidisciplinary team and, where possible, the therapists themselves may enable families like Isabella's and the multidisciplinary team to work together to achieve the best care for the child or young person with a chronic condition.

🔑 Key points

- Families may use CAM for comfort or symptom management for the child or young person with chronic illness. This should be in conjunction with liaison and advice from medical professionals.
- Discussion of the range of therapies available and referral to experts in CAM will enable families to become 'partners in care'.

Health promotion

The case study describes the improvement in Isabella's condition. However, it has not been an easy time for Isabella and her family as it is evident that caring for a child with a chronic illness can impact on family functioning as a whole. Before discharge, the continuing care needs of Isabella and her family should be addressed. Health promotion is necessary to ensure the appropriate future management of Isabella's eczema. When children are ill, parents have an overwhelming need to obtain information regarding their child's condition and want to be involved as partners in care (Fisher, 2001). Using a partnership approach, the children's nurse can negotiate a programme of care with the family. This can be a diverse role as it involves having prior knowledge of the family situation, their coping mechanisms, and their ability and willingness to be involved in particular aspects of care. It also requires the children's nurse to be aware of family support mechanisms.

Hopia *et al.* (2004) suggest that parental involvement in care can be achieved if the children's nurse:

- Explains the child's illness, diagnosis and prognosis
- Assesses the confidence and competence of the family to manage their child's condition
- Offers a plan of care that has been negotiated with the child and family
- Ensures parental and child understanding of the illness and treatment plan
- Involves the child and family in the decision making process
- Allows the child and family to express their views

Having a greater understanding and control of Isabella's physical condition can help improve psychological and social well-being. The condition of atopic eczema was discussed with Isabella and her family and a plan of care was initiated with the support of the health care team. When planning a care regimen, it is important to consider the patient's lifestyle as this helps with adherence with treatment.

Conclusion

Eczema is a common childhood atopic condition that is associated with other atopic diseases such as asthma and hay fever. It is a condition that can lead to deterioration of the physical, psychological and social functioning of a child and family. Physical symptoms can result in altered external appearance of the skin, pain, discomfort and insomnia, as well as the itch scratch cycle. Poor educational achievement, poor socialisation and emotional turmoil can prevail if the condition is not managed effectively. This can counter-impact on family life as a whole, affecting marital relationships, socio-economic function of the family and parents' ability to cope.

During an acute exacerbation of eczema, pain management and diversion therapy are essential elements of care. Family support and guidance with coping strategies is paramount. There are several options available that can help treat and prevent exacerbations of the condition. These include non-soap products, emollients, topical steroids and use of wet wraps. Thorough assessment of the skin is necessary to ensure an appropriate treatment regimen is planned. Ongoing follow-up and support of the child and family is essential to monitor the effectiveness of the treatment regimen. Children's nurses need to promote parental involvement in their child's care to ensure their understanding of the condition, which will allow them to recognise signs and symptoms, encourage adherence to treatment plans and involve them in the decision making process. Spiritual and cultural requirements need to be considered in relation to all aspects of care. Liaison with schoolteachers and the school nursing team is essential to promote emotional health and well-being. Providing ongoing support and follow-up, and involving the multidisciplinary team in the process, will enable the child and family to adapt to living with chronic illness, helping them on the way to achieve a good 'quality of life'.

Test your knowledge

- Outline the signs and symptoms of eczema.
- List the priorities that need to be considered when assessing the needs of children and young people with eczema.
- Consider the physical symptoms of eczema and write down how these can have an impact on the child, young person and family from a social and psychological perspective.

Acknowledgement

We would like to thank *Paediatric Nursing* for their kind permission to reproduce the table by Gaskell (2005).

Useful websites

http://www.bad.org.uk/about/
http://www.bdng.org.uk/
http://www.bma.org.uk/ap.nsf/Content/LIBAlternativeMedicine
http://www.eczema.org/

Recommended reading

Corlett, S. & Whitson, A. (1999) Play and culture. *Paediatric Nursing*, **11** (7), 28–29.
Done, A. (2001) The therapeutic use of story telling. *Paediatric Nursing*, **13** (3), 17–20.
Robinson, S., Kendrick, K. & Brown, A. (2003) *Spirituality and the Practice of Health Care.* Basingstoke, Palgrave McMillan.
Schaffer, H.R. (2004) *Introducing Child Psychology.* Oxford, Blackwell Publishing.

References

Aldridge, D. (2000) *Spirituality Healing and Medicine: Return to the Silence.* London, Jessica Kingsley Publishers.
Baker, C. & Wong, D. (1987) QUESTT: a process of pain assessment in children. *Orthopaedic Nursing*, **6** (1), 11–21.
Bash, A. (2004) Spirituality: the emperor's new clothes? *Journal of Clinical Nursing*, **13**, 11–16.
Beltrani, V.S. (1999) Managing atopic dermatitis. *Dermatology Nursing*, **11** (3), 171–176.
British Association of Dermatologists (2004) www.bad.org.uk/public/leaflets/atopiceczema.asp Accessed 4/12/06.
Burr, S. & Penzer, R. (2005) Promoting skin health. *Nursing Standard*, **19** (36), 57–65.
Carr, E.C.J. & Mann, E.M. (2000) *Pain: Creative Approaches to Effective Management.* Basingstoke, Hampshire, Palgrave.

Chen, M.Y. (1999) The effectiveness of health promoting counselling to family care givers. *Public Health Nursing*, **16** (2), 125–132.

Chou, K.R. (2000) Care giver burden: a concept analysis. *International Pediatric Nursing*, **15** (6), 398–407.

Cuijpers, P. (1999) The effects of family interventions on relatives' burden: a meta-analysis. *Journal of Mental Health*, **8**, 275–285.

Department of Health (1992) *Patient's Charter*. London, HMSO.

Erikson, E.H. (1963) *Children and Society* (second edition). New York, W.W. Norton & Co.

Fisher, H.R. (2001) The needs of parents with chronically sick children: a literature review. *Journal of Advanced Nursing*, **36** (4), 600–607.

Fisher, P. (2004) *Homeopathy National Eczema Society Fact Sheet* available at: http://www.eczema.org/factsheets/Homeopathy.pdf Accessed November 2005.

Gariepy, N. & Howe, N. (2003) The therapeutic power of play: examining the play of young children with leukaemia. *Child Care Health Development*, **29** (6), 523–537.

Gaskell, S. (2005) Taking the sting out of needles: education for staff in primary care. *Paediatric Nursing*, **17** (4), 24–28.

Gould, D. (2001) Childhood eczema. *Primary Health Care*, **11** (7), 43–49.

Govier, I. (2000) Spiritual care in nursing: a systematic approach. *Nursing Standard*, **12** (14), 32–36.

Hardwick, P. & Bigg, J. (1997) Psychological aspects of chronic illness in children. *British Journal of Hospital Medicine*, **57** (4), 154–156.

Hawkins, C. (2005) The effects of atopic eczema on children and their families: a review. *Paediatric Nursing*, **17** (6), 35–39.

Hindley, D., Galloway, G., Murray, J. & Gardener, L. (2006) A randomised study of 'wet wraps' versus conventional treatment for atopic eczema. *Archives of Disease in Childhood*, **91** (2), 164–168.

Hopia, H., Paavilainen, E. & Astedt-Kurki, P. (2004) Promoting health for families of children with chronic illness. *Journal of Advanced Nursing*, **48** (6), 575–583.

Karstadt, L. & Woods, S. (1999) The school bullying problem. *Nursing Standard*, **14** (11), 32–35.

Knafl, K.A. & Deatrick, J.A. (1986) How families manage chronic conditions: an analysis of the concept of normalisation. *Research in Nursing and Health*, **9**, 215–222.

Lawton, S. (2004) Effective use of emollients in infants and young people. *Nursing Standard*, **19** (7), 44–50.

Lui, H. & Murphy, J.R. (2003) Hygiene hypothesis: fact or fiction? *Journal of Allergy and Clinical Immunology*, **111** (3), 471–478.

Mantle, F. (2001) Hypnosis in the management of eczema in children. *Nursing Standard*, **15** (51), 41–44.

McSherry, W. (2000) *Making Sense of Spirituality in Nursing Practice: an Interactive Approach*. London, Churchill Livingstone.

Melnyk, B.M., Feinstein, N.F., Moldenhouer, Z. & Small, L. (2001) Coping in parents of children who are chronically ill: strategies for assessment and intervention. *Pediatric Nursing*, **27** (6), 548–559.

Narayanasamy, A. (2001) *Spiritual Care: a Practical Guide for Nurses and Health Care Practitioners* (second edition). Wiltshire, Quay Books.

National Eczema Society (2003) *Eczema Facts*. London, National Eczema Society www.eczema.org.uk Accessed 4/12/06.

National Institute for Clinical Excellence (2004) *The Frequency of Application of Topical Corticosteroids for Atopic Eczema. Technology Appraisal 81*. London, National Institute for Clinical Excellence.

NIH Panel on Definition and Description (1997) Defining and describing complementary and alternative medicine. *Alternative Therapies,* **3** (2), 49–57.

Olweus, D. (1994) Bullying at school: basic facts and effects of a school-based intervention programme. *Journal of Child Psychology Psychiatry,* **35** (7), 1171–1190.

Patterson, G. (2005) The bully as a victim? *Paediatric Nursing,* **17** (10), 27–30.

Robinson, S., Kendrick, K. & Brown, A. (2003) *Spirituality and the Practice of Health Care.* Basingstoke, Palgrave McMillan.

Royal College of Nursing (2001) *Managing your Stress: a Guide for Nurses.* London, Royal College of Nursing.

Royal College of Nursing (2002) *Clinical Practice Guidelines. The Recognition and Assessment of Acute Pain in Children. Technical Report. Guideline Objectives and Methods of Guideline Development.* London, Royal College of Nursing.

Savins, C. (2002) Therapeutic work with children in pain. *Paediatric Nursing,* **14** (5), 14–16.

Springhouse, P.A. (2003) *Pain Management Made Incredibly Easy.* New York, Lippincott Williams and Wilkins.

Thorne, S., Paterson, B., Russell, C. & Schultz, A. (2002) Complementary/alternative medicine in chronic illness as informed self-care decision making. *International Journal of Nursing Studies,* **39** (7), 671–683.

Townley, M. (2002) Mental health needs of children and young people. *Nursing Standard,* **16** (30), 38–45.

Twycross, A., Moriarty, A. & Betts, T. (1998) *Paediatric Pain Management. A Multidisciplinary Approach.* Oxford, Radcliffe Medical Press.

Wadonda-Kabonda, N. (2004) Association of parental eczema, hay fever and asthma with atopic dermatitis in infancy: birth cohort study. *Archives of Disease in Childhood,* **89** (10), 917–921.

Webster, A. (2000) The facilitating role of the play specialist. *Paediatric Nursing,* **12** (7), 24–27.

Welsh Assembly Government (2005) *National Service Framework for Children, Young People and Maternity Services in Wales.* Available at: http://www.wales.nhs.uk/sites3/Documents/441/EnglishNSF%5Famended%5Ffinal%2Epdf Accessed 5/12/06.

5 Empowering Children, Young People and their Families

Mandy Brimble

Introduction

Advances in medical technology have resulted in increased life expectancy for many children with chronic illness (Carson, 2001). The growing redirection of health care service provision from acute to community and primary care settings (Audit Commission, 1993; National Heath Service Executive, 1996) has resulted in an increased number of children with chronic illnesses being cared for by their parents in partnership with health and social care professionals, locally or in their own homes. This has provided professionals with an opportunity to enhance the quality of life for this client group, with the implementation of health promotion advice and strategies (Sindall, 2001). The *National Service Framework for Children, Young People and Maternity Services* core standards (Department of Health, 2004a) highlights that all children, young people and their parents/carers should have access to services that promote health and well-being.

Aim of the chapter

This chapter considers the challenges and issues surrounding the delivery of health promotion strategies by children's nurses, and the uptake of this advice by those in our care. Exploration of a chronic illness scenario will illustrate how these challenges may be exacerbated in terms of the receptiveness of the child, young person and family and their ability to change behaviour.

It is not the intention of this chapter to provide a detailed critique or in-depth theoretical discussion of health promotion models or the condition of childhood asthma, which is used in the case study. For a broader overview of health promotion, the reader may wish to access Naidoo and Wills (2000), Scriven and Orme

(2001), Ewles and Simnett (2003) and Tones and Green (2004), full references for which can be found at the end of this chapter.

The aim of this chapter is to develop the readers' knowledge base to enable them to conceptualise how health education and promotion can be used to inform and empower children/young people with a chronic illness and their families.

Intended learning outcomes

- To define the concepts of health promotion and empowerment
- To apply fundamental theoretical approaches to a case study in order to illustrate aspects of promoting health and well-being in the context of chronic illness
- To explore strategies used by health care professionals, in particular children's nurses, in the empowerment of children, young people and families
- Through a chronic illness case study, to examine barriers that may affect the uptake of health promotion advice and identify strategies to overcome these

Health promotion

The World Health Organization (WHO) (1946) defined health as 'a state of complete physical, mental and social well-being, and not merely the absence of disease or infirmity'. Although this definition can be criticised for conveying a somewhat unachievable ideal, it does describe health in positive terms, underlining the notion of health as a holistic concept. In today's multicultural and diverse society, it is important for nurses to recognise that there are many factors that can influence our individual ideas and health beliefs, for example culture, social class (Naidoo & Wills, 2000).

The reader should note that although health education and health promotion are terms that are often used interchangeably, they are two different concepts. Generally, health promotion activities contain a component of health education (Naidoo & Wills, 2000). Health education is primarily preventative and aims to increase knowledge, thus enabling informed choice in addressing issues that affect health and well-being. There are currently many health education campaigns aimed at the general population, for example smoking cessation and healthy eating, and although some individuals will act on these campaigns, many do not.

Test your knowledge

Why is it that despite having good quality information about the benefits of healthy eating, many people choose to ignore it? Identify reasons from a child, young person and adult perspective.

Key point

The reason for inaction by large sections of the population, despite having the necessary information, is that knowledge does not necessarily change attitude or behaviour. The effectiveness of health education activities is likely to be linked to an individual's perception of whether their 'locus of control' is primarily internal or external. Basically, this refers to an individual's view of their own strength and ability in influencing their life versus the influence that external factors have on them.

It is clear, therefore, that health education alone is not widely effective in increasing the health of the population, thus highlighting the importance of other components of health promotion. Just as health is a complex and multifaceted concept so is health promotion and can, therefore, have a variety of meanings for individuals (Tones & Tilford, 2001). Health promotion is defined as 'the process of enabling people to increase control over and to improve their health' (WHO, 1984, p. 4). This definition highlights the enabling or empowering facet of health promotion and underlines the role of the health professional in not merely education of clients but facilitation of the conversion of knowledge into health enhancing actions. This aspect of health promotion is likely, therefore, to involve increasing the individual's concept of their internal locus of control.

Key point

Within a chronic disease scenario, 'health' in terms of the WHO definition can sometimes never be achieved. Therefore, it is more likely that the aim of health promotion strategies will be to allow the child or young person to perform their social roles and achieve their personal potential.

Reflection

Before reading the following passage, consider your own notion of health promotion and make a note of your key thoughts.

The Ottawa Charter (WHO, 1986) presents health promotion as an 'enabling' concept, which can assist individuals and/or groups to establish a state of well-being. Enabling is an essential aspect of health promotion and WHO identifies several elements that potentially influence lifestyle choice, for example empowerment, autonomy, egalitarianism, partnership and collaboration. The importance of health promotion in relation to chronic disease care is discussed by Sindall (2001), who highlights it as a vehicle for preparing individuals to cope with chronic illness, should they experience it, and as a means of improving quality of life for the patient within the confines of the disease or condition.

Reflection

Reflect on why and how you could use health promotion strategies in relation to children and young people with chronic illnesses. Make notes of your thoughts.

🔑 **Key point**

It is the health professionals' responsibility to ensure that communication with all clients is in a format and at a level that is easy to understand. Children's nurses require knowledge of child development to be able to assess a child or young person's developmental stage and skills to interact appropriately with them, at all levels.

Delivery of health promotion advice and health education strategies to children and young people is likely to pose a challenge to children's nurses as some issues may be complex and will have to be dissected and presented carefully, for example children who are in the pre-operational stage (Piaget, 1963) will not have an understanding of internal body parts. Therefore, justification for behaviour change that focuses on damage to such organs or body systems will be at best ineffective and at worst frightening for the child. In addition, as children and young people are somewhat reliant on their carers for provision of healthy diet or lifestyle options, it will be necessary to fully engage the family/carer in order to facilitate any behaviour change. Finally, because the factors that influence the uptake of health promotion advice are multifaceted, the practitioner needs to be skilled in assessment of the client's individual situation in order to utilise appropriate strategies.

Within a chronic illness scenario, these challenges increase in complexity, as the disease or condition may greatly influence the child or young person's ability or motivation to adopt healthier behaviours. For example, a ten-year-old who is obese and confined to a wheelchair, due to disability, will be unable to increase their exercise levels significantly. The motivation and ability to change the diet will be affected by a historical relationship with food, which at ten years of age is likely to be well established, and an overall view of the future will influence motivation to lose weight. Another significant factor that will affect desire to lose weight is the opportunity to interact with peers, such as pride in appearance and/or fitting in with the group. Likely progression of disease and/or prognosis could also impact on children's or young people's overall view of their general health and desire to improve it. Issues for such children, relating to reliance on their family/carers for healthy diet and lifestyle options, are likely to be long-standing, rather than confined to infancy and the young childhood period.

Empowerment

Empowerment is a concept that has been widely discussed in relation to the promotion and achievement of good health. In fact, Tones and Green (2004) state that it is the most important component of health promotion strategies.

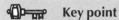 **Key point**

The concept of empowerment was analysed by Rodwell (1996) and defined, in simple terms, as 'the process of enabling or imparting power transfer from one individual or group to another'.

There are two main forms of empowerment: individual and community. There are many political and individual factors that influence both forms of empowerment but as nursing care focuses primarily on individuals this chapter will concentrate on enabling children, young people and families to take control over and make decisions about their lives, rather than how nurses may influence the political agenda in order to empower communities.

Individual empowerment involves a partnership approach, whereby the care provider aims to assist clients to develop the knowledge, skills and attitudes that will enable them to be proactive in gaining control over their life, health and health care (Tones & Green, 2004). An example of empowering versus non-empowering health promotion behaviour in a ward setting is given below.

A nurse who gives information on and discusses a healthy diet with a child/young person and/or family and then:

- Supports them in making healthy food choices but allows negotiation to take place (empowering)
- Makes menu choices on their behalf, without consultation (non-empowering)

Test your knowledge

What type of knowledge, skills and attitudes do you think may be required by the children's nurse in order to empower:

(1)   children
(2)   adolescents
(3)   parents?

Make a note of your thoughts.

Individual empowerment is associated with psychological characteristics such as self-concept, self-esteem, self-assertiveness and perceived locus of control. It can also be influenced by the possession of life skills, for example coping strategies (Katz *et al.*, 2000). For children and young people, the ability to become empowered will be linked to their developmental stage. Naidoo and Wills (2000) state that methods by which care givers can promote the acquisition of these psychological characteristics and life skills are advocacy, negotiation, networking and facilitation. The empowerment of children, young people and families in coping with chronic illness, specifically during periods of hospitalisation, has been researched by Coyne (1997; 2006) who highlights adaptation to the illness, facilitation of coping strategies and involvement in decision making in order to promote self-esteem as key factors. Chapter 9 highlights some of the impact of chronic illness upon young people's self-esteem and coping.

Approaches to health promotion

There are many models of health promotion that can be applied to a wide variety of scenarios, with varying degrees of success, depending on numerous internal and external factors. This chapter will use the work of Ewles and Simnett (2003), who have identified a framework of five approaches to health promotion that are universal to most models. This will assist the reader to gain knowledge and understanding of the principles of health promotion. The approaches to health promotion identified by Ewles and Simnett (2003), together with a summary of each, are shown in Table 5.1.

Table 5.1   Approaches to health promotion.

Approach	Aim	Health Promotion Activity	Important Values
Medical	Freedom from medically defined disease and disability	Promotion of medical intervention to prevent or ameliorate ill health	Patient compliance with preventative medical procedures
Behaviour change	Individual behaviour conducive to freedom from disease	Attitude and behaviour change to encourage adoption of 'healthier' lifestyle	Healthy lifestyle as defined by health promoter
Educational	Individuals with knowledge and understanding, enabling well informed decisions to be made and acted upon	Information about cause and effects of health-demoting factors Exploration of values and attitudes Development of skills required for healthy living	Individual right of free choice Health promoter's responsibility to identify educational content
Client centred	Working with clients on their own terms	Working with health issues, choices and actions that clients identify Empowering the client	Clients as equals Clients' right to set agenda Self-empowerment of client
Societal change	Physical and social environment that enables choice of healthier lifestyle	Political/social action to change physical/social environment	Right and need to make environment health enhancing

Source   Ewles & Simnett, 2003, pp. 45–46.

The last of these approaches, the societal change approach, will be primarily excluded from this chapter, which aims to focus on individual interactions between the children's nurse and the child/young person or family, rather than community and/or Government approaches via legislation, rules and regulations. However, in relation to the issues identified, some brief examples will be given.

Key points

- It is important to note that health promotion advice that involves behaviour change must include a client centred and educational approach (in certain cases, medical intervention may also be used).
- Other strategies need to be deployed in assisting clients to change behaviour, because merely informing clients that a specific behaviour is undesirable is likely to invoke negative responses such as aversion, defiance, rationalisation or reconciliation (Croghan, 2005).
- It is necessary first to provide information (education) relating to how the undesirable behaviour is likely to affect clients and/or those around them and then work with them to make small changes that will motivate them to sustain and extend these changes.
- Health promotion involving behaviour change is an evolving process that commences with the nurse as an external motivator who provides knowledge and facilitates skills, thus empowering clients by helping them to identify internal motivators that enable them to sustain the change.

Of the approaches listed by Ewles and Simnet (2003), being client centred is a fundamental aspect of children's nursing, as it encompasses the principles of family focused care. This is a concept that underpins our interactions and care for children, young people and families. However, the true meaning of family focused care has been and continues to be debated (Smith *et al.*, 2002; Franck & Callery, 2004). The case study that follows, and the interventions discussed, aim to give the reader an understanding of how the concept of family focused care may be delivered within a chronic illness scenario.

Key points

- Children and young people with chronic illness, their families and other carers often become experts on their particular condition and have a more comprehensive understanding of the condition itself, how it affects the patient and which treatment or interventions are most effective and appropriate (DoH, 2001; Fox, 2005).

- In family focused care, the nurse, child and family truly work in partnership, each taking equal responsibility for care planning, making decisions and care delivery.
- However, it must not be assumed that 'expert parents' wish to undertake the majority of care whilst the child/young person is in hospital – they may view this situation as a welcome opportunity for respite from the daily burden that this level of care imposes on them.
- An empowered parent should feel confident to negotiate care roles, including refusal to undertake any if they wish to act in a parental role only, rather than a care giver.

Read part 1 of the case study below and answer the questions that follow. This will enable you to start to consider areas of health promotion within a chronic illness scenario and apply the identified approaches to these areas. Throughout the chapter, following each part of the case study, there will be a discussion of the approaches and strategies that could be used to address emergent issues.

  Case study 5.1

Megan was a normal delivery, born full term to Sarah, aged 19 years, who smokes 20 cigarettes a day. Sarah is a lone parent with a supportive maternal family network. Currently she does not work. At six months of age, Megan presented in the A&E department with a history of poor feeding and a wheezy chest. On this occasion, she was admitted to the children's medical ward, prescribed bronchodilators and her condition improved. She did not require any further pharmacological intervention on discharge. Since this time, she has been a healthy child with no respiratory symptoms. At age six years, Megan was admitted to hospital with an inspiratory wheeze and diagnosed as asthmatic. She was prescribed bronchodilators and inhaled steroids via an MDI (measured dose inhaler) and spacer, as recommended for children over five years of age (NICE, 2002). Before discharge, Megan and Sarah were seen by the respiratory nurse specialist who assessed, and deemed competent, their administration of medication.

Over the last two years, Sarah has consulted their GP on many occasions about Megan's condition. Sarah is aware that her smoking impacts upon Megan's condition and has previously discussed this with the GP, health visitor, school nurse and practice nurse. However, to date, Sarah has not been able to give up smoking.

Now aged eight years, Megan has been admitted to hospital with an acute exacerbation of her asthma. On admission, her height is 127 cm (50th centile) and she weighs 50 kg (above the 99.6th centile). Her observations are: temperature 36.8 centigrade, pulse 140 beats per minute, respirations 40 breaths per minute, oxygen saturations 91%.

Test your knowledge

- What do you consider are the two main health promotion issues?
- Identify from Ewles and Simnett (2003), the approaches to health promotion you consider are appropriate for these issues.
- What skills are required to enable the practitioner to effectively promote healthy behaviour for Megan and Sarah?
- What would normal temperature, pulse, respirations and oxygen saturations be for a child who is eight years of age?

Your answer to question 1 should have been parental smoking and obesity, and you should have identified that all five approaches were appropriate to address these issues. As stated earlier, societal change will not be discussed in this chapter. However, examples of this approach are the ban on smoking in public places to discourage smoking and protect non-smokers from second-hand smoke, the ban on cigarette advertising at sporting events and it being illegal to sell cigarettes to children less than 16 years of age.

Parental smoking

The remaining four approaches to health promotion will now be examined in relation to assisting Sarah to give up smoking. This will improve Megan's environment and consequently her condition and the future health of her mother. To empower Sarah to help her to stop smoking, we need to take a *client-centred* approach. Sarah has already identified that she wishes to give up smoking but has, so far, been unsuccessful. Some parents do not smoke in the house because they are aware of the risks to their child from second-hand smoke, such as exacerbation of asthma, respiratory and ear infections (Scientific Committee on Tobacco and Health (SCOTH), 2004), and because parental smoking sets a 'bad example', which may lead to a child taking up smoking later in life through learned behaviour. However, although avoidance of smoking in the home reduces a child's exposure to second-hand smoke (Hovell *et al.*, 2000), it is ineffective in terms of the harmful substances that are still present in the environment and, therefore, giving up completely is preferable (Jarvis *et al.*, 2000).

According to Lancaster *et al.* (2001), simple advice from a health professional can be the sole motivation for a client attempting to give up smoking. This research emphasises the importance of nurses having the health promotion skills and knowledge to deliver this advice effectively and in an empowering manner. Unfortunately, in Sarah's case, the information/advice given by the GP, health visitor, school nurse and practice nurse had been unsuccessful, a common situation because even those motivated to give up can make numerous attempts before they achieve their aim, due to the difficulty in overcoming an addiction. Randall (2006) states that all health professionals have a role in helping clients to give up smoking but, in view of clear evidence relating to the effects of second-hand smoke on children, emphasises that children's nurses are ideally placed to take a key role.

As Sarah has already demonstrated an insight into the harm she is likely to be causing Megan, it would be easy to assume that she has adequate information relating to the effects of second-hand smoke. However, to be effective and client centred, the practitioner needs to explore Sarah's current level of knowledge and understanding before offering any further advice or intervention. In terms of the nursing process, this is equal to undertaking an assessment before devising a plan of care. Once the assessment process is complete, the practitioner can then begin to formulate a plan in partnership with the individual. It is, therefore, important that the nurse clearly understands the condition or behaviour about which they are advising.

To empower Sarah to undertake the required *behaviour change*, it may be necessary to provide *education* to supplement and extend her current level of knowledge. To help Sarah transfer this knowledge into action, her motivational level will need to be explored to assess her attitude towards the behaviour change. It is possible, for example, that Sarah is using cigarette smoking to help relieve the stress she experiences as sole carer of a child with chronic illness. Having identified relevant internal and external factors that impact on Sarah's ability to quit smoking, an individualised behaviour change plan can be formulated. An intervention that is sometimes successful in smoking cessation is one-to-one or group support, which involves counselling and/or group therapy. One-to-one counselling could be face to face or via helplines such as those run by the Department of Health.

It may also be necessary to help Sarah develop some life skills such as coping strategies or relaxation techniques for her to be successful in quitting smoking. It is clear, therefore, that in this particular scenario the *educational* and *behaviour change* approaches are closely linked and interdependent.

A *medical* approach could also be used, for example nicotine replacement therapy (NRT). Lancaster *et al.* (2001) state that not all smokers are nicotine dependent but if they are (i.e. smoke their first cigarette within an hour of waking and smoke more than 15 per day), NRT is likely to be effective, increasing the success rate by approximately one and a half to two times (Silagy *et al.*, 2001). In addition, certain components of antidepressant medications have been shown to be effective in treating nicotine dependence and are licensed in some countries.

Despite much publicity regarding alternative therapies, systematic reviews have found that interventions such as acupuncture and hypnotherapy have limited success in aiding smoking cessation (White *et al.*, 2001; Abbot *et al.*, 2001).

Obesity

Magnusson (2005a) states that being overweight or obese is almost always the result of a negative energy balance, that a greater number of calories are consumed than expended. Childhood obesity can cause hypertension, is associated with type 2 diabetes, increases the risk of coronary heart disease, increases stress on the weight-bearing joints, lowers self-esteem and affects relationships with peers.

There are various methods of determining if an individual is obese, for example waist circumference, skin fold measurements and calculation of Body Mass Index (BMI). According to Kiess *et al.* (2001), BMI is the accepted method of determining obesity in children, a belief reiterated by Whitlock *et al.* (2005) who found that, for children particularly, BMI allows a better correlation of measurements from childhood to adolescence and into young adulthood.

Calculation of BMI is achieved by dividing weight (in kilograms) by the square of the height (in metres). In other words the algebraic expression for BMI is:

$$BMI = Kg/m^2$$

Using the weight and height measurements given for Megan, we can calculate her BMI as follows:

$$50 \text{ kgs} \div 1.27 \text{ m}^2 = 31.00006$$

There are BMI categories for adults and children/young people (up to 20 years of age). Adult bandings are unsuitable for children due to changes in body fat as children grow. In addition, girls and boys differ in their body fatness as they mature. BMI for children, known as BMI for age, is calculated using centile charts published by the Child Growth Foundation (CGF, 1997) and based on the work of Cole *et al.* (1995; 2000).

Whether an adult or gender and age specific means of BMI assessment is used, Megan would be classified as obese. For her to be on the 50th centile of a traditional percentile chart (see Figure 5.1) and, therefore, in proportion, she would need to weigh 26 kg. This correlates with the children's BMI chart (as shown below) in that a weight of 26 kg would give a BMI of 16.12, which is on the 50th centile. If one used adult banding classifications, then a BMI of 16.12 would be in the underweight range, thus illustrating the importance of age and gender appropriate means of assessment.

Magnusson (2005b) reports that guidelines developed in Scotland state that weight loss is not the best target for obese children, as they are still growing, and that interventions should be aimed at weight maintenance. For Megan, therefore, the desired outcome would be that she remains at 50 kg until she reaches 14 years of age. This would mean that if she continues on the 50th centile for height and is 160 cm tall at 14 years of age, then her weight and height will be in proportion. In addition, these measurements would give a BMI of 19.5, which is in the middle of the healthy range.

As with smoking cessation, all five approaches to health promotion can be used to address the prevention and/or treatment of obesity. However, the education, behaviour change and client centred approaches are most applicable to this case study. Before examining these approaches in detail, the relevance of the societal and medical approaches will be briefly discussed.

Societal approach

Obesity is now considered a global epidemic (WHO, 1997) and is therefore a grave cause for concern regarding the effects on the morbidity and mortality of

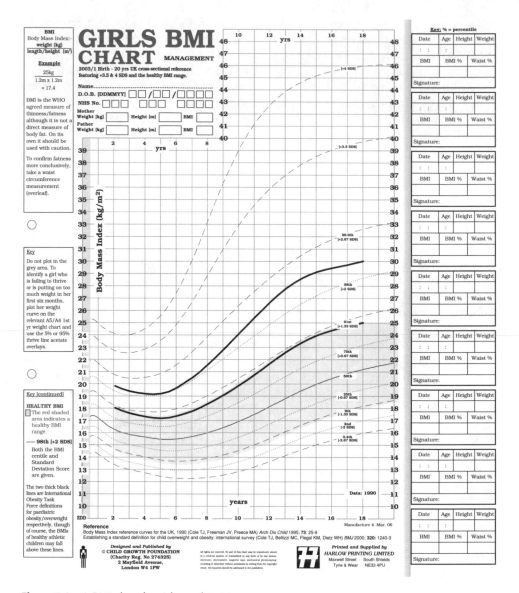

Figure 5.1   A BMI chart for girls aged 0–20 years.

the population and the financial impact on health service resources. The extent of the problem makes it necessary for a societal approach to be taken, in the first instance by using widespread health education to raise awareness of the problem and related issues. However, as eating habits are personal and likely to have been established in childhood, it is necessary to adopt an individual and client centred approach to affect behaviour change in treating obesity. If the current, widespread, health education approach continues, and this is targeted at children as they begin to form their eating habits, it is possible that in the long term a societal educational approach may be effective in actually preventing obesity occurring. This approach may also be successful in perpetuating effective parenting in relation to healthy eating, thereby substantially reducing obesity in future generations.

When targeting children who are currently overweight, that is treating the problem rather than preventing it, education aimed at parents and carers is an important factor. Madge and Franklin (2003) found that children who are concerned about their diet or weight are most likely to turn to their parents for advice.

Medical approach

The National Institute of Clinical Excellence (NICE) has approved the use of drugs in the management of adult obesity (NICE, 2001a; b). However, there is no guidance in relation to the use of these drugs in children, but this approach is being explored. A randomised controlled trial (RCT) of the effects of the drug Metformin on obesity in children showed a significant statistical reduction in BMI (Freemark & Bursey, 2001). In addition, there is an ongoing RCT of Orlistat use in treating obese 12–17-year-olds funded by the National Institutes of Health (NIH, 2005).

Cosmetic surgery, to reduce weight, in the form of liposuction is becoming increasingly popular, particularly in the US. However, removal of fat in this way does not decrease the risk of developing heart conditions, hypertension or diabetes (Klein et al., 2004) and carries significant risk of death through infection or blood clot. Although such radical measures may improve a child or young person's body image and subsequently their self-esteem, this form of cosmetic surgery may lead to a misconceived perception of a 'quick fix' to weight issues, as opposed to sustained personal effort to address the problem.

Individual educational, client-centred and behavioural change approaches

From their updated Cochrane review, Wilson et al. (2003) conclude that there is a lack of good quality evidence relating to the effectiveness of specific interventions to prevent and treat childhood obesity. For example, trials have primarily been undertaken in the US in circumstances that may not make their findings transferable to the UK, small sample groups are used, there is a high drop-out rate, and the reports produced are difficult to understand.

However, the review does state that there is some evidence that current UK Government initiatives can play a part in treating and preventing childhood obesity. These are multifaceted programmes, which may be school or family based, and promote physical activity, diet modification and targeting of sedentary behaviours to reduce childhood obesity. The review highlights that family based behaviour modification programmes, where parents take primary responsibility and act as agents of change, may help children to lose weight. More recent work by Magnusson (2005b) also reviews effective interventions and reinforces the findings of Wilson *et al.* (2003). In addition, Magnusson (2005b) points out many other factors that may influence the effectiveness of interventions, for example although parents may readily accept responsibility for diet, they do not have quite the same attitude in relation to physical activity and expect schools to play a greater part in this area. She also highlights research by Hart *et al.* (2003), which shows that parents from lower socio-economic backgrounds need more education regarding diet and nutrition. In relation to children/young people with chronic illness, their condition may restrict their physical activity in terms of their mobility, energy levels, pain experiences and health risk issues.

Another barrier to dietary changes underlined by Magnusson (2005b) is the confusion created by the variety of messages conveyed by the Government, media and food manufacturers, which leads to parents being unsure of which strategy to follow when addressing overweight or obesity in their children, for example low fat versus low calorie, good/bad types of fat. In relation to both prevention and treatment of excess weight and obesity, current legislation and trends towards comprehensive but understandable food labelling may help to empower individuals to make informed healthy eating choices.

The prevention and treatment of childhood obesity is clearly complex. In the absence of conclusive evidence of effective interventions, it is necessary to implement those that have at least been indicated as such and do not cause harm, thus upholding the *Nursing and Midwifery Council Code of Professional Conduct* (NMC, 2004, section 1.4) and the ethical principle of non-maleficence. (See Chapter 7 for a discussion on this ethical principle.)

A *behaviour change* approach in relation to increasing physical activity, diet modification and avoidance of sedentary behaviour is therefore required to address Megan's weight issues. The intervention is likely to be *educational* in the first instance and, having explored Sarah and Megan's current level of knowledge and motivational level, should be individualised and therefore *client centred.*

A logical approach to making information client centred and more meaningful and relevant to a client is an individualised plan or programme. In addition, the use of graphics or symbols that link information in the plan to specific health education, for example the 'five a day' campaign, may help to consolidate this knowledge.

Clearly, it is important that children's nurses work very closely with dietitians and paediatricians in delivering this information to Sarah and Megan while maintaining a central role in relation to the intervention. This approach upholds the ideal proposed by Casey *et al.* (1997) for effective multidisciplinary teamworking; promotes continuity of care and effectiveness, since the children's nurses will have already established a relationship with the child and family during the hospital admission (Croghan, 2005); and helps ensure that encounters with new people are minimised during hospitalisation. Lack of continuity in health professional input is a factor that can affect mental health and cause temporary regression in areas such as speech, educational attainment or behaviour (Taylor *et al.*, 1999). These potential problems should be discussed with parents so that if they do occur, parents are prepared for them. In addition, the child's school nurse or health visitor should be advised of the admission so that they are similarly prepared.

Many factors can trigger asthma, for example exercise, temperature and humidity, stress, food allergies or intolerances and certain drugs (Jordan & White, 2001). It is very important therefore, at this stage, to fully explore the factors that appear to trigger Megan's asthma. If exercise is an issue, then behaviour change in relation to increasing physical activity may need to be managed with particular care. By fully exploring this area and designing an individualised activity plan, any concerns that Sarah and Megan may have in relation to exercise induced asthma can be discussed. Any misconceptions should then be dispelled, thereby overcoming such barriers to the uptake of health promotion advice.

Test your knowledge

What specific information could be included in an individualised diet and activity programme for Megan?

 Case study 5.2

Megan is now an in-patient on the children's ward. During a conversation with a student nurse, Sarah confides that she has not been administering Megan's preventative inhaled medication. She does not want Megan to take steroids because she is already overweight and does not wish this problem to be exacerbated. Sarah believes that taking steroids will result in Megan gaining even more weight. (See Chapter 6 for a discussion on ethical issues relating to the dilemma of the nursing student.)

Appropriate medications, delivered via a mask and spacer were unsuccessful in alleviating Megan's symptoms. Therefore, these are now being administered via a nebuliser. Unfortunately, Megan has displayed some difficult behaviour when receiving treatment in this way and it has been necessary for the nurses and Sarah to restrain Megan during the procedure.

Test your knowledge

- What do you consider to be the main health promotion issue?
- Identify approaches to health promotion you would consider to be appropriate regarding this issue.
- Which skills are now required to enable the practitioner to effectively promote healthy behaviour?
- Are there any legal issues relating to the restraining of children for medical / nursing procedures?

You will have recognised that non-compliance is the main health promotion issue, in terms of Sarah's resistance to oral steroids and Megan not wishing to comply with nebulised medication. Which approaches to addressing this issue did you identify as being appropriate? These issues can, as in the previous section, be addressed by the medical, behaviour change, educational and client-centred approaches.

Non-compliance

Failure to take medication within a chronic disease scenario is a common problem (Shuttleworth, 2004), particularly in relation to inhaled steroid therapy for asthma (Trueman, 2000; O'Connor, 2001). This is due to a number of factors, for example lack of understanding of the role of 'preventer' medication, fear of side effects and absence of immediate symptom improvement (compared to reliever medication). For Megan to benefit from the correct medical approach, as prescribed, it will be necessary for the practitioner to use an educational, client-centred approach to ensure that Sarah has all the necessary information to make an informed choice regarding compliance with the medical regimen, thereby achieving concordance and the desired behaviour change. Problems experienced during this admission concerning Megan's compliance with the administration of nebulised medication also need to be addressed. (In Chapter 9, compliance is discussed in more detail in relation to adolescent development.)

Steroids

An educational approach is needed to ensure that a full explanation is given to Sarah regarding the safety of low dose steroid therapy, and to reassure Megan and her about the small risk of side effects and exactly what they are. In addition, the practitioner needs to stress that the dangers of uncontrolled asthma far outweigh any risks of treatment (Latham, 2000). It is important that this information is conveyed in a non-judgemental, factual manner to prevent it being misinterpreted as 'scaremongering' to force compliance.

Once this additional information has been internalised and understood by Sarah, and possibly Megan, it may be possible to formulate an individualised self-management plan. This is a client-centred approach that involves keeping an asthma diary, with careful monitoring of peak flow measurements and adjustment of treatment as necessary, together with criteria for seeking further medical advice and/or help. This should enable Megan and Sarah to feel more confident in managing the condition and therefore empowered (Harrop, 2002).

Self-management plans for children have been discussed by Milnes and Callery (2003), who state that, although those already in use have been successful they remain, on the whole, a tool used primarily by parents and carers, and suggest they need further development to make them more child centred. Until there are further developments in this field, practitioners probably have to be content with empowering parents and carers rather than the child.

Restraint

Restraint of children for procedures or administration of medication has been frequently discussed in recent times, and although organisations such as the Royal College of Nursing (2003) have issued guidelines on this topic, there are still many grey areas in terms of the legal position. In addition to the possibility of accidental physical harm to the child, parent or health professional, Pearch (2005) highlights the possible detrimental effects such incidents may have on the mental health of all those involved, and stresses that restraint should only be used as a last resort. Alternatives such as distraction techniques, for example storytelling and guided imagery (see Chapter 4) are suggested and should be used in negotiation with the child and family to suit their individual needs (i.e. a client-centred approach). In this particular scenario, it may be possible to alter the administration technique slightly to give Megan more control over the situation, thereby empowering her. Many children object strongly to having a mask held over their face, and allowing Megan to hold the mask herself may be all that is required to promote cooperation and compliance.

Test your knowledge

- What developmental stage (according to Piaget) is Megan likely to be at?
- What appropriate educational tools could be used to inform Megan in relation to her asthma and treatment?

As Megan is eight years of age and has no learning difficulties, it is likely that she is at the concrete operational developmental stage (Piaget, 1963) and able to understand basic information regarding her condition and its management. Staff should aim, therefore, to explain information in an age appropriate manner and reinforce this with resources that are specifically designed for children with asthma, for example leaflets available from relevant organisations and suitable websites. Some hospitals have designed their own software packages that aim to increase the child's level of knowledge regarding their asthma (McPherson et al., 2002). These interventions should enable Megan to gain a better understanding of her condition and, as she becomes older, increase her level of participation in discussion and decisions about her care.

Being able to interact with other children who suffer from asthma, via forums such as appropriate Internet sites and projects such as Asthma Camps (Hodges, 2005), should help ensure that Megan does not feel 'different' or isolated from her peers, and potentially improve symptom control.

Colleagues in primary care play a vital role in managing patients' asthma in the community (Latham, 2000). It is essential, therefore, that in relation to the case study, the ward practitioner liaises effectively with the GP, practice nurse and school nurse to support Sarah and Megan. The school nurse is particularly important in this type of scenario, as recognised by the Department of Health (1999) who state that school nurses are expected to take the lead on health improvement initiatives to support children with medical needs. Research by Madge and Franklin (2003) demonstrated that asthma was the most common medical condition (411 out of 3000 pupils, 13.7%) in six schools surveyed, which illustrates the extent of school nurses' involvement in providing support to children with asthma, together with the scope available for implementing initiatives that are relevant to a large number of their caseload. Within this scenario, the school nurse should ensure that Megan's teachers are confident and competent in helping with administration of medication, know what usually exacerbates Megan's asthma and are alert to early signs and symptoms of an attack. Education about asthma to Megan's peers (with Sarah and Megan's agreement, so privacy and confidentiality is not compromised) may also be helpful in supporting her, dispelling myths and overcoming prejudice within the school environment. Yawn *et al.* (2000) discuss the use of computer based education in schools that have such aims.

 Case study 5.3

Eight months later, following a period of good health, the practice nurse sees Megan in asthma clinic. Her peak flow measurements are significantly reduced. Sarah reports that Megan is taking her 'preventer' medication regularly but it has been necessary for her to take her bronchodilators more frequently over the last two weeks. During the consultation, Megan proudly tells the practice nurse that their kitten, Sooty, will be a year old next week. Sarah also relates a funny story about their experience of pony trekking on a recent holiday in the country.

Test your knowledge

What factors do you think may have contributed to the recent exacerbation of Megan's asthma?

It is likely that Megan and Sarah have been exposed to high levels of pollen, horsehair and cat fur. Assuming that they have not consciously disregarded advice already given on avoidance of such allergens, one assumes that there is a gap in their knowledge. This may have occurred for two reasons. First, the health professionals involved in giving health promotion advice may have focused solely on the main issues, believing that the information provided was substantial and that any additional advice would detract from it. Unfortunately, this viewpoint results in a failure to undertake a truly holistic approach, despite the application of all relevant approaches to health promotion. Second, Sarah and Megan may have received, but forgotten, allergen avoidance advice, perhaps due to information overload or due to a lack of recent reinforcement.

Test your knowledge

- What practical measures could have been taken by the health professionals involved to ensure that Megan and Sarah were fully informed of potential allergens earlier?
- How can children's nurses ensure that families receive all relevant information about a disease or condition, together with health promotion advice, without overloading them?

Allergen testing could have been performed during Megan's hospital admission or followed up at clinic. Although a medical approach was used during that admission to promote compliance and concordance with prescribed medication, an assumption was made that non-compliance was solely responsible for the exacerbation of Megan's condition. As Sooty is now aged one, it is likely that he would have been with Megan and Sarah eight months ago. One must assume, therefore, that for some reason staff did not ask about pets when admitting Megan or that the information received was disregarded due to oversight or lack of staff knowledge. In this instance, optimum care has not been achieved because only a partially client-centred approach was used, which focused on only one aspect of behaviour change.

Failure to test for allergens earlier and/or discuss potential allergens has now led to a situation where, having become attached to Sooty over a period of months, Megan and Sarah may have to make the difficult decision to find a new home for their family pet.

Educational approaches to ensure that children, young people and their families receive comprehensive information about a disease, symptom control and health promotion will, as already discussed, need to be appropriate to their developmental age and their individual circumstances, that is client centred. These could include bullet points within an asthma diary so that, when it is used daily by the child and parent, important information is reinforced. Board games that are designed by medication/appliance manufacturers or ward staff could be used during clinics or admissions to convey information, in a fun way, to younger children. Anatomical dolls and mannequins are another resource that can be used, particularly by play specialists, with this age group. Older children and adolescents may prefer to access information via the Internet or use specially developed CD ROMs, as discussed by Shegog et al. (2001) and Kallstrom (2002). However, care needs to be taken when recommending the access of information via the Internet. First, not all sites are suitable or evidence based. Second, some clients may not have access to a computer at home. It is advisable, therefore, to provide details of recommended websites to clients and, if finances permit, provide computers and Internet access for clients' use in clinic waiting areas or on children's wards. It is important to note that all information given to clients, particularly those suffering from chronic illness, should be reinforced with written materials such as leaflets (Coyne, 1997).

Cuffwright (1999) examined parental perceptions of childhood asthma and emphasised that, due to the variability of the disease, opportunistic education should take place in whichever environment the health professional sees the child, that is not just in asthma clinics. Parental asthma education programmes, covering topics such as lay support services/groups, disease process, allergen/trigger avoidance and professional services, were studied by Trollvik and Severinsson (2005), and were shown to impact significantly on understanding, attitude and feelings of empowerment. Individual (for child and/or parent) and group (for families or just parents) educational strategies were examined. Both methods included information, counselling, use of home peak flow or symptom monitoring. Trollvik and Severinsson (2005) concluded that empowerment was particularly enhanced if programmes were undertaken in a group, with other parents.

This chapter has encompassed almost all of the principles outlined in the Department of Health Guidance for implementing the *NSF for Children Young People and Maternity Services* in relation to childhood asthma (DoH, 2004b). Principles have only been omitted if they are not applicable to the scenario discussed. Similar guidance will soon be available in Wales as, in response to the Welsh Assembly Government (2005) *National Service Framework for Children, Young People and Maternity Services*, the Children and Young People Specialist Service (CYPSS) project is setting standards for asthma via managed clinical networks (MCNs). Consultation on these standards was completed in September 2006, but at the time of writing, had not been published.

Conclusion

This chapter has utilised the work of Ewles and Simnet (2003) to illustrate how principles of health promotion may be applied in a chronic illness scenario. The individual interpretation of the term 'health' within the general population has been highlighted, together with how this may differ for those with long-standing and non-curable conditions. By addressing specific health promotion issues within a scenario, the aim was to demonstrate the use of relevant strategies by children's nurses to promote healthy behaviours to alleviate symptoms and improve the overall well-being of the child and family.

The effect of external and internal factors on the client's receptiveness to health promotion strategies has also been highlighted alongside suggestions for overcoming barriers to health promotion advice. Potential pitfalls have been outlined in relation to assessment and adaptation to changes in circumstance, thus reinforcing the need for a holistic approach.

The importance of education as a basis for health promotion, and its ineffectiveness if not used in conjunction with other approaches, has been discussed. Empowerment has been identified as the key component of health promotion. The facilitation of empowerment can be summarised as providing client-centred information, retention of this knowledge by the client, facilitation (by the practitioner) of skills development (in the client), which then enable them to effect and sustain health enhancing behaviour change.

Finally, the importance of children's nurses' specialist knowledge of child development and family focused interpersonal skills has been highlighted. The approaches to health promotion and strategies discussed in relation to the case study have illustrated that children's nurses working in the hospital environment should be as competent and confident in using such knowledge and approaches as their community counterparts. In doing so, opportunities to maximise the health potential of children and young people suffering from chronic illness will be fully utilised so that they, and their families, feel supported and empowered.

🔑 Key points

- Knowledge does not necessarily change attitude or behaviour.
- Empowerment is 'the process of enabling or imparting power transfer from one individual or group to another' (Rodwell, 1996) and has been identified as the most important component of health promotion strategies (Tones & Green, 2004).
- Health promotion advice that involves behaviour change must include a client-centred educational approach (in certain cases, medical intervention may also be used).
- Behaviour change is an evolving process that is primarily concerned with the nurse influencing the client's perception of their locus of control.
- Within a chronic disease scenario, 'health' in terms of the WHO definition can sometimes never be achieved. Therefore, it is more likely that the aim of health promotion strategies will be to allow the child or young person to perform their social roles and achieve their personal potential.

Useful websites

Asthma www.asthma.org.uk Accessed 31/07/06.
Health Promotion www.hj-web.co.uk/sheps/ Accessed 31/07/06.
Obesity www.nationalobesityforum.org.uk, www.aso.org.uk Accessed 31/07/06.
Smoking Cessation Support http://www.patient.co.uk/showdoc/40000776/ Accessed 31/07/06.
http://kidshealth.org/kid/stay_healthy/ Accessed 31/07/06.
http://www.givingupsmoking.co.uk/ Accessed 31/07/06.
http://www.talk4teens.co.uk/keepinhealthy.htm Accessed 31/07/06.
http://www.dh.gov.uk/PolicyAndGuidance/HealthAndSocialCareTopics/Tobacco/fs/en Accessed 31/07/06.
www.bbc.co.uk/schools/scienceclips/ages/9_10/keeping_healthy.shtml Accessed 31/07/06.

References

Abbot, N.C., Stead, L.F., White, A.R., Barnes, J. & Ernst, E. (2001) Hypnotherapy for smoking cessation (Cochrane Review), *The Cochrane Library, Issue 1*. Oxford, Update Software.

Audit Commission (1993) *Children First: a Study of Hospital Services.* London, HMSO.

Carson, A.R. (2001) Adult paediatric patients. *American Journal of Nursing,* **101** (3), 46–54.

Casey, A., Young, L. & Rote, S. (1997) Integrated nursing services for children. *Paediatric Nursing,* **9** (5), 8.

Child Growth Foundation (1997) Available at: http://www.patient.co.uk/showdoc/ 26738763/ Accessed 8/12/06.

Cole, T.J., Freeman, J.V. & Preece, M.A. (1995) Body mass index reference curves for the UK, 1990. *Archives of Disease in Childhood,* **73**, 25–29.

Cole, T.J., Bellizzi, M.C., Flegal, K.M. & Dietz, W.H. (2000) Establishing a standard definition for child overweight and obesity worldwide: international survey. *British Medical Journal,* **320**, 1240–1243.

Coyne, I.T. (1997) Chronic illness: the importance of support for families caring for a child with cystic fibrosis. *Journal of Clinical Nursing,* **6**, 121–129.

Coyne, I.T. (2006) Consultation with children in hospital: children, parents' and nurses' perspectives. *Journal of Clinical Nursing,* **15** (1), 61–71.

Croghan, E. (2005) An introduction to behaviour change among clients. *Nursing Standard,* **19** (30), 60–62.

Cuffwright, M. (1999) Childhood asthma: influencing parents' perceptions of disease. *Community Practitioner,* **72** (2), 25–26.

Department of Health (1999) *Saving Lives: Our Healthier Nation.* London, The Stationery Office.

Department of Health (2001) *The Expert Patient: a New Approach to Chronic Disease Management for the 21st Century.* London, Department of Health.

Department of Health (2004a) *National Service Framework for Children, Young People and Maternity Services: Core Standards.* London, Department of Health.

Department of Health (2004b) *National Service Framework for Children, Young People and Maternity Services: Asthma.* London, Department of Health.

Ewles, L. & Simnett, I. (2003) *Promoting Health: a Practical Guide* (fifth edition). Edinburgh, Baillière Tindall.

Fox, J. (2005) The role of the expert patient in the management of chronic illness. *British Journal of Nursing,* **14** (1), 25–28.

Franck, L.S. & Callery, P. (2004) Rethinking family-centred care across the continuum of children's health care. *Child: Care, Health & Development,* **30** (3), 265–277.

Freemark, M. & Bursey, D. (2001) The effects of metformin on body mass index and glucose tolerance in obese adolescents with fasting hyperinsulinemia and a family history of type 2 diabetes. *Pediatrics,* **107** (4), 763–764.

Harrop, M. (2002) Self-management plans in childhood asthma. *Nursing Standard,* **17** (10), 38–42.

Hart, K.H., Herriot, A., Bishop, J.A. & Truby, H. (2003) Promoting healthy diet and exercise patterns amongst primary school children: a qualitative investigation of parental perspectives. *Journal of Human Nutrition and Dietetics,* **16** (2), 89–96.

Hodges, B. (2005) Asthma camp. *Paediatric Nursing,* **17** (6), 20–22.

Hovell, M.F., Zakarian, J.M., Matt, G.E., Hofsetter, C.R., Bernert, J.T. & Pirkle, J. (2000) Effect of counselling mothers on their children's exposure to environmental tobacco smoke: randomised controlled trial. *British Medical Journal,* **321**, 337–342.

Jarvis, M.J., Goddard, E., Higgins, V., Feyerabend, C., Bryant, A. & Cook, D.G. (2000) Children's exposure to passive smoking in England since the 1980s: cotinine evidence from population surveys. *British Medical Journal,* **321**, 343–345.

Jordan, S. & White, J. (2001) Bronchodilators: implications for nursing practice. *Nursing Standard,* **15** (27), 45–52.

Kallstrom, T.J. (2002) Focus on asthma. Interactive asthma game by Starbright offers fun and education. *AARC Times,* **26** (10), 12–14.

Katz, J., Peberdy, A. & Douglas, J. (2000) *Promoting Health: Knowledge & Practice* (second edition). Basingstoke, Palgrave.

Kiess, W., Galler, A., Reich, A. *et al.* (2001) Clinical aspects of obesity in childhood and adolescence. *Obesity Reviews*, **2**, 29–36.

Klein, S., Fontana, L., Young, V.L. *et al.* (2004) Absence of effect of liposuction on insulin action and risk factors for coronary heart disease. *The New England Journal of Medicine*, **350** (25), 2549–2557.

Lancaster, T., Stead, L. & Shepperd, S. (2001) Helping parents to stop smoking: which interventions are effective? *Paediatric Respiratory Reviews*, **2** (3), 222–226.

Latham, S. (2000) Breathing space. *Nursing Standard*, **14** (44), 18–19.

McPherson, A., Forster, D., Glazebrook, C. & Smith, A. (2002) The asthma files. *Paediatric Nursing*, **14** (2), 32–35.

Madge, N. & Franklin, A. (2003) *Change, Challenge & School Nursing*. London, National Children's Bureau.

Magnusson, J. (2005a) Childhood obesity: diagnosis, prevalence and implications for health. *Community Practitioner*, **78** (2), 66–68.

Magnusson, J. (2005b) Childhood obesity: prevention, treatment and recommendations for health. *Community Practitioner*, **78** (4), 147–149.

Milnes, L.J. & Callery, P. (2003) The adaptation of written self-management plans for children with asthma. *Journal of Advanced Nursing*, **41** (5), 444–453.

Naidoo, J. & Wills, J. (2000) *Health Promotion: Foundations for Practice* (second edition). London, Baillière Tindall.

National Health Service Executive (1996) *Child Health in the Community: a Guide to Good Practice*. London, The Stationery Office.

National Institute for Clinical Excellence (2001a) *Orlistat for the Treatment of Obesity in Adults. Technology Appraisal Guidance No. 22*. London, NICE.

National Institute for Clinical Excellence (2001b) *Guidance on the Use of Sibutromine for the Treatment of Obesity in Adults. Technology Appraisal Guidance No. 31*. London, NICE.

National Institute for Clinical Excellence (2002) *Inhaler Devices for Routine Treatment of Chronic Asthma in Older Children (aged 5–15 years)*. London, NICE.

National Institutes of Health (2005) Clinical studies database. Safety and efficacy of Orlistat in African American and Caucasian children and adolescents with obesity-related co-morbid conditions. Protocol no 98-CH-0111. London, National Institute of Health. Available from: http://clinicalstudies.info.nih.gov/detail/A_1998-CH-0111.html Accessed 17/11/06.

Nursing and Midwifery Council (2004) *The NMC Code of Professional Conduct: Standards for Conduct, Performance and Ethics*. London, Nursing and Midwifery Council.

O'Connor, B. (2001) Inhaler devices: compliance with steroid therapy. *Nursing Standard*, **15** (48), 40–42.

Pearch, J. (2005) Restraining children for clinical procedures. *Paediatric Nursing*, **9**, 36–38.

Piaget, J. (1963) *The Origins of Intelligence in Children*. New York, W.W. Norton & Company, Inc.

Randall, S. (2006) Children and second-hand smoke: not just a community issue. *Paediatric Nursing*, **18** (2), 29–31.

Rodwell, C.M. (1996) An analysis of the concept of empowerment. *Journal of Advanced Nursing*, **23**, 305–313.

Royal College of Nursing (2003) *Restraining, Holding Still and Containing Children and Young People: Guidance for Nursing Staff*. London, Royal College of Nursing.

Scientific Committee on Tobacco and Health (SCOTH) (2004) *Second-hand Smoke: Review of Evidence since 1998*. London, Department of Health.

Scriven, A. & Orme, J. (2001) *Health Promotion: Professional Perspectives* (second edition). Hampshire, Palgrave.

Shegog, R., Bartholomew, K., Parcel, G., Sockrider, M.D., Masse, L. & Abramson, S.L. (2001) Impact of computer-assisted education program on factors related to self-management behavior. *The Journal of the American Medical Informatics Association*, **8** (1), 49–61.

Shuttleworth, A. (2004) Improving drug concordance in patients with chronic conditions. *Nursing Times*, **100** (24), 28–29.

Silagy, C., Mant, D., Fowler, G. & Lancaster, T. (2001) Nicotine replacement therapy for smoking cessation (Cochrane Review), *The Cochrane Library, Issue 1*. Oxford, Update Software.

Sindall, C. (2001) Health promotion and chronic disease: building on the Ottawa Charter, not betraying it? *Health Promotion International*, **16** (3), 215–217.

Smith, L., Coleman, V. & Bradshaw, M. (2002) *Family-centred Care: Concept, Theory & Practice*. Basingstoke, Palgrave.

Taylor, J., Muller, D.J. & Wattley, L. (1999) *Nursing Children: Psychology, Research and Practice* (third edition). Cheltenham, Stanley Thornes.

Tones, K. & Green, J. (2004) *Health Promotion: Planning & Strategies*. London, Sage.

Tones, K. & Tilford, S. (2001) *Health Education. Effectiveness, Efficiency and Equity* (third edition). London, Chapman and Hall.

Trollvik, A. & Severinsson, E. (2005) Influence of an asthma education program on parents with children suffering from asthma. *Nursing and Health Sciences*, **7**, 157–163.

Trueman, J.F. (2000) Non-adherence to medication in asthma. *Professional Nurse*, **15** (9), 583–586.

Welsh Assembly Government (2005) *National Service Framework for Children, Young People and Maternity Services*. Cardiff, Welsh Assembly Government.

White, A.R., Rampes, H. & Ernst, E. (2001) Acupuncture for smoking cessation (Cochrane Review), *The Cochrane Library, Issue 1*. Oxford, Update Software.

Whitlock, E.P., Williams, S.B., Gold, R., Smith, P.R. & Shipman, S.A. (2005) Screening and interventions for childhood obesity. *Pediatrics*, **116** (1), 125–144.

Wilson, P., O'Meara, S., Summerbell, C. & Kelly, S. (2003) The prevention and treatment of childhood obesity: effectiveness bulletin. *Quality & Safety in Health Care*, **1** (12), 65–74.

World Health Organization (1946) *Constitution*. Geneva, World Health Organization.

World Heath Organization (1984) *Health Promotion. A Discussion Document on the Concept and Principles*. Copenhagen, World Heath Organization.

World Health Organization (1986) Ottawa Charter for Health Promotion. *Journal of Health Promotion*, **1**, 1–4.

World Health Organization (1997) *Obesity, Preventing and Managing the Global Epidemic: Report of the WHO Consultation of Obesity*. Geneva, World Health Organization.

Yawn, B.P., Algatt-Bergstrom, P.J., Yawn, R.A. *et al.* (2000) An in-school CD-ROM asthma education program. *Journal of School Health*, **70** (4), 153–159.

6 Ethical Issues

Peter Mcnee and Maggie Furness

Introduction

This chapter will examine two of the ethical theories commonly used in the teaching of nursing ethics, followed by an exploration of four ethical principles. This is not an exhaustive list of principles and other authors use additional principles, which will not be included here. Similarly, beneficence and non-maleficence will be considered separately and not in this instance together as used by Beauchamp and Childress (2001). It is intended that this chapter will offer the reader a basic understanding of nursing ethics that will be useful in the care of children and young people with chronic illness.

This chapter will apply the identified ethical theories and principles to clinical situations through the use of some of the practice case histories examined in other chapters of this book. It will raise and explore ethical dilemmas that can potentially occur in the care of children and young people with chronic illness.

Aim of the chapter

The purpose of this chapter is to explore some of the ethical theories and principles that can be used in practice. The study of these should help provide a possible framework for ethical decision making. The care of children and young people with chronic illness can present professionals and carers with ethical dilemmas. There is no easy answer or clear solution, but knowledge of ethics will empower the reader and enable decision making. Case studies from other chapters in the book will be used to apply these theories and principles to practice. This text does not include a critique of philosophical methods of decision making that may be found in other published works, for example Seedhouse (1998).

The aim of the chapter is to examine ethical theories and principles and their application to clinical practice through case study and clinical practice examples.

Intended learning outcomes

- To examine the ethical theories of utilitarianism/consequentialism and deontology, rights, duty and obligation, in relation to delivering nursing practice to children, young people and families with chronic illness
- To explore the ethical principles of autonomy, beneficence, non-maleficence, justice and veracity and their application to practice
- To analyse some of the ethical dilemmas arising within this book
- To explore the use of ethical theories and principles as a possible framework to aid ethical decision making in practice

---

⏱ Time out

- Consider why it is important to study ethics.
- Produce your own definition of ethics and a rationale for its application and relevance to your practice.

Why study ethics?

The study and use of ethics is an essential tool for children and young people's nurses because there is an ethical component to all aspects of care in any setting, whether or not this becomes a dilemma (Brykczynska, 1994). Care is improved by a comprehensive knowledge of ethics and its application to an individual situation (Fletcher, 1979). The study of ethics provides a challenge and is something that takes time to learn and understand before it can become useful. The application of ethical principles needs to be incorporated into everyday practice to ensure that children, young people and their families receive optimum care.

A definition of ethics

Before examining the ethical theories and principles that may be used in decision making, it is necessary to define ethics or morals. Versey and Foulkes (1990) define ethics or moral philosophy as the examination of what is good and evil, and state that it is, in a literal sense, a practical study of the actions of human beings as members of social groups. Children's nurses are one such social group. How then do individuals within such a group achieve moral competence and the ability to make decisions which they can recognise as ethical? Some theorists would suggest that this morality is learnt through observation of society and by conforming to moral rules and codes of behaviour. This does not mean that individuals always behave as they ought to, or even that they know how they should behave. (See Kohlberg's theory of moral development for further reading/study.)

Introduction to ethical theories

In reading various texts, it can be observed that the relationship between the theories of teleology, consequentialism, utilitarianism, and deontology and the principles of ethics can be confusing. This may arise from the fact that the study of ethics is a very old subject and the language used by theorists such as Bentham (1748–1832), Kant (1724–1804) and Mill (1806–1873) has changed over time. These ethical terms will be discussed later and applied to practice situations.

Additionally, the concepts surrounding ethical theories and principles are complex and need careful reading to gain understanding. The realm of ethics is far removed from the normal practice area of children and young people's nurses, but is an essential knowledge base to aid ethical decision making. There is only one solution to the acquisition of this knowledge; these theories and principles have to be learnt, just like, for example drug calculations, for they are equally important. In the study of ethics, nurses should set out to learn the underlying theories and principles of personal and social morality (Thompson *et al.*, 2000).

There is a division between the theories of normative and non-normative ethics. General normative or prescriptive ethics forms and defends a system of moral principles, which decide what actions are right or wrong. Applied normative ethics are used in making concrete decisions in daily life to resolve particular moral problems in the care of children and young people.

Non-normative descriptive and scientific ethics fall into two categories, namely descriptive ethics, which is a factual investigation of moral behaviour and beliefs, and meta-ethics, which is an analysis of the meaning of ethical terms, for example 'rights', 'obligations', 'virtue', and 'responsibility'. They are applied to try to find out what factually and/or conceptually is the case, not what ought to be the case. In contrast to normative ethics, non-normative ethics has little practical application (Tschudin, 2003).

Consequentialism, utilitarianism, and deontology and non-consequentialism are all normative theories, which tend to look for moral absolutes, so avoiding relativism, in other words that which is good is simply what the nursing community defines as good. These theories are the most frequently used and have influenced moral thinking. Examples are given later in the chapter.

Theory of consequentialism

The theory of consequentialism is the starting point for learning about the two theories of ethics discussed in this chapter. Consequentialism is also called teleology from the Greek meaning 'end' or 'purpose'. In this theory, the rightness or wrongness of an action depends upon its consequences. The morally right action is that which produces the best consequence or outcome (Hendrick, 2000). In other words, for children and young people's nurses the correct or moral thing to do is that which produces the optimum outcome for each child or young person. In the care of children and young people with chronic illness, the relevant outcome may be the control of disease, relief from pain, promotion of health or the prolongation of life (Brykczynska, 1994). The outcome may also depend upon the teleological theory used. The best known consequentialist theory is the theory of utilitarianism or utility.

Utilitarianism

The theory of utilitarianism, as espoused by Bentham (1748–1832), Mill (1806–1873) and Smart and Williams (1989), amongst others, seeks the promotion of the greatest good for the greatest number. It focuses mainly on the consequences of an action. In modern terminology, it is called consequentialism or teleology: right in terms of the good introduced from the consequences of an action.

Early ethical theories, which make the quest for pleasure and the avoidance of pain the basis for making moral choices, have been called hedonistic. Later applications of utilitarianism were also hedonistic, and sought to base moral judgements on their usefulness or practical value in adding to our pleasure, diminishing our pain, and so adding to the sum total of human happiness (Thompson *et al.*, 2000). Examples will be discussed in the case studies.

Utilitarianism is particularly associated with Jeremy Bentham (1748–1832) and John Stuart Mill (1806–1873). Bentham defined the greatest happiness principle; put simply, it seeks the greatest good for the greatest number, the least pain, and the greatest happiness, focusing mostly on the consequences of an action. Mill refined this principle by using measuring criteria for happiness and noting the complexity of moral decision making. Bentham's felicific calculus for measuring happiness was replaced by a cost benefit analysis of the consequences of actions towards the greatest good–right in terms of the good introduced by the consequences of an action (Smart & Williams, 1989). Utilitarians do not regard their actions as inherently good or bad, but as a means to an end (Hendrick, 2000). In the context of caring for children and young people with chronic illness, it is the outcome that matters and not how it is achieved. Modern philosophers such as Frankenna (1973) have recognised a difference between act and rule utilitarianism.

Act utilitarianism

Act utilitarianism considers the consequences of an act. Using past experience, act utilitarianism tries to predict possible outcomes for various courses of action (Thompson *et al.*, 2000). The principle of utility is the ultimate standard of rightness and wrongness for all utilitarians. The act utilitarian justifies actions not using rules but appealing directly to the principle of utility (Beauchamp & Childress, 2001). The action of a children and young people's nurse must achieve the optimum balance of good over bad with everyone considered.

Rule utilitarianism

This form of utilitarianism does not judge an action as right or wrong because of the predicted or actual consequences, but judges an action correct if it was based upon a general rule, which if followed should lead to the best consequences (Thompson *et al.*, 2000).

Obedience to certain rules is fundamental to morality, but there are flaws with rules. Rule utilitarianism considers the consequences of adopting certain rules (Beauchamp & Childress, 2001). A nurse's actions are considered morally right if they are following the rules, for example the Nursing and Midwifery Council (2004) *Code of Professional Conduct*. These rules, if followed, will usually produce the best possible outcome.

Case study from Chapter 5: respiratory

Megan's case study outlines a range of issues associated with non-compliance with treatment and the need to access a range of services to control the symptoms of asthma. Megan is first seen at six months of age and treated for a wheeze that did not require ongoing medication at discharge. In treating Megan, we see a morally right action producing the best consequences for the child and family, in that Megan's symptoms have been resolved and she has been successfully discharged home. At six years of age, Megan is admitted to hospital again, where a diagnosis of asthma is made. She is prescribed appropriate medication and the respiratory nurse specialist deems her inhalation technique competent. In terms of service provision, again we see a morally right action. Services have been configured to produce the best outcomes for children with asthma. In-patient beds are available for treatment and a nurse specialist is available to provide the appropriate health education and promotion. At eight years of age, again Megan is admitted to hospital. On this occasion, it is apparent that there are clear ethical issues facing the children's nurse.

Reflection

Reflecting back on Megan's case study, what do you consider are the ethical issues and challenges arising from it?

Medication

- First, Megan's mother, Sarah, is not administering Megan's preventative medication due to concerns about Megan's weight.

- Second, Megan needs to be restrained to administer her medication.
- Third, non-compliance with treatment raises a number of issues for the student nurse in whom Sarah confides.

Confidentiality

It is the duty of all children's nurses to act in the best interests of the child. There is also a need to ensure confidentiality in the information that we receive from those in our care. What should the student nurse do? If the student nurse was to withhold the information provided by Sarah, she would be acting against the best interests of Megan, as Megan has been admitted with an exacerbation of her asthma and has had repeated GP visits related to her condition. The student nurse would also be colluding with Sarah in relation to the non-compliance in Megan's treatment. This would be a morally unjustified act, as potentially there could be severe consequences for Megan's health and well-being. Following the theory of consequentialim, the morally right action to take is to disclose the information provided by Sarah to senior nursing staff and the doctors involved in Megan's care. Obviously, there is a role here for negotiating care and discussing with Sarah the anxieties that have led to the non-administration of medication. It is within the parameters of the role of the children's nurse to attempt to achieve the best outcome and consequences for both Megan's family and the professionals involved in Megan's care.

Restraint

Restraint is a difficult and complex issue within children's nursing. It raises a number of legal, professional and ethical issues. In terms of consequentialism, the nurses restraining Megan need to consider the best outcomes for the alleviation of her symptoms. Clearly, the administration of her medication is in her best interest as it will treat and alleviate her symptoms. The consequences of the nurse's actions will produce a morally justifiable outcome. However, the distress caused to Megan by restraining her may exacerbate her symptoms and negate the benefits of the treatment. Therefore, the action of restraint becomes morally unjustifiable as the outcomes will not provide a benefit for Megan. It has often been said of ethics that there are no right or wrong answers. In terms of consequentialism, what is important is the morally justifiable outcome. For the children's nurse, again, the role of negotiation is important. Megan would need to be prepared for the administration of nebulisers by involving other members of the multidisciplinary team including the play specialist. Restraint should always be an action of last resort and only used if other avenues have been exhausted. Restraint can be used to achieve the necessary outcome of administering the nebuliser as long as it remains in Megan's best interest and provides the best outcome.

Case study from Chapter 9: chronic renal disease

In Chapter 9, Thomas is presented as a fifteen-year-old boy who has been diagnosed with chronic renal failure since the age of five years. Thomas' condition is now beginning to deteriorate as a consequence of his non-compliance with a conservative management regime. A number of reasons are presented as contributing to this situation, including the influence of his peers. This is a common issue encountered across a range of chronic illnesses. In terms of the wider clinical issues, the utilitarian approach considers the cost and benefits of a potential intervention.

Key issue

In Thomas' case, a regional specialist centre has managed his care over a number of years. This ongoing care is expensive, particularly during a time where value for money, clinical effectiveness and cost effectiveness are all issues within the modern NHS. The question is then posed:

If Thomas is unwilling to comply with conservative treatment, he will require closer monitoring and an increase in the resources of the multidisciplinary team managing his care, and potentially he may require renal transplantation. Should these services be provided to a potentially non-compliant patient?

Utilitarianism looks to provide the greatest good for the greatest number. If Thomas continues on his current conservative management regime, resources could be applied to children and young people who are compliant with treatment or diverted to children and young people with other chronic illnesses. This is a pertinent issue, particularly in times of health care rationing. Withholding these interventions from Thomas will ultimately lead to deterioration in his condition. Therefore, this act is against utilitarian principles as the greatest good would not be achieved for Thomas, his family or the health care professionals involved in his care.

Clearly, no children's nurse or health care professional is going to refuse Thomas further care provision. In terms of rule utilitarianism, children's nurses are bound by their code of conduct which clearly states that at all times we must act in the best interest of our patients (NMC, 2004). In this scenario, it is incumbent upon the children's nurse to negotiate with Thomas to help ensure his compliance and participation to achieve the best health outcomes in his care delivery; this may involve the children's nurse liaising with the wider multidisciplinary team.

Key points

When caring for children and young people the following points should be considered. It is incumbent on the children's nurse to:

- Do the greatest good for the greatest number
- Ensure that children and young people experience the least possible pain and suffering
- Adhere to Bentham's happiness principle and focus on the legal, professional and ethical consequences of any action taken

---

Theory of deontology

Having started with the theory of consequentialism, we now examine the theory of deontology, which has a very different approach.

Deontology, from the Greek *deon* meaning duty, argues that what makes an action right or wrong is clearly defined by rules. Our moral duties and rights are guided by rules (Thompson *et al.*, 2000). Deontology is often described as duty ethics. It may require doing what is right regardless of the consequences. For this reason, it is also sometimes called non-consequentialism (Tschudin, 2003).

The theory of deontology was advanced by Kant (1785) cited in Thompson *et al.* (2000). It advocates determining what is right by considering the intrinsic features of an action, for example duty, often independently from its consequences. It is mostly concerned with the determination of duties and obligations using moral principles and rules, for example respect for the individual and telling the truth. According to Kant, actions are right if they conform to a moral law and are not to be judged by the consequences. Kant propounded the categorical imperative, a principle that should govern all moral behaviour. It may be formulated in various ways. These are:

- So act that the principle of your action can become a universal law for all rational beings.
- So act as if the principle of your action were to become by your will a universal law of nature.
- So act as to treat humanity, whether in your own person or in that of any other, in every case as an end, never as a mere means.

Another aspect of deontological theory is rights theory. Rights may be defined as a justified claim to have or receive something, or to act in a certain way. There is an obvious link between 'rights' in this sense, and obligations and duties. They could be said to be different sides of the same deontological coin. Using rights theory, the morality of an action can be judged by whether or not it falls within the scope of a right. There are different means of categorising rights, for example:

- Positive rights – rights to do something or have someone else do something
- Negative rights – which are the forbearance or omission to act by others

However, the most important distinction to be made between rights is that of natural or human rights and legal rights. Natural or human rights are sometimes said to be self-evident, for example those in the American Declaration of Independence, and are the most important moral rights, overriding all conflicting rights and being shared equally by all humans by virtue of their humanity. They include positive and negative rights, examples being the right to life and the right not to be tortured.

Legal rights are those rights allowed by law, either by express legislation or based on legal principles, and upheld by the courts. They are necessarily narrower in scope than natural or human rights, being confined to the legal jurisdiction in which they are formulated, and being concerned with more parochial matters, such as property rights.

Rights theory is often employed in an effort to promote the interests of minorities, such as a counter to utilitarian arguments. The United Nations (1989) declared that the child has a right to express an opinion and to have that opinion taken into account in decision making affecting the child. This was an expression of a natural or human right. However, subsequent legislation in the UK Children Act (1989; 2004) and the Human Rights Act (1998) has specifically provided for the wishes and feelings of the child to be taken into account in decisions affecting the child. Accordingly, it is now a legal right when applying deontological theory, that children and young people's nurses have a duty to take account of the moral and legal rights of the child, such as the right to family life and those explicit in their *Code of Professional Conduct* (NMC, 2004).

Case study from Chapter 4: eczema

In this case study, Isabella has eczema and so far treatment has been ineffective. The problems encountered by the child and family are compounded by their recent move to the UK, Isabella's reduced diet and nutritional intake and possibly by the use of alternative treatments. In this case study, a number of health care professionals have been involved in Isabella's care including the paediatrician, nurse specialist, health visitor and school nurse. All professionals involved have a duty of care.

In terms of deontology, it is the role of the individual to perform their pre-ordained duty (Muir & Gordon, 2000). On a simplistic level, this can be seen in the referral process that has led to Isabella receiving care as an in-patient. Also, we can see that the family is struggling to manage Isabella's condition, with her mother losing sleep and feeling isolated and unsupported. To help to resolve this situation, the multidisciplinary team have liaised in order to provide effective treatment and support, thus fulfilling their duty.

In the UK, Isabella and her family have a number of rights, including free access to health care at the point of delivery. One of the main principles of the Children Act (1989) is that the rights of the child are paramount. Her mother Merelee is entitled to receive appropriate and evidence based care to ensure the effective treatment of Isabella's condition. Merelee also expresses the need for Isabella to interact and play with other children. Again, the Children Act (1989) highlights the need to take children's views into account in any decisions surrounding care. Here, the children's nurse has fulfilled her duty by ensuring the involvement of the play specialist in an attempt to engage Isabella in activities with other children. The United Nations (1989) *Convention on the Rights of the Child* also identifies the need to actively consult with and facilitate children's participation in their care. By providing a multidisciplinary approach to the care of Isabella and the support of Merelee, the children's nurse is fulfilling the principles of deontology.

⊄⊐⟨ₚ   Key points

In deontology:

- What makes an action right or wrong is defined by rules.
- Our moral duties and rights are guided by rules.
- Deontology is often described as duty ethics.
- In some instances, doing what is right is the correct course of action regardless of the potential consequences.

Ethical principles

Kant (1724–1804) argued that the concept of 'person' is fundamental to ethics and is a formative principle of ethics (Thompson *et al.*, 2000). If there is no idea of a person who has rights and responsibilities, then ethics cannot work. A person must be treated as an end and never as a means to an end. Therefore, 'persons' are to be treated with respect, whatever their age or cognitive ability. If a person has rights and responsibilities, there must be in this person some degree of morality or self-determination, which is exercised freely. Kant calls this moral independence or autonomy. He argues that the principle of autonomy is necessary, both theoretically and practically, for a working system of ethics.

Respect for persons, as a principle, informs codes of ethics such as the International Council of Nurses (ICN) (1973) *Code for Nurses* and the NMC (2004) *Code of Professional Conduct: Standards for Conduct, Performance and Ethics.*

Ethical principles are fundamental moral rules that are used to justify actions (Fletcher *et al.*, 1995). A principle, as suggested by Thompson *et al.* (2000), is a starting point for moral reasoning, and refers to the basic questions the nurse must ask. Principles are guides to give direction. They are pointers but do not tell nurses where they will finish, or what will happen along the way. Thiroux (1995) argues that principles can act like a compass, giving direction but not a road map.

They are not rigid like theories, but flexible without being too specific. They do not provide answers but help direct thinking to achieve an agreement about what ought to be done.

Some of the best known ethical principles are those described by Beauchamp and Childress (2001). They used the *Belmont Report* (Presidents Commission for the Study of Ethical Problems in Medicine and Biomedical Research, 1981), which was the outcome of the National Commission for the Protection of Human Subjects of Biomedical and Behavioural research. The *Belmont Report* stated that respect for persons, beneficence and justice should be the ethical principles governing research. Beauchamp and Childress (2001) added non-maleficence, making four principles.

(1)   Respect for autonomy
(2)   Beneficence
(3)   Non-maleficence
(4)   Justice

These four principles are general guidelines that leave plenty of room for judgement in particular cases.

 Time out

- What do you understand by the term autonomy?
- What is the role of the children's nurse in relation to autonomy?

Principle of autonomy

There are many views of autonomy, a word that comes from the Greek *autos* (self) *nomous* (rule of law) (Dworkin, 1988). It is a term associated with ideas such as self-determination, self-government, self-mastery, voluntariness and choosing one's own moral position (Beauchamp & Childress, 2001). Autonomy can be defined as the capacity to think, decide, and act on the basis of such thought and decision freely and independently and without let or hindrance (Gillon, 1985). To be an autonomous person, therefore, means being able to live one's own life according to a set of self-chosen rules and values. A cardinal principle of autonomy means recognising children and young people as persons who are entitled to such basic human rights as:

- The right to know
- The right to privacy
- The right to receive care and treatment (Thompson *et al.*, 2000)

In relation to a capable person's autonomy, Hendrick (2000) refers to an individual's ability to come to his/her own decisions and requires nurses to respect the choices patients make concerning their own lives. Respect for autonomy also means the protection of those incapable of autonomy because of illness, injury, mental disorder or developmental age.

Respect for a child or young person's autonomy, and the right to consent to or refuse treatment, are now widely accepted as central values in health care (DoH, 2004; WAG, 2005). *The Patient's Charter* (1991) also acknowledged this. There are potential difficulties associated with the exercise of autonomy and consent for children, which will not be discussed here. (See reference list for suggested further reading.)

The principle of autonomy according to Seedhouse (1998) can be defined in three ways:

(1) Autonomy as a single principle. This view of autonomy suggests that there is a basic principle that asserts that the wishes and needs of children and young people ought to be respected.
(2) Autonomy as a right. The child or young person's ability to choose should be acknowledged and the choice made should be respected, as a right.
(3) Autonomy as a quality. The basic intrinsic quality of children and young people. Simply to be autonomous is to be able to do something, rather than nothing.

Autonomy, therefore, means some element of choice for the child or young person and their families. The choice may be wide-ranging, for example to receive care or to refuse care. However, one child's choice may conflict with another's interests, for example one child may want a night light on, but it may keep the other children awake. A further example would be an adolescent who wishes to watch a '15' rated film but is unable to because there are much younger children within the same clinical area. Freedom of choice may not be possible because of circumstances:

●   If a child is unconscious and therefore a choice must be made on his/her behalf. Someone acts in the best interests of the child at this time, that is parents, doctor or nurse caring for the child.
●   The child is vulnerable in another way, unable to communicate well, for example deaf, dumb, blind, physically or mentally ill. These children must have their autonomy protected and have a competent person to make choices for them. This could be called preference utilitarianism, indicating what the child may have chosen.

Autonomy may not be possible because somebody in a position of power is withholding choice from the child or young person, for example children in young offender institutes or oppressive regimes in a global context. Those in power can control the child's choice, and that may mean that there is a limited choice or none at all, which means they have lost their autonomy. Children's nurses must be very careful if a child or young person's autonomy is unprotected or lost, because then that child is at risk of harm.

Nursing has many definitions but may be said to encompass the care of the sick, frail and vulnerable child. It covers the provision of comfort, services and care in any situation, whether in the hospital or community, employing the virtue of selfless caring. There is an onus on the children's nurse, for these reasons, to become the guardian of autonomy for the child, young person and their family.

When examining the professionalism of nursing, some criteria ought to be considered, such as autonomy. It is sometimes difficult for the children's nurse to be autonomous. If nurses are to achieve autonomy, they must also become accountable for their practice. This may arise from personal moral standards or from a code of ethics or professional code, such as NMC (2004) *Code of Professional Conduct; Standards for Conduct, Performance and Ethics.*

The idea of autonomy is central to the NMC (2004) code. The thing that distinguishes a 'person' is the fact that he/she is a rational human being. The code includes the obligation that the nurse respects the independence of the child/young person and family and respects their involvement in the planning and delivery of care. This invokes the ethical principle of autonomy and it is implicit in the reference to patient involvement, that the child/young person is given sufficient and truthful information to make that involvement meaningful and provide autonomy, while incorporating the ethical principle of keeping trust.

Case study from Chapter 8: oncology

In this case study, Katie is presented as a three-year-old girl with a diagnosis of acute lymphoblastic leukaemia. Katie has been treated with chemotherapy and has acquired an infection that necessitates transfer to a children's high dependency unit. Katie's mother, Claire, is 17 years of age and is supported by her own parents. This case study is a good example of the provision of care for a non-autonomous patient or client. As Katie is only three years of age, she is reliant on Claire to make key decisions for her and consent to treatment on her behalf. It is the role of the children's nurse to protect the autonomy of both Katie and Claire, who could both be considered vulnerable.

The children's nurse should facilitate the decision making process to enable Claire to make autonomous decisions. Autonomy is a central concept of health care rights (Charles-Edwards & Glasper, 2002). It is the role of the children's nurse to safeguard this position and prevent paternalism, which has been a feature of health care in recent years. Marriott (2004) advocates the need to focus on the needs of children rather than professional groups. In the decision making process, it is important to involve and encourage children with chronic illness to make decisions about their care. In Katie's case, the facilitation of this process is geared towards Claire acting in the best interests of her child. Some authors have identified that autonomy and childhood have often been perceived as mutually exclusive (Glasper & Richardson, 2006). This has been based on society's view of children as incompetent to make effective decisions for themselves. In Katie's case, it is important that Claire is supported in the difficult decisions that she will have to make about Katie's care.

In this case, the children's nurse can assure Katie's autonomy by supporting Claire as she makes difficult and complex decisions. One of the key aspects of this decision making process is the consent to ongoing invasive treatment. There is recognition that, wherever possible, children should be involved in the process of gaining consent to treatment. Edgar *et al.* (2001) identify five preconditions for consent to be legally and ethically gained: that the individual is competent to do so; that the individual is fully informed; that they understand the information that has been presented to them; that they give consent voluntarily; and that they authorise the intervention or procedure. Clearly, there are limitations to Katie's understanding of her illness and she cannot give consent due to her age. However, her autonomy and her right to self-determination should still be upper-most in the minds of those professionals involved in her care.

Key points

- An essential attribute of professionalism is autonomy: the ability to make independent decisions.
- Knowledge of ethics equips the nurse, so far as possible, to make such decisions.

Ethical principle of beneficence

Beneficence has been explained in many ways, but can be defined as a principle that generates an obligation to act in ways that promote the well-being of others, or a moral injunction to do good (Rumbold, 1999). As the point of nursing action is to promote the well-being of others, for example children and young people, it follows that such actions accord with the principles of beneficence (Edwards, 1996).

Beneficence is a major part of a nurse's professional duty and requires nurses to benefit children and young people. It has been said to be the cornerstone of nursing ethics (Tschudin, 1996) and is enshrined in the NMC (2004) *Code of Professional Conduct*, for example to act in such a manner as to safeguard and promote the well-being of patients (Hendrick, 2000). The principle of beneficence generates significant obligations towards all children and young people who may be affected, directly or indirectly by a nurse's conduct. Beneficence poses several questions for the nurse:

- What may count as a benefit?
- Who decides what is in the children and young people's best interests?
- Whom do nurses have to benefit, that is to whom do they owe a moral obligation?

Reflection

Consider the three questions above, reflect upon your own clinical experiences and identify some answers based upon clinical care.

What do the words benefit, well-being and interests mean? They all mean 'good' that the children's nurse is expected to promote both physically and psychologically (Edwards, 1996). This may include the prevention of disease, the restoration of health, and a reduction in pain and suffering (Davis & Aroskar, 1991).

Who must nurses benefit? There is a primary duty towards children and young people on their own wards, neighbouring wards (Edwards, 1996), other nurses, patients, relatives, public and themselves (NMC, 2004).

Beneficence demands that the children's nurse respects the rights of the children and young people, for example to informed consent. Strict justice may have to be compromised, as attention to the special needs of children and young people with chronic illness may result in less attention being given to other children and young people in a busy ward setting. Conversely, special regard for the rights of children and young people has to be balanced against consideration of the common good, as in a case where children and young people have to be quarantined to protect others in an epidemic.

Acting beneficently, immunisations for children and young people may inflict some degree of pain or discomfort but have longer-term health benefits. A surgical procedure may also be viewed as causing harm in order to promote a positive outcome. Beneficence also requires an assessment and balancing of 'trade-offs' in situations where decisions are often made against a background of uncertainty.

Case study from Chapter 10: cystic fibrosis

In the case study, it becomes clear that Sophie is at a crossroads in her life as she is about to undergo the transition to adult services. A number of children with chronic illness will experience this change, which can have a major impact on the confidence of young people in the management of their conditions. Sophie has got a job and a circle of friends in whom she has not confided about her condition. Sophie has been admitted to hospital for the treatment of a chest infection and nutritional input. During this stay in hospital, the nurse specialist discusses and guides Sophie through the transition process. In this way, the children's nurse is acting beneficently as she is allowing Sophie time and space to reach a decision of her own choosing about when to transfer to adult services.

Issues

National Service Frameworks (DoH, 2004; WAG, 2005) advocate the need for children/young people to be listened to and their views taken into account when care decisions are made. In this scenario, it is the role of the multidisciplinary team to make effective and ethical decisions. This can often result in a need to make fateful decisions that they may have to justify (Botes, 2000). To act beneficently, there is a responsibility to do good (Charles-Edwards & Glasper, 2002). Not to support Sophie in her decision about transition would be a breach of duty and therefore counter to the beneficent view. Breaches of duty have been seen in a number of high profile cases across the NHS, including the cases of

Beverly Allitt (DoH, 1994) and the Bristol hearts scandal (Kennedy, 2001). Above all, the children's nurse within the case study must be guided by the thoughts and actions of Sophie and support her in making autonomous and effective decisions to ensure a good outcome.

⌁⏦ Key points

- To act beneficently, there is an obligation to act in a way that promotes the well-being of children/young people, or a moral injunction to do good.
- As the role of the nurse is to do good and promote health and well-being, nursing actions correspond to the principles of beneficence.
- Beneficence is a major part of the duty of care of the children's nurse.

Ethical principle of non-maleficence

Non-maleficence may be defined as the avoidance of harm to the interests of others, or at least the minimisation of the risk of harm befalling individuals. The principle of non-maleficence generates obligations not to harm others. This differs from beneficence in the sense that it imposes few obligations on others (Edwards, 1996).

The principle of non-maleficence requires that nurses have a duty not to harm children and young people, nor to subject them to risk of harm (Rumbold, 1999; Hendrick, 2000; Beauchamp & Childress, 2001). As with beneficence, it is enshrined in the NMC (2004) *Code of Professional Conduct*, although there is no explicit mention of the word harm, for example nurses must ensure that no act or omission on their part in their sphere of responsibility is detrimental to the interests, condition or safety of patients and clients (Edwards, 1996).

What counts as harm to an individual child and young person with chronic illness, may not be harm at all to another person. Harm may be physical, pain, disability and death. Harm may also be psychological, such as mental stress. Beauchamp and Childress (2001) give a broad definition of harm which includes the following:

- Thwarting or defeating of interests
- Self-harm
- Actions of another party
- Intimidation
- Undue influence or pressure
- Misleading or misinforming children and young people
- Abuse
- Assault
- Exploitation

Non-maleficence is less morally demanding than beneficence and generates fewer obligations. It does not demand positive action, and only requires that the children and young people's nurse does not harm anybody (Hendrick, 2000).

Beneficence and non-maleficence are closely related. Both promote the moral objectives of medicine and nursing – beneficence to help those who are sick and suffering, and non-maleficence to prevent harm, preventing deterioration of existing illness, damage or disease (Gillon, 1985). Frankenna (1973) puts the two principles together. Beauchamp and Childress (2001) treat them as separate principles, but recognise that they are entwined. Many nursing or medical interventions that aim to benefit a child or young person may at the same time result in some degree of harm. Beneficence and non-maleficence have to be weighted together and the benefits and harms balanced against each other.

Sometimes, the principles of beneficence and non-maleficence conflict and there is a dilemma as to which one should have priority. For Gillon (1985), the claim that non-maleficence should normally override beneficence is untenable. Nevertheless, in some situations, non-maleficence should override beneficence. If the risks of a procedure or treatment are very high and serious, it will be morally indefensible to carry out the procedure if the benefit is small. On the other hand, there is the example of immunisation programmes. If non-maleficence was to be prioritised, it would mean that nobody could be immunised because of the risk to a minority who may suffer side effects. Rumbold (1999) says that this is illogical, because the benefit to the wider community carries more moral weight.

The principles of beneficence and non-maleficence provide a moral foundation for the obligations set out in the NMC (2004) *Code of Professional Conduct*. The code gives some guidance on using ethical principles to underpin practice. Practically, children and young people's nurses could link these with other concepts such as accountability and responsibility.

Case study from Chapter 3: diabetes

In this case study, Taleisha has recently been diagnosed with type 1 diabetes. Initially, this has been managed well, but following Taleisha's transfer to secondary school it becomes apparent that Taleisha is not administering all of her insulin. Taleisha is also upset by the apparently protective nature of her parents limiting her freedom.

Issues

The key issue within this case study is to minimise any harm caused by the non-administration of insulin. The role of the children's nurse here is to facilitate an open dialogue between Taleisha, her parents and members of the multidisciplinary team to ensure compliance with treatment. Harm can befall a number of people within this scenario. Taleisha's parents are experiencing some stress over the management of her condition and to ignore this would negate the principle of non-maleficence and would be working outside the NMC (2004) *Code of Professional Conduct*. If the nurse were to ignore Taleisha's non-compliance with treatment, she is likely to experience a further deterioration in her condition. To ensure that the principle of non-maleficence is upheld, the children's nurse must provide continued access to services for Taleisha and her family. Taleisha must be allowed time to discuss her thoughts and feelings about her condition and treatment regimen. Above all, the children's nurse must negotiate a way forward, empowering Taleisha to take control of the management of her condition, thus ensuring her autonomy and upholding the identified principle.

Key points

- In any nursing action it is important to avoid harm, whether that is on a physical, spiritual or psychological level.
- Where harm cannot be totally avoided, it should be minimised at all costs.
- Non-maleficence generates a clear obligation not to harm others.

Ethical principle of justice

Justice as defined by Beauchamp and Childress (2001) is divided into four parts:

(1) Justice as fairness, that is to say, one acts justly towards a child or young person when one has given them what is due or owed, what he or she deserves or can legitimately claim.

   Justice is concerned with the fair distribution of benefits, risk and costs. The idea is that children and young people in similar positions should be treated in a similar manner.

(2) Distributive justice, that is pertaining to an equal distribution of benefits and harms for children and young people.

   Distributive justice refers widely to the distribution of rights and responsibilities in society, including, for instance, civil and political rights.

(3) Justice and equality, the presumption that children and young people should be treated equally, unless there is a difference between them that is relative to the care in question.

   Justice and equality, according to Aristotle, means treating equals equally and unequals unequally. In other words, whatever respects are relevant, children equal in those respects should be treated the same.

(4) Justice as desert, concerned with equal distribution and may also be referred to as material or needs principles. Various philosophers have proposed the following principles as a valid material principle of distribution justice:

   (a) to each child and family an equal share
   (b) to each child and family according to need
   (c) to each child and family according to effort
   (d) to each child and family according to contribution
   (e) to each child and family according to merit
   (f) to each child and family according to free market changes

   Adapted from Beauchamp and Childress (2001)

Thompson *et al.* (2000) describe the principle of justice as the duty of universal fairness, equal opportunity for children and young people. Equity is the equality of outcomes for groups such as children. Rawls (1997) describes justice as fairness. The distribution of burdens and benefits should be considered from the point of view of the least advantaged in society, for example poor children should share the benefits in society equally with all others. Benefit to the least advantaged becomes the 'norm' for decision and policymaking. Brykczynska (1994) says that the principle of justice provides equal opportunities and access to treatment for all children.

Justice incorporates the ideals of fairness, equality and non-discrimination. The application and relevance of this principle for children and young people's nurses may be shown in discussions about the allocation of resources and nursing priorities and time allocation.

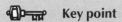 **Key point**

Justice is concerned with the fair distribution of benefits, risk and costs. The idea is that children and young people in similar positions should be treated in a similar manner.

A nursing ethic

With respect to nursing, the meaning of the term ethics has been considered and explained in various ways. Rowson (1990) defined ethics as thinking and reasoning about morality, and morality as respect for a person's autonomy or self-rule. This suggests a dutiful view of ethics consistent with deontology. Another definition is provided by Thompson *et al.* (2000), namely that ethics refers to science, or a study of morals, or moral philosophy. They also suggest that 'an ethic' can refer to the morals of a group, such as a 'nursing ethic'.

On a more practical level, ethics is often seen to focus on the study and practice of what is right and good for people. Thompson *et al.* (2000) suggested that ethics teaches humankind the practice of duties in human life and the reasons for what they should do and what they should leave undone. In the nineteenth century, nursing ethics were entirely concerned with duty and there was a demand for unquestioning obedience from nurses. At about that time, Nightingale wrote of the need for those with practical knowledge of nursing's real moral dilemmas to engage in common study with those of other disciplines, including those with some skill in asking pertinent ethical questions and exploring their implications. This remains true for children and young people's nurses today. To achieve this, individual nurses will need to use their professional and personal life experiences, and social and cultural influences, which have shaped their previous moral upbringing and current moral status.

It is suggested by Jameton (1990) that in order to understand the terms 'culture' and 'morality', they must be considered more closely. Culture can be said to cover the basic aspects and ideas of a society. It also covers settings of life, traditions and work, and it gives explanations for conduct. Morality, which forms part of a culture, assists with the formation of societal beliefs and conduct and also provides laws, standards, ideals and statements of value.

In the absence of ethical theories, society determines whether or not an act is moral on the basis of what is acceptable to it (relativism). Thus, within the nursing community, by tradition nurses are not allowed to run in the ward. However, an exception to this general rule is in an emergency, when it is perfectly correct to run. Even then, nurses must not run fast, because they will consequently be out of breath on arriving at the emergency and limited in their ability to help. Tradition dictates they must simply 'walk quickly'.

Increasingly, nurses are spurning traditional practices in favour of new thinking, leading to rational rather than traditional actions. The nursing profession then examines the resulting practices to assess their morality. This illustrates the need for the application of ethical theory and principles to nursing practice.

Morality, whether learned by observation, intuition or the application of theories and principles, may be influenced by society and also by situations. (See also *Situation Ethics*, Fletcher, 1979.) The individual needs a moral sense, and the ability to grasp and make moral judgements. This is sometimes called conscience, and may be said to be a prerequisite for social existence. The moral growth of a nurse may depend upon the extent of his/her autonomy, that is an individual making his/her own decisions rather than having them determined by outside forces. Thus, ethical rules must be freely arrived at and be reasonable rather than enforced.

In the context of children's nursing, nursing ethics may be defined as a moral code that they apply when caring for children and young people with chronic illnesses and their families. Nursing ethics may also be construed as a set of moral standards by which nurses live and work. These ethics or moral standards should not be confused with other codes, for example NMC (2004), which may include ethical and behavioural guidance. The grounding for the nursing ethic may be a personal moral code, a professional code (NMC, 2004) or a moral framework such as Cooper's (1988) covenantal relationship, triple contract or covenant theory (Veatch, 1981). When a comparison is made between models, mutuality and reciprocity are found to be common to all. These suggestions for grounding the nursing ethic echo the two basic principles of Trusted (1987), namely keeping trust and benevolence.

Having reflected upon the nursing ethic, it is now possible to consider how a framework for ethical decision making may help children and young people's nurses in practice with issues surrounding chronic illness.

Definition of an ethical dilemma

Thompson *et al.* (2000) define an ethical dilemma as a choice, of whatever kind, between two equally unsatisfactory alternatives. This may involve a conflict between moral principles and values where there are no rules or precedents to follow. This has been established within the case studies presented in this chapter.

Ethical dilemmas demand the attention of children and young people's nurses and other members of the multidisciplinary team. They are not confined to the obvious ethical dilemmas such as decisions about abortion, euthanasia, transplants and research on humans, but also arise every day in nursing and medical decisions, for example:

- What nurses and doctors should tell children and young people and their families regarding their diseases and treatments
- On a larger scale, decisions about resource allocation, for example how much of society's money should be spent on health care, and how much should be spent on the provision and delivery of children and young people's services

To decide upon a particular course of action is to decide that it is better than, or preferable to, the available alternatives; this means making value judgements. Such judgements involve ethical choices, but not every ethical decision or value judgement requires conscious thought, and sometimes can be made intuitively using long held beliefs, commitments and habits.

Sometimes intuition fails and gives no clear answer, or it may deceive and give the wrong answer. Furthermore, there is the risk that intuition can vary from person to person. Intuition is therefore unreliable, making it essential to use another method of ethical decision making using a framework or a model such as the NMC (2004) *Code of Professional Conduct.*

Ethical decision making

Ethical decision making is not some kind of hidden process but is a problem-solving process similar to many others. Demystifying ethics and using common sense will enable the solving of an ethical problem (Thompson *et al.*, 2000).

All ethical decisions and judgements are made within a cultural tradition. From traditions come the formation of the idea of what is moral, and how and when moral decisions should be made. MacIntyre (1981) suggests that these traditions could arise from a historical background. Perhaps both individuals and societies are actors in a play, in which they act out previous life experiences, which in turn influence their subsequent behaviour.

Within the society of a hospital, ethics is employed as a moral guideline, and may be used to make comparisons between personal and professional moral benefits. The value for nurses of using nursing ethics is that by looking at these areas, they may improve their powers of observation and pursue insights into morality by clarifying cultural traditions. This enables them to make clearer decisions, having established moral beliefs, and also gives them the power and ability to make autonomous decisions, as seen in the case studies presented within this book.

One of the purposes of an ethical education for nurses is to enable them to justify their decisions. There are a number of different situations in which nurses may be required to justify their decisions. For example, the most obvious is when a nurse must defend their decision to the doctor. This is of great importance, because such defence goes to the root of their professional autonomy and accountability (NMC, 2004).

In addition to doctors, nurses have to justify their decisions to children/young people and their families, nursing colleagues and managers. It is possible that they may also have to justify their decisions to the general public, for example when deciding to stand up for what they believe at a subsequent public enquiry or in care proceedings.

All the above have a common objective, namely the promotion of improved practice and care of children and young people with chronic illness. Nurses need the confidence and assurance when making decisions that can only be engendered by ethical knowledge and education.

Nurses ought to be encouraged to think about why and how they deliver care and the possible consequences of their actions. It is in this area that children and young people's nurses need help and guidance but they do not need another set of rules, because they are inappropriately rigid with respect to complex situations and reduce autonomy by providing a ready-made answer. However, nurses do need a framework with which they can determine what is best and most appropriate. An ethical model or framework could be said to be a systematic construction and evaluation of arguments that can be used when making ethical decisions.

Benjamin and Curtis (1992) argue that frameworks are important for two reasons. First, a framework may provide common ground for resolving dilemmas, or at least a starting point for developing a satisfactory resolution. Second, it can provide the individual with personal integrity and continuity when they are making decisions.

There are a wide variety of ethical models and frameworks for use when attempting to make ethical decisions, which can range from a simple set of steps to a complex grid of many layers. Their common feature is that they all require significant thought and analysis before reaching a conclusion, albeit this may be achieved in different ways. Readers are directed to Davis and Aroskar (1991), Beauchamp and Childress (2001), Husted and Husted (1991) and Seedhouse (1998) for information on a number of ethical models and frameworks that can be applied to the ethical dilemmas described in this book.

A simple model to follow involves the achievement of an ethical education to facilitate ethical decision making:

(1) *Learning* ethical theories, principles and models to establish a sound theoretical knowledge base for use in practice
(2) *Discussing* ethical theories, principles and models to improve understanding and comprehension for use in practice
(3) *Applying* ethical theories, principles and models to case histories to demonstrate comprehension and for use in practice
(4) *Using* ethical theories, principles and models for practical decision making in any setting

A suggested model for ethics in practice/decision making

The model illustrated in Figure 6.1 is intended to guide practitioners through ethical dilemmas they may encounter in clinical practice. The model aids the decision making process in attempting to apply ethical theories and principles to clinical scenarios, thus allowing the individual practitioner to consider the potential outcomes of their own professional actions. To illustrate the use of the model, a case study from earlier in the chapter is now discussed and the model applied.

In Chapter 9, Thomas is presented as a fifteen-year-old boy with chronic renal disease. The identified ethical dilemma is Thomas' non-compliance with treatment. This is clearly a problem as it impacts upon his ongoing health and well-being. On a wider scale, it also has an impact on the resources needed to care for Thomas from the multidisciplinary team, and potentially the deviation of those resources from other children. The ethical theory that has been applied to this situation is utilitarianism, which advocates the greatest good for the greatest number. Here we see that the tenets of this theory may not be achieved as Thomas, his family and the multidisciplinary team may all be affected by his decision not to comply with treatment. A variety of principles may also be applied to this situation, including autonomy, in terms of Thomas' ability to make his own decisions; beneficence, in terms of the role of the children's nurse in being obliged to act in ways to promote the well-being of others; non-maleficence again relating to the role of the children's nurse in avoiding the risk of harm to Thomas or minimising that risk, whilst facilitating his own autonomous decision making processes.

Once the practitioner has identified the appropriate ethical theory and principles it is incumbent on them to find solutions. In Thomas' case, this is around negotiation and partnership, in attempting to find a way forward to ensure that Thomas is compliant with his treatment to assure his ongoing health and well-being. When applying this model in practice, it would be beneficial to identify a

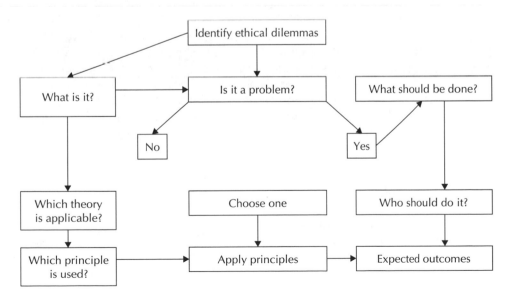

Figure 6.1   A model for ethics in practice/decision making.

range of possible outcomes and the ethical implications of each action, and their impact on the individual child or young person, their families and the children's nurse responsible for their care.

Conclusion

The aim of this chapter was to identify and apply a range of ethical theories and principles to clinical practice. For the application of ethics to be pertinent to individual nurses, they must have a clear understanding of the guiding theory and principles. Within the case studies we have used to aid the discussion, we have seen that children and young people with chronic illness experience a range of difficulties and dilemmas as they pass through the care setting, whether this is within the acute or community setting. Children's nurses are constantly involved in the decision making process within a range of clinical settings. We have seen that there are no easy solutions to a number of ethical dilemmas; the onus is on individual nurses to be aware of the ethical dimensions of the care that they deliver to ensure that at all times they do no harm and act within the legal, professional and ethical boundaries of their role.

Key points

- There is no such person as a moral expert.
- Children's nurses must make their own ethical decisions and must not blindly follow the dictates of others.
- In particular, they must recognise that the doctor or any other member of the multidisciplinary team is potentially no more morally competent than themselves.
- Children's nurses must appreciate that not all ethical dilemmas have solutions, but nevertheless be equipped to make the best possible decision.
- The study and application of ethical principles to the often difficult decisions made during the care trajectory of children and young people with chronic illness will enhance the decision making capabilities of individual children's nurses and allow them to contribute to the decision making process and support the child, young person and their family.

Useful websites

Kohlberg's theory of moral development
http://psychology.about.com/od/developmentalpsychology/a/kohlberg.htm Accessed 29/11/06.

UK clinical ethics network
www.ethics-network.org.uk

📖   Recommended reading

Beauchamp, T.L. & Childress, J.F. (2001) *Principles of Bio-Medical Ethics* (fifth edition). Oxford, Oxford University Press.

References

Beauchamp, T.L. & Childress, J.F. (2001) *Principles of Bio-Medical Ethics* (fifth edition). Oxford, Oxford University Press.

Benjamin, M. & Curtis, J. (1992) *Ethics in Nursing.* Oxford, Oxford University Press.

Botes, A. (2000) An integrated approach to ethical decision making in the health team. *Journal of Advanced Nursing,* **32** (5), 1076–1082.

Brykczynska, G.M. (ed.) (1994) *Ethics in Paediatric Nursing.* London, Chapman & Hall.

Charles-Edwards, I. & Glasper, E.A. (2002) Ethics and children's rights: learning from past mistakes. *British Journal of Nursing,* **11** (17), 1132–1140.

Children Act (1989) London, The Stationery Office.

Children Act (2004) London, The Stationery Office.

Cooper, M.C. (1988) Covenantal relationships: grounding for the nursing ethic. *Advances in Nursing Science,* **10** (4), 48–59.

Davis, A.J. & Aroskar, M.A. (1991) *Ethical Dilemmas and Nursing Practice* (third edition). Norwalk, Appleton & Large.

Department of Health (1994) *The Allitt Inquiry.* London, HMSO.

Department of Health (2004) *National Service Framework for Children, Young People and Maternity Services.* London, the Stationery Office.

Dworkin, G. (1988) *The Theory and Practice of Autonomy.* Cambridge, Cambridge University Press.

Edgar, J., Morton, N.S. & Pace, A. (2001) Review of ethics in paediatric anaesthesia: consent issues. *Paediatric Anaesthesia,* **11**, 355–359.

Edwards, S.D. (1996) *Nursing Ethics: a Principle-based Approach.* Basingstoke, Macmillan.

Fletcher, J. (1979) *Situation Ethics.* London, S.C.M. Press.

Fletcher, N., Holt, J., Brazier, M. & Harris, J. (1995) *Ethics Law and Nursing.* Manchester, Manchester University Press.

Frankenna, W.K. (1973) *Ethics* (second edition). Englewood Cliffs, N.J. Prentice Hall.

Gillon, R. (1985) *Philosophical Medical Ethics.* Chester, John Wiley.

Glasper, E.A. & Richardson, J. (2006) *A Textbook of Children and Young People's Nursing.* London, Churchill Livingstone.

Hendrick, J. (2000) *Law and Ethics in Nursing and Health Care.* Cheltenham, Nelson Thornes.

Human Rights Act (1998) London, The Stationery Office.

Husted, G.L. & Husted, J.H. (1991) *Ethical Decision Making in Nursing.* St. Louis, Mosby Year Book.

International Council of Nurses (1973) *Code for Nurses: Ethical Concepts Applied to Nursing.* Geneva, ICN.

Jameton, A.I. (1990) Culture morality and ethics twirling the spindle. *Critical Care Nursing Clinics of North America* (12), 3.

Kennedy, I. (2001) *Learning from Bristol: the Report of the Public Inquiry into Children's Heart Surgery at the Bristol Royal Infirmary 1984–1995.* London, the Stationery Office.

Macintyre, A. (1981) *After Virtue* (second edition). London, Duckworth.

Marriott, S. (2004) Right from the start. *Nursing Management,* **11** (6), 16–18.

Muir, J. & Gordon, K. (2000) Home care for ventilated children: an analysis of the application of ethical reasoning. In: *Textbook of Community Children's Nursing*. (eds J. Muir & A. Sidey), pp. 130–139. London, Baillière Tindall.

Nursing and Midwifery Council (2004) *Code of Professional Conduct Standards of Performance & Ethics*. London, Nursing and Midwifery Council.

The Patient's Charter (1991) London, The Stationery Office.

Presidents Commission for the Study of Ethical Problems in Medicine and Biomedical Research (1981) *Protecting Human Subjects: the Belmont Report*. Washington, DC, US Government printing office.

Rawls, J. (1997) *A Theory of Justice*. Cambridge, Harvard University Press.

Rowson, R. (1990) *An Introduction to Ethics*. Harrow, Scutari Press.

Rumbold, G. (1999) *Ethics in Nursing* Practice (third edition). Edinburgh, Baillière Tindall.

Seedhouse, D. (1998) *Ethics: the Heart of Health Care* (second edition). Chichester, Wiley & Sons.

Smart, J.J.C. & Williams, B. (1989) *Utilitarianism: For and Against*. Cambridge, Cambridge University Press.

Thiroux, J.P. (1995) *Ethics, Theory and Practice* (fifth edition). New Jersey, Prentice-Hall.

Thompson, I.E., Melia, K.M. & Boyd, K.M. (2000) *Nursing Ethics* (fourth edition). Edinburgh, Churchill Livingstone.

Trusted, J. (1987) *Moral Principles and Social Values*. London, Routledge & Keegan.

Tschudin, V. (1996) *Nursing the Patient with Cancer*. London, Prentice-Hall.

Tschudin, V. (2003) *Ethics in Nursing: the Caring Relationship* (third edition). Edinburgh, Butterworth Heinemann.

United Nations (1989) *Convention on the Rights of the Child*. Geneva, UN.

Veatch, R.M. (1981) *A Theory of Medical Ethics*. New York, Basic Books.

Versey, G. & Foulkes, P. (1990) *The Collins Dictionary of Philosophy*. London, Collins.

Welsh Assembly Government (2005) *National Service Framework for Children, Young People and Maternity Service in Wales*. Cardiff, Welsh Assembly Government.

7 Continuing Care Needs

Melda Price and Sian Thomas

Introduction

Due to developments in medical care and technology, the survival of children with complex needs and chronic illness has become more prevalent (Jardine *et al.*, 1999; Emond & Eaton, 2004). The first part of this chapter will explore the impact of changing service boundaries and the development of children's nursing roles on children/young people and their families. An analysis of assessment methods and models of delivery of continuing care and support will follow this.

A case study approach will be used to follow the care pathway of a child with a neurological degenerative condition, Batten's disease, in a variety of settings. This condition manifests itself in various supportive care issues that can be applied to a number of neurological conditions, and these will be discussed throughout the chapter.

Aim of the chapter

The aim of this chapter is to explore the context of care for children and young people who require continuing care support in the community setting.

Intended learning outcomes

- To discuss the importance of multidisciplinary and partnership working across boundaries of care
- To explore discharge planning and its application to the child and young person

- To discuss the challenges of joint working in planning appropriate services by exploring models of needs assessment
- To examine aspects of assessment and care delivery for children and young people with continuing care needs
- To explore the relationships between the child/young person and their family and the key worker-children's nurse

Complex health needs

When planning the care of children and young people with complex needs, the *National Service Framework for Children and Young People* (DoH, 2003; WAG, 2005) recognises the importance of family centred care. Children who need complex care can be described as children who require jointly commissioned health, education and social care (Lenton *et al.*, 2004). The role of parents as parents foremost and carers second, is vital. The child and family should be central in negotiating packages of care, and these should be agreed between health, social services and education (if the child is school-aged).

Within the literature, there is no agreed definition for children with complex health care needs as these are often identified as a group who are 'technology dependent' (Muir & Dryden, 2000), that is a child or young person who uses one or more medical devices to compensate for the partial failure or loss of a body function. Alternatively, Kirk (1999) classifies this group of children as having 'specialised health care needs'. Other authors have described children requiring complex care packages as those who are not technology dependent but require jointly commissioned health, education and social services, because they require greater resources than those available within individual services (Lenton *et al.*, 2004).

It is difficult to estimate the number of children requiring long-term complex health care but anecdotally this is an increasing population. Glendinning *et al.* (2001) acknowledge that this group of children are sometimes hidden in other illness categories, for example adolescent health statistics or disability, but suggest that there may be up to 6000 technology dependent children living at home in the UK. These children are quite diverse, with variance in cause, age of onset, duration, severity and frequency of use of technology. Research confirms that a large number of these children are very young (Roberts & Lawton, 2001). Brett (2004) suggests that children with complex medical needs have an increased survival rate due to supportive care such as gastrostomy feeding, home oxygen and ventilation. It is also difficult to define disability, the subject of many debates since the 1960s, which has led to the adoption of the *International Classification of Impairments, Disabilities and Handicap* by the World Health Organization (WHO, 1980).

Case study 7.1

Background information

David is eight years old and lives with his parents and two-year-old brother on a farm in a rural area of North Wales. His mother is the main carer and feels quite isolated as her husband works long hours managing the farm. The family is Welsh speaking and David attends a mainstream Welsh primary school. David was diagnosed with late infantile Batten's disease at the age of four years. Over a period of a few months, his walking became increasingly unsteady and he continually fell over. Also, at this time, David had his first convulsion, which was initially thought to be a febrile convulsion. David was admitted to his local hospital where he was investigated for a focus for the infection that might have caused a febrile convulsion. However, it was found to be neurological in nature and he was diagnosed with epilepsy. Due to his deterioration in walking and continuation of convulsions he required more specialised care and was referred to a consultant paediatric neurologist. As they live in North Wales, the nearest specialist centre for paediatric neurology is at a children's hospital, 60 miles away, in England.

Hospital admissions and travelling long distances for assessment and treatment present many practical difficulties for parents. There are a variety of factors impacting on the family at this time, for example siblings, distance, travel and financial circumstances. As Welsh is David and his family's first language, staff caring for them need to consider this during the admission and assessment process. David may only have had limited exposure to the English language and consequently may not be able to understand and express himself as well in English as in Welsh, which could significantly influence the accuracy of the assessment.

Reflection

- Reflect upon the children and young people you have cared for whose first language is not English.
- Consider the social, emotional and environmental factors that may impact on these children and their families.

David has a right to be able to communicate in his first language and in Wales the Welsh Assembly Government (2000) encourages the bilingual provision of public services. This means that Welsh health care organisations consider the following in delivering a service to David and his family:

- Welsh speaking staff available to provide health services through the medium of Welsh
- Procedures or systems that facilitate service provision through the medium of Welsh
- Welsh speaking officers are in one location to assist other staff when required
- The use of and access to professional translators

These requirements (WAG, 2000) are to support individuals to be able to express themselves in their mother tongue, whilst also aiming to ensure that those individuals whose first language is not English receive the same standard of care. An English health care provider delivers David's tertiary care and therefore the Welsh Government standard does not apply. As a lead children's hospital, it regularly provides tertiary care to children and their families from North Wales and to children from a number of minority ethnic groups. The hospital staff aim to offer services to support the child and family by allocating a nurse who can communicate in Welsh (if available) to care for David, and by making sure that all staff communicate carefully and organise interpreters as appropriate. The hospital also provides written information in the language of choice when requested.

 Case study 7.2

Following assessment by the paediatric neurologist, and a skin biopsy, David was diagnosed with Batten's disease, but his two-year-old brother tested negative to Batten's disease. Batten's disease is an inherited disorder and has an autosomal recessive characteristic. Before the diagnosis, David's parents had been trying for another baby and, therefore, they were offered genetic counselling.

Test your knowledge

Return to Chapter 1 and revise the genetics of autosomal recessive conditions.

- In an autosomal recessive disorder, what incidence is there for each pregnancy?
- If one parent is the carrier, what chances are there that the child would be affected?

Batten's disease is a metabolic disease that causes neurological degeneration (see Table 7.1). All metabolic diseases commonly have a malfunction with an enzyme that causes chemical imbalance (Gilbert, 2000) resulting in signs and symptoms related to the system affected. In Batten's disease, the affected enzyme is the neuronal ceroid lipofuscinose (NCL). The onset of the condition is gradual and not easily recognised (Maria, 2002). It is estimated that in the UK the incidence is approximately 1:200 000 (Great Ormond Street Children's Hospital NHS Trust, 2005). Although a metabolic condition, management is collaboratively provided

Table 7.1   Types of Batten's disease.

Diagnosis	Symptoms	Prognosis
Infantile (Santavourie or Finnish) type Diagnosed at 1 year of age	Convulsions and mental deterioration. Milestones tested by routine checks are below the norm. Walking ability becomes progressively unsteady. Head circumference fails to increase within normal parameters and microcephaly becomes obvious in a year or two.	The prognosis is poor, with deterioration and death usually occurring between 3–5 years of age and very occasionally up to 8 or 9 years of age.
Late Infantile Batten's (Jansky-Bielchowsky) type Develops between 2–4 years of age	Convulsions occur that are difficult to control. Child's walking becomes clumsy and ataxic and fine motor movements are affected. Many skills learnt previously deteriorate. Also visual loss and mental deterioration occurs.	The prognosis is poor with death occurring at about 10 years of age.
Juvenile Batten's (Speilmeyer-Vogt) type Diagnosed between 6–10 years of age	First sign is deterioration in vision, followed by a slowing in mental abilities and convulsions. Muscular coordination, walking difficulties occur and eventually paralysis.	Prognosis is poor with death occurring at 15–25 years of age.
Adult (Kufs disease) type Can develop around puberty (13–15 years of age)	Personality problems occur initially with unpredictable behaviour that can be mistaken for normal adolescent behaviour. Problems with balance and ataxia also occur.	People with this condition survive into middle age.

Adapted from Gilbert, 2000.

by a paediatrician, paediatric neurologist and a paediatrician specialising in childhood metabolic diseases.

Reflection

Reflect upon the children with neurological degenerative disorders that you have cared for in practice. Make a list of their conditions.

Some examples of neurodegenerative conditions are given in Table 7.2.

Due to the devastating nature of a diagnosis of a life-limiting condition such as Batten's disease, David and his family will need support. The communication of bad news to families requires careful planning and consideration, and needs to be delivered by a health professional with good communication skills in a calm well prepared environment. Specialist nurses, community children's nurses, social

Table 7.2 Neurodegenerative conditions.

Examples of neurodegenerative conditions: Mucopolysaccharidoses	Lipid storage diseases	Leukodystrophies
Morquio	Tay-Sachs	Adrenoleukodystrophy
Hunter	Gaucher	—
Hurlers	Neuman-Pick	—
Sanfilipo	—	—

services or voluntary organisations, for example Contact a Family (CaF), can provide support to families, which is vitally important given that families are known to experience stress and grief arising from their child's condition (Fawcett *et al.*, 2005), as discussed in detail in Chapter 3.

 Case study 7.3

David's eating and drinking has gradually deteriorated and he is losing weight. When David swallows fluids, he frequently splutters, and is finding it increasingly problematic to swallow food and drink. He has also suffered from several chest infections and now requires admission to hospital to investigate whether these are being caused by inhalation of fluids and food into his lungs.

Reflection

Consider children you have cared for with feeding difficulties. What are the common symptoms associated with this and why?

Children with Batten's disease or similar neurodegenerative disorders frequently have feeding and swallowing difficulties, and may develop gastro-oesophageal reflux (GOR). GOR is associated with chronic vomiting leading to inadequate weight gain, recurrent cough or wheeze following feed aspiration, blood streaked vomit due to oesophagitis, and feed refusal due to the severe pain on feeding (Sullivan & Rosenbloom, 2002). GOR is often difficult to manage and may be treated medically or surgically. The child's nutritional requirements may not be met despite every effort being made by the child and carers. This in turn results in poor bone and tissue growth, decreased muscle strength (with consequent reduction in the ability to cough), decreased cerebral function with possible exacerbation of neurological impairment, disturbances of the immune system and poor circulation, with delayed healing of pressure sores (Sullivan & Rosenbloom, 2002).

In addition to a poor ability to chew and swallow, there are various reasons why children with neurodegenerative disorders do not achieve adequate food intake, including:

- Limited communication skills preventing the child from requesting food when hungry
- A lack of mobility hindering the child from seeking snacks independently
- Poor hand function hindering self-feeding
- Weak head and trunk control with extensor posturing limiting self-feeding opportunities

---

Test your knowledge

Make a list of care practices you have seen used for children who are disabled and have difficulties with feeding.

Children with neurodegenerative disorders may find fluid difficult to tolerate in the mouth and therefore the speech and language therapist or the dietitian may recommend a feed thickener. This can be added to any liquid and allows the fluid to be more easily controlled in the mouth. Another method of supporting children who can only manage to consume small amounts of food and drink is to increase the energy intake of the foods consumed, which can be achieved by adding cream to puddings, butter to mashed vegetables or toast, sauces to savoury dishes and offering creamy desserts.

The physical and emotional burden on parents and carers of children with severe feeding and swallowing difficulties is constant. Eating is not only beneficial for physical growth and development but is also a central part of social activity. Mealtimes for this group of children can be prolonged and stressful due to severe oro-motor dysfunction causing feeding difficulties, which often extends the time it takes to complete their meal. Despite the time and care taken, the child may still be malnourished due to the high calorie expenditure usage to complete the feeding process. The nurse should assess the impact of psychological and emotional factors on the child and family (refer to Chapter 4 to reinforce your knowledge about meeting children's psychological needs). Failure to establish a safe, effective feeding method that is satisfying and rewarding to both the child and parents can disrupt the bond between them. Poor nutrition in early life can affect health and development of the child in later life, in addition to the immediate risk of morbidity and mortality (Barker *et al.*, 1989). Families and schools need expert advice on how to make mealtimes safe, nutritionally adequate and enjoyable. A children's nutrition nurse, community children's nurse, community dietitian, school nurse, health visitor or specialist health visitor can provide this advice.

It is beneficial to the child to establish a routine and ensure that all carers who feed the child use a consistent approach. In some areas, there is a coordinated approach to dealing with feeding problems through the establishment of multidisciplinary feeding teams (Sullivan & Rosenbloom, 2002) who hold joint clinics. Where a team approach is not available, the parents, child and dietitian should work with the speech and language therapist, referring to other professionals as necessary, to meet the child's needs.

Reflection

- What would be the individual roles of the multidisciplinary feeding team?
- In David's case, which professionals would need to be in this team?

The specialist multidisciplinary feeding team should include:

- A paediatric gastroenterologist for clinical management of the gastrointestinal aspect of the condition
- A paediatric neurologist to manage the neurological aspect of the condition
- A paediatric dietician to provide advice on dietary requirements
- A speech and language therapist who would focus on assessment and observation of feeding skills
- A children's nutrition nurse to provide education, care and advice to children and families on the management of enteral feeding
- A paediatric psychologist to advise on the behavioural aspects

    Key point

No one profession is adequately equipped to single-handedly manage the feeding difficulties of a child with disability.

    Case study 7.4

After a detailed assessment, it was decided that David would require admission to hospital for insertion of a gastrostomy tube to meet most of his nutritional requirements.

Children with a degenerative condition such as Batten's disease may reach a stage where their poor swallow reflex is classed as unsafe, and the need for enteral feeding methods are explored. Ethical and professional issues regarding the parents' and child/young person's consent to the insertion of the gastrostomy tube should be considered. For consent to be valid and informed, the child and/or parent must be capable of taking that decision, acting voluntarily (not under pressure or duress) and given sufficient information to enable a decision to be made (DoH, 2001).

Guidance from the Department of Health suggests that:

'Children under 16 are not presumed to be legally competent to make decisions for their health care. However, the Courts have stated that under 16-year-olds will be competent to give valid consent to an intervention if they have sufficient understanding and intelligence to enable him or her to understand fully what is proposed.' (Gillick competence) (DoH, 2001, p. 5)

Thus, Gillick competence is a term used in English medical law to describe the ruling made by the House of Lords relating to the rights of children under the age of 16 years to consent to treatment without their parents' knowledge, but the term Frazer competence (after Lord Frazer who made the ruling) is preferred. However, even if children and young people are not able to give legal consent, it is important to involve them in the process. Consideration of their developmental age and understanding is important when explaining procedures or providing information. They should be involved in decision making, be informed about what is going to happen and given choices about, for example, the timing of procedures. The beneficence of the child and the advocacy role of the nurse in providing information and support for the parents to make an informed decision are key skills required of the children's nurse. (Refer to Chapter 6.)

Refer to the Department of Health website for further information on consent: http://www.doh.gov.uk/

Reflection

Reflect upon the ethical and professional dilemmas that the children's community nurse may need to contemplate (refer to Chapter 6 if necessary).

Enteral nutrition is the method of supplying nutrients to the gastrointestinal tract and is the term used to describe nasogastric, gastrostomy and jejunostomy feeding (Holden & MacDonald, 2000). The feeding options need to be fully discussed with the family, outlining the advantages and disadvantages of each method (see Table 7.3). Some children and their families find enteral feeding socially unacceptable, which emphasises that this is not always the best solution for every child or young person.

Reflection

- Consider the different types of feeding routes you have observed in practice.
- What were the advantages and disadvantages of each method?
- How did the child and family cope with the feeding method and regime?
- Make a note of your reflections.

Transition to home care

To enable parents and carers to effectively care for a medically stable, technology dependent child at home, a robust and comprehensive training programme needs

Table 7.3   Advantages and disadvantages of enteral feeding methods.

Method	Description	Advantages	Disadvantages
Nasogastric	Feeding tube that enters the gastrointestinal tract via the nose	Easily inserted Method of first choice Short-term feeding	Easily visible Causes discomfort to nasopharynx May block or be easily removed Tube re-insertion is distressing to child and family Risk of aspiration
Gastrostomy	Direct long-term access to stomach via a soft plastic tube or button that is flush to the skin	Easily hidden under clothes Suitable for long-term feeding	Requires general anaesthetic May increase reflux if present before surgery Risk of: skin irritation, infection, granulation tissue, leakage, gastric distension Stoma will close within few hours if accidentally removed
Nasojejunal	Nasal feeding tube enters the jejunum via the gastrointestinal tract	Short-term feeding Less risk of aspiration than nasogastric feeding	Difficult to insert Risk of perforation Abdominal pain and diarrhoea if continuous feeding is not used Discomfort to nasopharynx
Jejunostomy	Delivers feeds via a tube inserted directly into jejunum or via the stomach through gastrostomy tube Suitable for children with persistent GOR	Reduced risk of aspiration Long-term feeding	Risk of perforation Feed needs to be infused constantly Risk of bacterial overgrowth Dumping syndrome can occur

Adapted from Holden & MacDonald, 2000.

to be developed and implemented as one aspect of the pre-discharge care. The training programme should provide information about theoretical and practical aspects of the role and should include opportunities for supervised practice before a suitably qualified practitioner undertakes an assessment of competence.

 Case study 7.5

During David's admission, the nursing staff realised the pressure that his family was under due to his high level of nursing care needs. The nursing staff discussed this with his family and the consultant. A multidisciplinary discharge meeting was organised to discuss David and his family's needs. It was identified from this meeting that David's family required additional financial, social, psychological and health care support at home, and a referral was made for a continuing health care package.

Discharge planning is a process during which the child and family's needs are identified and negotiated in order to prepare them for transition of care from hospital to home. Effective discharge planning takes time to do well and requires good collaboration between hospital and community services (Hewitt-Taylor, 2005). The Department of Health (1996; 2004) stated that planning for any child to go home should begin on admission. However, coordinating a smooth transition from hospital to home for a child or young person with long-term care needs is often challenging and diverse. This process is often hindered due to a lack of clarity about which service is responsible, who funds the care and poor collaboration between services (Noyes, 2002; Ludvigsen & Morrison, 2003; Edwards, 2004). The care of a child or young person should be seamless (Smith & Daughtrey, 2000), and the key to this is a multi-professional team not restricted by organisational boundaries and with clear roles and responsibilities. Effective partnerships are the only way of delivering fully integrated services (DoH, 2003; 2004). Factors relating to discharge planning are outlined in Table 7.4.

Reflection

- Reflect on your practice area and consider why a child with complex care needs might have a delayed discharge from hospital.
- Write down the factors the nurse should consider in preparation for David's discharge.

Planning of complex care packages via continuing care remains a challenge for families and professionals. The term continuing care is used to describe the care that a client needs over an extended period as the result of a disability, accident or illness to address their physical, social and psychological health needs. The child or young person may require services from both health and social care, which may be provided in the hospital or community setting. Irrespective of the child's locality, age, diagnosis or impairment, the aim is for an integrated care pathway, which through a joined up planning and service delivery process will aim to link the child and family with the appropriate community and hospital based services, social services, education and the voluntary sector (Limbrick, 2003; ACT, 2004). Unfortunately, the Audit Commission (2003) found that the needs of individual families were not fully considered when organising services and Myers (2005) reiterates the need for services that enable families to make choices that meet their needs and their child's. Getting this assessment process right is one of the most important factors in delivering an effective service that meets the needs of families, children and young people (DoH, 2003).

Parents may find the responsibilities of caring for their child at home overwhelming (Hewitt-Taylor, 2005) and following extended stays in hospital, a period of adjustment is required to empower parents to be the main carers for their child's needs at home (Hewitt-Taylor, 2005). Government policies and guidelines have been developed in order to guide services to meet the supportive needs of families in a cost effective way (DoH, 1995; 1996; 2000a; 2004; WAG, 2005).

Table 7.4   Issues to be considered in discharge planning.

Factors that delay children with complex health needs being discharged from hospital	Factors that need to be considered in preparation for home care
Time taken for planning	Key worker role Communication and liaison between multidisciplinary/multi-professional teams or services Collaboration between health, social care and education agencies are vital
Priority given by health care staff/management to discharge planning	Establish funding for respite care package
Recruitment of community staff with relevant experience	Understanding of child's condition – implications for home management, for example medical/social/financial needs, home adaptations required
Issues around who will fund the respite care in the community	Clinical skills training for parents and/or carers
A lack of collaboration between services	Organisation of equipment and/or supplies Health and safety issues
—	Identification of level of nursing and social care support required
—	Development of an action plan for professionals with clear lines of responsibility

Continuing care policy

The continuing care policy (DoH, 1995) was originally developed for the assessment of clients over 18 years of age. Some health and social services have developed eligibility criteria for children and young people from the model adopted for the older age group. This has proved inadequate and has caused disparities between different areas of the country (Widdas *et al.*, 2005). This policy is focused primarily on adult services and requires further development of explicit criteria for children's services (DoH, 1996). This has been devolved locally. Any professional can instigate a referral for continuing care but this must include an assessment of care from the carer and all professionals involved in the management of the child. There are a number of categories to the eligibility criteria that need to be identified in the application. Each category being applied for needs to be clarified before a decision for the funding of an appropriate care package can be agreed upon. Conflict about the amount and type of care can often occur, which is distressing for parents. The children's NSFs (DoH, 2003; WAG, 2005) have suggested joint funding as an improved method of approaching continuing care for children.

Framework for assessment of children in need

The framework for assessment of children in need and their families (DoH, 2000a) was introduced by the Government to assist local authorities to identify the needs of children in order to offer appropriate support. The guidance has been produced primarily for the use of professional and other staff who will be involved in undertaking assessment of children in need and their families under the Children Act (DoH, 1989) and following the *Every Child Matters* initiative (DfES, 2003). It stresses the need for a corporate approach to children's services by emphasising the importance of effective joint working by health, social services, education, housing and leisure. The social services department has lead responsibility to ensure that initial and core assessments are carried out according to the *Framework for the Assessment of Children in Need and their Families* (DoH, 2000a; b).

National Service Framework for Children, Young People and Maternity Services

More recently, England and Wales have developed NSFs for children, young people and maternity services (DoH, 2003; WAG, 2005), which set out the quality of services that children, young people and their families have a right to expect and receive. Scotland and Ireland are also developing children and young people's strategies. The NSF places children and their families at the centre of service delivery, with services designed to meet their particular needs. It sets standards for children's health, and the key actions identified in the documents are to be delivered over the next ten years. For this to happen, it is crucial that planning is coordinated across the various organisations and that there is a commitment to joint working between all agencies that deliver services to children and young people.

It is beneficial for the family to be given written copies of any assessment and resulting action or plan, in order that this may be shared with other professionals. It is also helpful if the family gives consent, within the agreed rules of confidentiality, for the information about their child to be shared between agencies so that parents can avoid having to continually repeat this information. A parent consultation highlighted that parents wanted to see more sharing of information between agencies to avoid having to repeat themselves at each assessment and appointment (WAG, 2003). Supporting this aim is one of the key actions in the NSF; that a hand-held record is offered to all children with disabilities and complex health needs (WAG, 2005).

Carers' assessments

Parents or carers are also entitled to a carer assessment to identify how they might best be supported in their caring role (DoH, 2000a). The literature highlights the financial stress on families, as the mother's income often has to be sacrificed so that she can be the main carer for her child with complex health needs. Financial problems can cause additional stress to families who may well be experiencing increased costs resulting from their child's condition. These include special food purchases, travel to hospital, car parking and increased purchases of bed linen and clothing. The key worker or social worker can support them through the application process for financial assistance and benefits. Social services departments are the lead agencies for developing local plans for carers. The Department of Health (2005a; b) has recently published draft policy guidance on the *Carers and Disabled Children Act* (DoH, 2000b). This Act will enable carers to receive support in their own right as well as the child.

Reflection

- Who should be involved in David's multidisciplinary discharge meeting and what are their key responsibilities?
- Make a list of your thoughts and compare these to Table 7.5.

Everyone who has significant ongoing involvement in the care of the child or young person should be invited to attend the discharge planning meeting or provide a report, in order to coordinate a seamless discharge plan. The key worker is generally identified at this meeting to take a lead role in future care coordination (Stephens, 2005). The role of the key worker is important as they have knowledge of local services and can liase between hospital, community and home, and work closely with the other members of the multidisciplinary team.

Identifying an appropriate care package

Where appropriate, it is advisable that the community children's nurse or other professional with experience of assessing continuing care packages provides advice. This will be a key focus of the multidisciplinary meeting and, where possible, this should be discussed with the family before the meeting. Agreement about an appropriate care package is often subjective, based on the complexity of the child's needs and family support structure. Emond and Eaton (2004) suggest that children's nurses and doctors develop care packages for which they have little evidence or experience. However, a continuing care needs assessment dependency tool (Escolme & James, 2004) is a beneficial means of quantifying this through a holistic assessment. David and his family will be referred to a social worker, and following a joint assessment David's care needs can be identified and a package of care agreed by health and social services. According to Murphy (2001a; b), it is important to establish funding for the care package as early as possible.

Key worker role

A key worker can be described as a named person who the family can approach for advice about, and practical help with, any problem related to the child with

Table 7.5   Multidisciplinary team members and associated responsibilities.

Multidisciplinary team members	Responsibilities
Parents	24-hour care
Paediatric neurologist (specialist)	Appointments to monitor condition and provide medical support
Community paediatrician (local service)	Health assessments of needs for support in school
General practitioner (local service)	Support to family, ongoing prescriptions for medications and enteral feeding
Named nurse – ward (specialist)	Key worker before discharge (to be discussed later in chapter)
Paediatrician (local acute hospital)	Local medical support and liaison with paediatric neurologist
Community children's nurse (if available – local service)	Local support to family on nursing care issues and key worker role following discharge; referral to continence advisor for continence supplies
Special needs health visitor (if available – local)	Support to family; advice on local services
Dietitian (specialist)	Enteral feeding advice, planning dietary requirements
Nutrition nurse (specialist)	Organising enteral feeding supplies and regular monitoring and problem solving advice on nursing care of enteral feeding; direct access to paediatric gastroenterologist
Epilepsy nurse specialist (specialist)	Advice and support on management of epilepsy; direct access to paediatric neurologist
Occupational therapist (local)	Local assessment of need for adaptations and activities of living at home and school
Physiotherapist (local)	Assessment of mobility, advice on seating, wheelchair positioning and exercises to maintain posture and mobility
School nurse (local)	Support at school; advice on care provision, medication issues, enteral feeding and continence
Teacher (local)	Educational support
Social worker (local)	Social support, referral for respite, coordination of package of care, joint working with health; advice on benefits, disability living allowance, mobility allowance, carers' allowance
Family health visitor	Support and advice; two-year-old sibling may need nursery placement to reduce family stress

disability (Greco *et al.*, 2004). The provision of 'key workers' who work across health, education and social services has been recommended in policy guidance and, most recently, the NSF for children (DoH, 1997; 2003). Research has shown that less than a third of families with children with severe disabilities have a key worker but those who do show benefit in terms of relationships with, and access to, services and an enhanced quality of life (Gatford, 2004). Key worker services provide the most benefit to families when they are effectively managed and when health, education and social services are all committed to the service and provide adequate resources (Gatford, 2004; Stephens, 2005).

Community children's nursing services

Community children's nursing services have been developed since the 1950s, with teams originally in Birmingham and St Mary's Paddington that were further expanded in the 1990s (Eaton, 2001; Whiting, 2006), but despite this, some areas of the UK do not have dedicated community children's nursing services. The role of the community children's nursing team includes:

- Coordination of discharge from hospital to home
- Teaching aspects of practical care to parents and children (injections, nasogastric feeding)
- Direct nursing care
- Support to families and children dying at home
- Teaching other professionals
- Education of children and parents with specific medical problems (diabetes, asthma)
- Safeguarding issues
- Multi-agency communication and collaboration
- Coordination and supervision of support staff

For further information on the role and development of community children's nursing services see Whiting (2005).

Reflection

- Reflect on your own area of clinical practice.
- What community children's nursing services are available?
- What care do these nurses provide?

For further information on the Directory of Community Children's Services and to identify whether there are community children's nurses in your area of the UK, refer to the Royal College of Nursing website: http://www2.rcn.org.uk/cyp/forums/rcn_professional_forums/community_children_nursing/directory

Provision of equipment for home care

Ideally, funding for all aspects of care should be agreed before discharge home. However, obtaining equipment and supplies has been identified as a significant stress factor for families (DoH, 1997; 2004). The provision and maintenance of equipment needs to be formally agreed before discharge. Supplies are sometimes difficult to obtain in the community or the child's condition may be unpredictable and parents sometimes need to travel long distances to a specialist centre. Parents are often unclear which professional provides which piece of equipment and they often need to collect bulky supplies at short notice. In David's case, this is further complicated by his community care provision being delivered by a different health care trust. This is time consuming and expensive and adds considerably to the stress of caring for a child with complex continuing care needs. These issues have been identified in the Welsh and English children's NSFs (DoH, 2003; WAG, 2005), which recommend that the supply of equipment and consumables should be organised to minimise disruption. Table 7.6 outlines responsibilities for provision of equipment.

Reflection

Consider who should provide the equipment that David would require on discharge:

- Wheelchair
- Bed
- Specially adapted eating utensils
- Special seating
- Enteral feeding pump and supplies
- Gastrostomy tubes and extension sets
- Medications

Table 7.6 Provision of equipment.

Provision of community equipment Equipment	Professional
Wheelchair	Physiotherapist or occupational therapist
Bed	Health trust
Specially adapted eating utensils, for example spoon, fork etc.	Occupational therapist
Special seating	Physiotherapist or occupational therapist
Feeding pump and supplies Gastrostomy tubes	Nutritional nurse specialist or community children's nurse
Medication	Pharmacist

Case study 7.6

During a home visit by the epilepsy outreach nurse, it was noted that David's condition had deteriorated. His seizures had become more difficult to manage and his parents required instruction on how to administer buccal midazolam. The nurse arranged an appointment for David to be reviewed by the local community paediatrician to avoid the family travelling to the regional centre.

Buccal midazolam is administered when a child has convulsive status epilepticus, a common neurological medical emergency with high morbidity and mortality (Scott *et al.*, 1999). In the past, rectal diazepam was administered, but many difficulties were experienced in carrying out the procedure at home and at school. In a survey of 33 parents by Wilson *et al.* (2004), 83% of parents preferred using midazolam to rectal diazepam. They found the midazolam was successful and easy to administer. However parents require training on the procedure and only when they feel confident and competent should they be allowed to administer the medication themselves (Wilson *et al.*, 2004). Parents will also need support and the community children's nursing team can offer this locally.

 Case study 7.7

The major features of Batten's are progressive loss of vision, motor and intellectual deterioration and seizures (Evans, 1987). David's condition has gradually deteriorated over the last year and he is now unable to walk, requiring a wheelchair. He has problems with incontinence and his seizures are controlled by a variety of anti-convulsive drugs. He has poor vision, very limited speech and requires 24-hour supervision and care to meet his daily needs due to severe disability and increasing learning difficulties. The community paediatrician reviews David and he is referred to the social worker, who will visit to assess for respite care and provide financial advice and support. David's parents have been finding the continual care exhausting. Mum is the main carer because dad is unable to provide much support as he works long hours on their farm. The key worker is concerned about mum's well-being and the impact that this may be having on the younger child. A referral is also required for an occupational therapist assessment to consider the need for home adaptations as the family are finding it increasingly difficult to carry David upstairs to his bedroom and access for his wheelchair is proving problematic.

Respite care

It is well documented that provision of care for a child with complex health needs within the family is challenging and will have a significant impact on family life, including sleep disruption, restriction in social activity, leading to isolation and marginalisation; it may leave families housebound (Murphy, 2001a; Roberts & Lawton, 2001; Lenton *et al.*, 2004). Parents are often required to learn complex nursing skills and they may feel physically exhausted from constant caring (Kirk, 1999). Equipment is often cumbersome, which has a negative impact on social outings, and family activities can be severely restricted as social plans can be altered at very short notice as a result of the child's health status. The family home often requires adaptation, which jeopardises home comforts, and there is a lack of privacy attributed to the input of health professionals (Kirk, 1999; Murphy, 2001a).

Evidence suggests that the daily routines and continual responsibilities associated with the medical care of a child with complex health needs can result in physical and emotional overburden on the carer (Bradley *et al.*, 1995; Thomlinson, 2002) and these families are at greater risk of deterioration to the family structure and marital problems. Mothers who care for medically fragile children at home are at risk of illness, especially if support and resources are limited or unavailable. They are reported to be at risk of poorer mental health status, which can compromise the quality of care they provide to their children and family (Thyen *et al.*, 1999). Other studies support this, reporting an increase in family illness (Patterson *et al.*, 1994), reduced family functioning (Diehl *et al.*, 1991) and difficulties with the mother's relationship with other children (Jennings, 1990). Even though parents attempt to protect the siblings, the literature generally acknowledges that having a child with complex health needs within the family will have a detrimental effect on siblings, citing behavioural changes, increased responsibility beyond years and feelings of neglect as issues of concern (Clarke, 1994; Dobson & Middleton, 1998).

Over recent years an improved understanding of the burden of care and the pressures faced by the family of a child with complex health needs has led to an appreciation that these families deserve a break from caring if they are to continue with the demands of the role (Murphy, 2001b). Therefore, it is not surprising to find that the most consistently cited need for the child with complex health needs is respite, which meets the needs of parents and provides additional opportunities for the child with 'special needs'. Even though families generally acknowledge the need for respite, for some, the concept suggests an inability to cope with the caring situation, which consequently develops into guilt. Hence it is suggested that respite care needs to be promoted more positively as a supportive service for the family (Millar, 2002). Research suggests that families want a spectrum of respite services offering flexibility, choice, high standards and continuity of care (Millar, 2002). Families should be offered choice, information on options and continuity of care that meets their child's needs (Mencap, 1994).

Respite provision for this group of children can be fraught with difficulties, primarily as a consequence of their complex nursing needs, with a recognised shortfall of highly specialised care. The Department of Health (2003) has noted the need to improve respite care options for families in England. Many studies report difficulties in families gaining access to respite care and believe the services to be poorly coordinated and fragmented. Consistent problems that families encounter from these services include delays in their provision, with parents having to fight to receive support (Jennings, 1990; Beresford, 1995; Petr *et al.*, 1995; Chamba *et al.*,

1999). The literature also reveals that parents are concerned about the quality of respite care on offer and that most services are designed for children with developmental problems rather than complex health needs. Social service facilities are inappropriate for meeting the needs of children requiring nursing intervention and therefore the only respite generally available to the child with complex health needs is either at a children's hospice or in their own home. Kirk (1999) suggests that this group of families prefer home based care to the institutional respite services provided by a hospice as the service is more flexible; the child remains within a familiar environment and it is less disruptive to the family as it avoids the need to transport large amounts of equipment. Other home based respite includes volunteer schemes such as Family Link, where a volunteer is matched to a family, but in practice it is extremely rare as there are difficulties in recruiting experienced volunteer carers to this group of children. The literature verifies that there is no consistency in the amount and type of provision and it appears to bear no relationship to the extent of health need, although this varies across the country (Clarke, 1994; Jardine & Wallis, 1998; Kirk & Glendinning, 1999; Townsley & Robinson, 1999).

Home adaptations

Referral to social services for adaptations to the family home for wheelchair access and activities of living requirements need accurate assessment by an occupational therapist. Although not applicable to England, in some areas adaptations can cause financial difficulties if major adaptations and building works are means tested, resulting in some parents only receiving part funding. Support and advice can be gained from Contact a Family (CaF) (see website details at end of chapter) who have useful fact sheets for families on all aspects of care provision. Access, mobility and care issues will also need consideration by the child's school.

 Case study 7.8

David's condition is stable. He is now receiving respite two days a month at the children's hospice, which is 50 miles from his home. David is awaiting a statement of his educational needs to provide him with further support at school. The community children's nurse visits on a weekly basis to assess David's condition and provide support to the family. His younger sibling now has a placement in a local nursery three days a week.

Education

Reflection

Reflect on what support you think David might require at school.

Due to David's deterioration and increased health care needs, he requires assessment for support in school. The schoolteacher highlighted this at the multidisciplinary discharge planning team meeting, and good communication and multi-agency partnership will ensure early referral for a statement of special educational need statutory assessment. The *Special Educational Needs Code of Practice* (DfES, 1999) suggests partnership working when assessing special educational needs.

Children with degenerative medical conditions require special consideration when educational support is being organised. Maintaining educational input is important to the child and family (DfES, 2001) and close liaison between health professionals and parents will be necessary, particularly where medication and medical equipment are provided (DfES, 2001). For David to access school, he will need support from a classroom assistant who is trained to care for all his needs. This will include mobility around and to school, accessing the curriculum, gastrostomy feeding, continence and hygiene, and observation for deterioration in condition. This support will be agreed between health, social services and education (DfES, 2001). The specialist nurse or community children's nurse will be involved in training David's support worker. Consideration should be given to the risk assessment of the school environment to ensure David is safely and competently cared for. A risk assessment will also need to be undertaken for transport to school and the school environment in relation to equipment and emergency procedures.

Support for families

As already discussed, caring for a child with complex health needs on a daily basis can be a fatiguing process both psychologically and physically for parents (Hewitt-Taylor, 2005). Health professionals and voluntary organisations should provide the necessary support. Over the past decade, in response to the demand for caring for children and young people with complex care needs in the community (RCN, 2000), a number of community children's nursing teams have been set up across the UK. These teams have demonstrated different models of working with children with complex needs in a variety of environments such as the home, school, respite and hospice setting (Eaton, 2001). As David's condition deteriorates, the multidisciplinary team and key worker will need to support the family by providing a regular review and assessment of David's condition, parental coping and services he and his family will require. Respite care should be provided and this service needs to be creative and flexible to meet the needs of both the child and family.

Conclusion

This chapter has explored the issues surrounding the requirements for a child with complex care needs in the community. The emphasis of care has been on collaborative working and the support and empowerment of families to enable them to care for their child safely.

The roles of the community children's nurse, the multidisciplinary team and the essential role of the key worker have been considered in relation to a coordinated, seamless and safe discharge. Continuing care needs of a child with complex health requirements have been described and the important responsibility of parents in this process has been explored.

Key points

- Effective multi-agency and inter-professional working and communication is paramount to enable a coordinated package of care to be delivered to minimise the burden of caring for a child with a life-limiting condition.
- It is essential that packages of care spanning health, social care and education are implemented in negotiation with the child and family.
- To support the child and family in the home, school or respite, resources need to be provided and coordinated.
- Care provision should include the holistic needs of the child and family; this includes direct care at home and in school education programmes, respite provision and financial support.
- The role of the community children's nurse is important as the key worker for children and families.

Useful websites

www.bris.ac.uk/Depts/NorahFry
www.cafamily.org.uk
www.davidkessler.org/
www.dfes.gov.uk/everychildmatters
www.direct.gov.uk/EducationAndLearning/Schools/Special EducationalNeeds/
www.doh.gov.uk
www.familyfund.org.uk
www.jrf.org.uk
www.scope.org.uk
www.gosh.nhs.uk/factsheets/families/F050308/index.html

Support groups

The Batten's Disease Family Association
BDFA
Heather Houses
Heather Drive
Tadley
Hants
RG26 4QR
www.bdfauk.freeserve.co.uk

References

Association for Children with Life Threatening Conditions and their Families (ACT) (2004) *Charter for Children with Life Threatening Conditions and Their Families*. Bristol, ACT.

Audit Commission (2003) *Services for Disabled Children: a Review of Services for Disabled Children and Their Families*. London, Audit Commission.

Barker, D.J.P., Winter, P.D., Osmond, C., Margetts, B. & Simmonds, S.J. (1989) Weight in infancy and death from ischaemic heart disease. *Lancet*, ii, 577–580.

Beresford, B. (1995) *Expert Opinions: a National Survey of Parents Caring for a Severely Disabled Child*. Bristol, the Policy Press.

Bradley, R.H., Parette, H.P. & Van Bierliet, A. (1995) Families of young technology-dependent children and the social worker. *Social Work in Pediatrics*, 21, 23–27.

Brett, J. (2004) The journey to accepting support: how parents of profoundly disabled children experience support in their lives. *Paediatric Nursing*, 16, 8.

Chamba, R., Ahmad, W., Hirst, M., Lawton, D. & Beresford, B. (1999) *On the Edge: Minority Ethnic Families Caring for a Severely Disabled Child*. Bristol, the Policy Press.

Clarke, A. (1994) Support for families with children with special needs. *Health Visitor*, 67 (10), 357.

Department of Health (1989) *The Children Act*. London, HMSO.

Department of Health (1995) *NHS Responsibilities for Meeting Continuing Health Care Needs*. London, HMSO.

Department of Health (1996) *Child Health in the Community: a Guide to Good Practice*. London, HMSO.

Department of Health (1997) *Government Response to the Reports of the Health Select Committee on Health Services for Children and Young People, Session 1996–1997. Health Services for Children and Young People in the Community, Home and School*. London, The Stationery Office.

Department of Health (2000a) *Framework for the Assessment of Children in Need and their Families*. London, The Stationery Office.

Department of Health (2000b) *Carers and Disabled Children's Act*. London, The Stationery Office.

Department of Health (2001) *Seeking Consent: Working with Children*. London, The Stationery Office.

Department of Health (2003) *Getting the Right Start: The National Service Framework for Children and Young People and Maternity Services*. London, The Stationery Office.

Department of Health (2004) *Achieving Timely 'Simple' Discharge from Hospital – a Toolkit for the Multidisciplinary team*. London, The Stationery Office.

Department of Health (2005a) *Supporting People with Long Term Conditions. An NHS and Social Care Model to Support Local Innovation and Integration*. London, The Stationery Office.

Department of Health (2005b) *Complex Disability Exemplar: National Service Framework for Children and Young People and Maternity Services*. London, The Stationery Office.

Department for Education and Skills (1999) *The Special Educational Needs Code of Practice*. London, The Stationery Office.

Department for Education and Skills (2001) *Access to Education for Children and Young People with Medical Needs*. London, The Stationery Office.

Department for Education and Skills (2003) *Every Child Matters Next Steps*. London, The Stationery Office.

Diehl, S., Moffitt, K. & Wade, S.M. (1991) Focus group interviews with parents of children with medically complex needs: an intimate look at their perceptions and feelings. *Children's Health Care*, 20 (3), 170–178.

Dobson, B. & Middleton, S. (1998) *Paying to Care: the Cost of Childhood Disability.* York, York Publishing Services.

Eaton, N. (2001) Models of Community Children's Nursing. *Paediatric Nursing,* **13** (1), 32–36.

Edwards, E.A. (2004) Sending children home on tracheostomy dependent ventilation: pitfalls and outcomes. *Archives of Disease in Childhood,* **89** (3), 251–255.

Emond, A. & Eaton, N. (2004) Supporting children with complex health care needs and their families – an overview of the research agenda. *Child: Care, Health and Development,* **30** (3), 195–199.

Escolme, D. & James, C. (2004) Assessing respite provision: the Leeds nursing dependency score. *Paediatric Nursing,* **16** (2), 27–30.

Evans, O.B. (1987) *Manual of Child Neurology.* New York, Churchill Livingstone.

Fawcett, T.N., Baggaley, S.E., Wu, C., Whyte, D.A. & Martinson, I.M. (2005) Parental responses to health care services for children with chronic conditions and their families: a comparison between Hong Kong and Scotland. *Journal of Child Health Care,* **9** (1), 8–19.

Gatford, A. (2004) Time to go home: putting together a package of care. *Child: Care, Health and Development,* **30** (3), 251–255.

Gilbert, P. (2000) *A–Z of Syndromes and Inherited Disorders* (third edition). London, Nelson Thornes Ltd.

Glendinning, C., Kirk, S., Guiffrida, A. & Lawton, D. (2001) Technology dependent children in the community: definitions, numbers and costs. *Child: Care, Health and Development,* **27** (4), 321–334.

Great Ormond Street Hospital for Children NHS Trust (2005) *Batten's Disease (Juvenile Form) Information for Families.* London, Great Ormond Street Hospital for Children NHS Trust.

Greco, V., Sloper, P., Webb, R. & Beecham, J. (2004) Care coordination and key worker schemes for disabled children: results of a UK-wide survey. *Child: Care, Health and Development,* **30** (1), 13–30.

Hewitt-Taylor, J. (2005) Caring for children with complex and continuing health needs. *Nursing Standard,* **19** (42), 41–47.

Holden, C. & MacDonald, A. (2000) *Nutrition and Child Health.* London, Baillière Tindall.

Jardine, E., O'Toole, M., Paton, J.Y. & Wallis, C. (1999) Current status of long-term ventilation of children in the UK: questionnaire survey. *British Medical Journal,* **318** (7179), 295–299.

Jardine, E. & Wallis, C. (1998) Core guidelines for the discharge home of the child on long-term assisted ventilation in the United Kingdom. *Thorax,* **53** (9), 762–767.

Jennings, P. (1990) Caring for a child with a tracheostomy. *Nursing Standard,* **4** (30), 24–26.

Kirk, S. (1999) Caring for children with specialised health care needs in the community: the challenges for primary care. *Health and Social Care in the Community,* **7** (5), 350–357.

Kirk, S. & Glendinning, C. (1999) *Supporting Parents Caring for a Technology-dependent Child.* Manchester, National Primary Care Research and Development Centre.

Lenton, S., Franck, L. & Salt, A. (2004) Children with complex health care needs: supporting the child and family in the community. *Child: Care Health and Development,* **30** (3), 191–192.

Limbrick, P. (2003) *An Integrated Care Pathway for Assessment and Support for Children with Complex Needs and their Families.* Worcester, Interconnections.

Ludvigsen, A. & Morrison, J. (2003) *Breathing Space: Community Support for Children on Long-term Ventilation.* Ilford, Barnardo's.

Maria, B.L. (2002) *Current Management in Child Neurology* (second edition). Hamilton, Decker.

Mencap (1994) *Respite Care.* London, Mencap.

Millar, S. (2002) Respite care for children who have complex special health care needs. *Paediatric Nursing*, **14** (5), 33–37.

Muir, J. & Dryden, S. (2000) Collaborative planning for children with chronic, complex care needs. In: *Textbook of Community Children's Nursing* (eds J. Muir & A. Sidey), pp. 216–222. London, Baillière Tindall.

Murphy, G. (2001a) The technology-dependent child at home. Part 1: in whose best interest? *Paediatric Nursing*, **13** (7), 14–18.

Murphy, G. (2001b) The technology-dependent child at home. Part 2: the need for respite. *Paediatric Nursing*, **13** (8), 24–27.

Myers, J. (2005) Community children's nursing services in the 21st century. *Paediatric Nursing*, **17** (2), 31–34.

Noyes, J. (2002) Barriers that delay children and young people who are dependent on mechanical ventilators from being discharged from hospital. *Journal of Clinical Nursing*, **11** (1), 2–11.

Patterson, J., Jernell, J., Leonard, B. & Titus, J. (1994) Caring for medically fragile children at home: the parent-professional relationship. *Journal of Pediatric Nursing*, **9** (2), 98–106.

Petr, C.G., Murdock, B. & Chapin, R. (1995) Home care for children dependent on technology: the family perspective. *Social Work in Health Care*, **21**, 5–22.

Roberts, K. & Lawton, D. (2001) Acknowledging the extra care parents give their disabled children. *Child: Care, Health and Development*, **27** (4), 307–319.

Royal College of Nursing (2000) *Community Children's Nursing. Information for Primary Care Organisations, Strategic Health Authorities and all Professionals Working with Children in the Community Settings*. London, Royal College of Nursing.

Scott, R.C., Besag, M.C. & Neville, B.G.R. (1999) Buccal midazolam and rectal diazepam for treatment of prolonged seizures in childhood and adolescence: a randomised trial. *The Lancet*, **353** (9153), 623–626.

Smith, L. & Daughtrey, H. (2000) Weaving the seamless web of care: an analysis of parents' perceptions of their needs following discharge from hospital. *Journal of Advanced Nursing*, **31** (4), 812–820.

Stephens, N. (2005) Complex care packages: supporting seamless discharge for child and family. *Paediatric Nursing*, **17** (7), 30–32.

Sullivan, P.B. & Rosenbloom, L. (2002) *Feeding the Disabled Child*. London, MacKeith Press.

Thomlinson, E.H. (2002) The lived experience of families of children who are failing to thrive. *Journal of Advanced Nursing*, **39**, 537–545.

Thyen, U., Kuhlthau, K. & Perrin, J.M. (1999) Employment, child care and mental health of mothers caring for children assisted by technology. *Pediatrics*, **103**, 1235–1242.

Townsley, R. & Robinson, C. (1999) What rights for disabled children? Home enteral feeding in the community. *Children and Society*, **13**, 48–60.

Welsh Assembly Government (2000) *Welsh in the Health Service. The Scope, Nature and Adequacy of Welsh Language Provision in the National Health Service in Wales*. Cardiff, Welsh Assembly Government.

Welsh Assembly Government (2003) *The National Service Framework for Children and Young People and Maternity Services Disabled Child Module Report. Parent Consultation*. Cardiff, Welsh Assembly Government / Contact a Family.

Welsh Assembly Government (2005) *The National Service Framework for Children and Young People and Maternity Services in Wales*. Cardiff, Welsh Assembly Government.

Whiting, M. (2005) 1888–2004: a historical overview of community children's nursing. In: *Textbook of Community Children's Nursing* (eds A. Sidey & D. Widdas). pp. 17–41. Edinburgh, Baillière Tindall.

Whiting, M. (2006) Public health, primary health care and the development of community children's nursing. In: *A Textbook of Children's and Young People's Nursing* (eds A. Glasper & J. Richardson). pp. 104–113. Edinburgh, Elsevier.

Widdas, D., Sidey, A. & Dryden, S. (2005) Delivering and funding care for children with complex needs. In: *Textbook of Community Children's Nursing* (eds A. Sidey & D. Widdas). pp. 249–261. Edinburgh, Baillière Tindall.

Wilson, M.T., Macloed, S. & O'Regan, M.E. (2004) Nasal/buccal midazolam use in the community. *Archives Disorders of Childhood*, **89**, 50–51.

World Health Organization (1980) *International Classification of Impairments, Disabilities and Handicap*. Geneva, World Health Organization.

8 Acute Emergencies

Peter Mcnee and Martina Nathan

Introduction

The purpose of this chapter is to explore some of the key factors that need to be considered for the assessment and management of children and young people with chronic illness who have an acute emergency either as a result of their chronic illness or an unrelated health problem. To illustrate these issues, a case study will be used to explore current care practices and organisation for a child with an oncology condition. It is expected that readers of this chapter will have a knowledge and understanding of the normal cell cycle, types of white cells, normal cell properties and blood cell production.

Aim of the chapter

This chapter aims to raise awareness of the problems facing children and young people with chronic illness and their families when an acute emergency occurs. Issues raised, such as the care environment and multidisciplinary care, will be relevant and transferable to a range of chronic conditions and should be able to be considered in the context of most acute emergencies.

Intended learning outcomes

- To critically examine the impact of acute emergencies on the child/young person with a pre-existing chronic illness and their family
- To explore the factors that may lead to acute emergencies in children and young people with chronic illness and the relevant treatment and management

requirements; a case study examining the care of a child with an oncology condition will be used to exemplify these factors

- To analyse the role of the children's nurse and the multidisciplinary team in supporting children, young people and their families during an acute phase of their chronic illness
- To explore the context of care in relation to the environment in which care is delivered and its impact on ongoing medical and nursing care

Acute emergencies

Children with a pre-existing chronic condition are at high risk of acute deterioration or suffering complications as a result of their illness. Due to this risk, clinical services have to be provided in acute and community settings that are responsive to the needs of this vulnerable population (Valentine *et al.*, 2001). The fact that the level of clinical dependency of children and young people nursed in general ward areas has increased over several years (Haines, 2005) mirrors the changes in service provision in the community sector, where more dependent children with chronic and complex health care issues are now cared for at home. Complications such as diabetic ketoacidosis, sickle cell crisis, status epilepticus, acute renal failure, circulatory instability, acute exacerbation of asthma and severe febrile neutropenia all require rapid access to skilled clinicians and appropriate environments to deliver the initial care required (DoH, 2001b). To facilitate this rapid access, a number of children are covered by an open-door policy where they can access the services they require when necessary. This flexibility and approach to treatment allows for care to be delivered around the needs of the individual child and young person rather than that of the organisation. This marks a cultural shift from organisational to person centred care (DoH, 2003). However, some centres prefer children to be assessed via a GP or an accident and emergency department before admission or transfer to the appropriate care environment. Other centres prefer children to be assessed in their assessment unit, as general wards may not have the staff available with the appropriate level of knowledge and skills to deal with an unexpected emergency admission. This is an important issue that needs to be discussed with parents at discharge as some parents in the stress of an emergency may take their child inappropriately to their usual admission ward.

 Case study 8.1

Katie is a three-year-old girl who was diagnosed five months ago with acute lymphoblastic leukaemia (ALL). She had a two-week history of lethargy, pallor, enlarged abdomen and poor appetite when she presented at the local GP surgery. A full blood count (FBC) was taken that showed a white cell count (WCC) = 12, haemoglobin (Hb) = 8.2, platelets = 90. She was referred to the local children's oncology/haematology unit where, following a bone marrow aspirate, she was diagnosed with ALL.

Katie is an only child and lives with her mother Claire, who is 17 years old, in a two-bedroomed council flat. She has no contact with her father, who lives abroad. Before Katie's illness, Claire worked part time in a local shop and Katie attended preschool. Claire's parents, Tom and Sarah, care for Katie sometimes, but both have work commitments.

Initially, Katie found it difficult to adapt to the hospital environment but is now less frightened as she has become familiar with the nursing staff and other children who attend the unit. As the treatment for ALL is essentially based on a randomised controlled trial, it was important to gain informed consent from her mother. Informed consent in this case involved a discussion of the parent's role, an examination of the decision to be made, the positive and negative aspects of available treatment, possible alternatives, and the exploration of parental preferences (Eiser *et al.*, 2005).

 Time out

Identify and document the childhood leukaemias that you are aware of and their presenting signs and symptoms.

Childhood cancer is rare, accounting for 2% of all cancers. Only 1 in every 650 children under the age of 15 years develops a cancer, with 1700 new cases of childhood cancer in this age group in the UK each year (UKCCSG, 2005).

Leukaemia is the most common childhood malignancy, accounting for 32% of total childhood cancer diagnoses (National Registry of Childhood Tumours, 2003). The most prevalent type of leukaemia is acute leukaemia, with acute lymphoblastic leukaemia (ALL) comprising four-fifths of all leukaemias. The peak incidence of ALL occurs between the ages of 2 and 5 years. Acute myeloid leukaemia is the next most common, also known as acute non-lymphoblastic leukaemia (ANLL). Chronic myeloid leukaemia (CML) accounts for only a small percentage, which differs from the adult population where it is much more common.

The above incidence relates to children under the age of 15 years. The incidence differs for young people and adults. As illustrated in Table 8.1, in the UK, leukaemia is far less common in this population, with lymphomas being the most common cancer.

For both age groups, leukaemia rates are higher in males than females, with a ratio of males to females 1.3:1, in the under 15-year age group. ALL is more common among white children than black children, with ALL being rare in North Africa and the Middle East.

Aetiology

When children and young people are diagnosed with cancer, parents often question if it is something they have done or failed to do that has caused the cancer.

Table 8.1   Average number and types of cases of blood cancer in 15–34-year-olds in the UK (1950–1999).

Types of blood cancer	Males	Females	Total
Total leukaemia	175	110	285
Myeloid	65	30	95
Lymphoid	110	80	190
Hodgkin's lymphoma	274	237	511
Non-Hodgkin's lymphoma	247	124	371
Myeloma	7	4	11

Source   Leukaemia Research Foundation, 2005.

The aetiology of childhood cancer is still not fully explained. Greaves (1997) suggests it is probably due to two events occurring, one pre-birth and the other post-birth. Therefore, the main factors thought to play a role in the cause of ALL are:

- Genetic
- Environmental

Genetic factors are presumed to play a significant role in the cause of acute leukaemia, due to the association between various chromosomal abnormalities and ALL, for example children with Trisomy 21 (Down syndrome) are up to 15 times more likely to develop leukaemia than the unaffected population of children (Dordelmann *et al.*, 1998).

Other pre-existing chromosomal abnormalities that increase the risk of ALL are:

- Fanconi's anaemia
- Ataxia telangiectasia
- Neurofibromatosis
- Schwachmann syndrome
- Klinefelter syndrome
- Bloom syndrome

Environmental factors

Dickinson (2005) believes that ALL is probably the result of genetic susceptibility and exposure to external risk factors at a time when the child is vulnerable. The high incidence of leukaemia following the atomic bombs in Japan demonstrated that ionising radiation is a cause of leukaemia. It is widely accepted, also, that if mothers are exposed to radiation during pregnancy, the baby's risk of developing leukaemia is increased (Doll & Wakeford, 1997). In a large case control study Draper *et al.* (2005) demonstrated that the risk of childhood leukaemia increased in children living in close proximity to high voltage power lines. The subject of magnetic fields has been put forward as a cause of leukaemia but this study did not include measurement of magnetic fields.

The issue of nuclear installations where 'clusters' of children nearby have been diagnosed with ALL has given rise to concern. Kinlen (1995) explains that 'clusters' may be due to 'population mixing', where families have moved into new areas, bringing an epidemic of common infections. It is the abnormal responses to these common infectious agents that may increase the risk of ALL. Greaves and Alexander (1993) consider that a 'delayed' exposure to infection in infancy gives rise to the abnormal response. Gilham *et al.* (2005) support this principle and demonstrate that exposure to other infants and children during the first few months of life can protect against the risk of developing ALL. Day care and crèches are promoted, as they will bring infants into contact with common infections.

Low serum immunoglobulin levels have been observed in approximately 30% of newly diagnosed children and young people with ALL. It is difficult to ascertain whether this is a cause of ALL or a consequence of the disease (Margolin *et al.*, 2006). Other possible factors considered in the aetiology of childhood leukaemia are infants born to mothers over the age of 35 years, infants not breastfed and parental occupation. Chapter 1 examines the influence of environmental factors upon a range of chronic diseases.

Pathophysiology

Cancer is a genetic condition (refer to Chapter 1) and is a Latin term meaning 'crab', which is probably linked to the erratic movement of cells, similar to that of crabs (Morgan, 2001). The properties of malignant cells are:

- Same chemical structure as normal cells
- Lack control mechanisms – apoptosis
- Critical change in growth
- Lack adhesiveness
- Reduced normal inhibition

Leukaemia is a Greek term meaning 'white blood'. It is a clonal disease and is the result of the malignant transformation of bone marrow progenitor cells during haematopoiesis. The classification of different leukaemias depends upon the cell lineage in which the mutation occurs. Malignant transformation along the lymphoid cell lineage is known as lymphocytic leukaemia.

The growth of immature white blood cells, called 'blasts', is characteristic of leukaemia. By failing to mature, the cells cannot function as normal white blood cells. The increased cell division (cell production greater than cell loss) results in blast cells overcrowding the bone marrow space and therefore failing to allow production of normal cells.

Presentation

The child or young person with ALL, as in Katie's situation, often presents with non-specific symptoms, which are insidious and subtle (Tomlinson, 2005), and can include:

- Bone/joint pain
- Limpness
- Fever
- Weight loss
- Bruising
- Headache
- Weakness
- Enlarged lymph nodes

ALL, however, can present as an acute illness with a short onset, for example flu-like symptoms. Katie's presentation with pallor and lethargy was due to her anaemia, as the normal haemoglobin for a child of this age should be 11–13 g/dl. Due to the overcrowding of blast cells in the bone marrow, normal red blood cells cannot be produced. An elevated leukocyte count (greater than 10 000 per mm^3) is commonly associated with leukaemia. Katie's enlarged abdomen is a result of hepatosplenomegaly (enlarged liver and spleen), which arises from extra-medullary disease spread. Hepatosplenomegaly occurs in approximately two-thirds of patients and is usually asymptomatic (Margolin *et al.*, 2006). Her poor appetite may have been due to lethargy and the disease process.

 Time out

Referring to the above list, provide a rationale for these presenting signs and symptoms for a child with ALL.

As clinical features of ALL can be non-specific, other diagnoses are often considered, for example viral illness, aplastic anaemia. For a definite diagnosis of ALL, a bone marrow aspirate (BMA) is required even though blast cells are usually present in peripheral blood counts. The aspirate site is usually the iliac crest. In children's oncology care, this procedure is usually carried out under a general anaesthetic (GA), but if the patient is respiratory compromised or has a mediastinal mass, it would need to be done under local anaesthetic (LA). The need for a chest X-ray on admission is therefore necessary. A lumbar puncture (LP) is usually performed at the same time, involving a sample of cerebrospinal fluid (CSF) being taken to examine whether the leukaemia cells have spread to the central nervous system (CNS). A count of more than 25% blast cells in the bone marrow will confirm a diagnosis of leukaemia. The BMA or trephine will be further examined to establish the type of leukaemia.

Prognosis

The following factors are examined to determine prognosis and stratify treatment:

- Cell morphology
- Immunophenotyping
- Cytogenetics

Cell morphology

This examines the appearance and structure of the cell.

Immunophenotyping

This examines the cell origin and stage of differentiation. Common ALL is known to have a common ALL antigen, CD10, on the cell surface and is known to be of early B cell lineage (Margolin *et al.*, 2006). Early B cell lineage subgroups have a better prognosis than mature B cell ALL and T cell ALL.

Cytogenetics

Children and young people with higher ploidy have the best prognosis. The worst prognosis occurs when the near-haploid ALL has an event free survival (EFS) less than 25% (Heerema *et al.*, 1999). Structural chromosomal abnormalities are also detected in ALL, with translocation being the most common and associated with a poor prognosis (Margolin *et al.*, 2006). The Philadelphia chromosome translocation t (9:22) remains the translocation with the worst prognosis, evident in 5% of childhood ALL.

Analysis of patients treated on MRC UKALL X exposed other recognised risk factors such as age, gender and presenting WCC. Hann *et al.* (2001) showed that girls have a better prognosis than boys, and that there is a poorer prognosis associated with increasing age (excluding infantile ALL) and increased WCC.

 Case study 8.2

Katie is being treated with cytotoxic chemotherapy. A central line, namely a Hickman line, was inserted on week five of her treatment.

During the next five months, Katie received treatment that included:

- Induction (first five weeks)
- Consolidation (three weeks)
- Interim maintenance (eight weeks)

Delayed intensification started at week seventeen. Whilst in hospital Katie was given cytotoxic agents, vincristine, steroids (dexamethasone) and L'asparaginase for the first two weeks as part of her induction treatment for ALL. This drug regime usually produces remission in 95% of children (Tomlinson, 2005). Intrathecal methotrexate was also given for CNS prophylaxis. For the first week of treatment, Katie was given an uricolytic agent and intravenous fluids to prevent tumour lysis syndrome (TLS), although Katie's risk of this was low as she had a low WCC. She was also commenced on prophylactic co-trimoxazole at the weekends to prevent the development of pneumocystis jiroveci pneumonia (PCP).

⏲ Time out

Make a list of the potential side effects of chemotherapy and a rationale for their causes.

Tumour lysis syndrome (TLS) occurs as a result of the excretory capacity of the kidneys' inability to cope with the large quantities of uric acid, potassium and phosphate that are emitted due to cancer cell death. Patients with bulky tumours, lymphomas, high WCCs are considered at high risk of developing TLS. Prophylactic measures include identification of risk factors, hydration, monitoring serum U/Es and uricolytic agents (allopurinol, rasburicase).

Pneumocystis jiroveci pneumonia (PCP) is caused by the pathogen *Pneumocystis jiroveci*. It can occur in immuno-compromised individuals, including children and young people, undergoing treatment for cancer (Parr, 2005). Sulphamethoxazole-trimethoprim (co-trimoxazole) is administered as a prophylactic measure whilst cytotoxic chemotherapy is administered.

Treatment

In the 1940s, cytotoxic chemotherapy was introduced as part of standard treatment for childhood cancer. Before this, surgery and radiation treatment were the only therapies available. Following the discovery of nitrogen mustard after World War 1, rapid drug development occurred in this area.

Cytotoxic chemotherapy means chemical therapy that is toxic to cells. Examples of cytotoxic agents and their actions are given in Table 8.2. These agents kill malignant and non-malignant cells as they move through the five phases of the cell cycle. Cytostatic agents hold cells in a specific phase of the cell cycle and arrest cell development (Young, 1999). Cytotoxic agents appear to be most effective in the proliferative phase of the cell cycle. They are classified according to their action within the cell cycle:

Table 8.2   Type and action of cytotoxic agents.

Type of cytotoxic agent	Action	Example
Alkylating agents	Disrupt DNA synthesis Reacts with DNA base forming cross-linking	Cyclophosphamide
Antimetabolites	Mimic metabolites that are essential for formation of nucleic acids	Methotrexate
Antitumour antibiotics	Prevent DNA synthesis by causing single or double strand breaks	Doxorubicin
Plant alkaloids	Interfere with normal microtubule formation and function in mitosis phase	Vincristine
Miscellaneous agents, for example asparaginase	L'asparaginase is an enzyme that acts by converting asparagines into aspartic acid and ammonia, inhibiting tumour cell protein synthesis	Asparaginase

- Cell cycle phase specific: agents that act specifically during one phase of the cell cycle. These agents are most effective in tumours with high growth fractions.
- Cell cycle non-phase specific: agents that are effective during all phases of the cell cycle, including the G0 (resting phase). These agents are most effective with tumours of low growth fraction.
- Cell cycle specific: agents that are effective while cells are actively in cycle but not dependent on cells being in a particular phase.

The efficacy of combinations of chemotherapy agents was first recognised over forty years ago in the treatment of acute lymphatic leukaemia (Young, 1999). The increase in patients achieving remission was significant but there was a more remarkable increase in the duration of remission.

The benefits of combination chemotherapy include:

- Prevention of multi-drug resistance
- Maximum cell kill within the range of toxicities
- No overlapping toxicities
- It can be administered at regular intervals
- The dosage of the agents can be maximised

Key point

Chemotherapy destroys not only cancerous cells but healthy cells as well. This causes certain common side effects such as alopecia, nausea and vomiting, and mouth ulcers, as well as more acute emergencies such as PCP and TLS.

Administration of chemotherapy

Cytotoxic chemotherapy is given by many different routes. The most common in childhood cancer are intravenous, oral, intrathecal and subcutaneous. Only staff with specific training and education should be involved in the preparation (pharmacists), checking and administration of cytotoxic chemotherapy. Administrators of chemotherapy need to be aware of treatment protocols, patient issues (RCN, 2005) and that the basis of good practice in administration of chemotherapy is safety and patient comfort (Hooker & Palmar, 1999). The importance of this is clearly demonstrated by the following case example.

In the UK in February 2001, a teenager died following the administration of vincristine by the intrathecal route (IT), rather than the intended intravenous route. The Department of Health (2001a) subsequently issued the circular *National Guidance on the Safe Administration of Intrathecal Chemotherapy*, with most of the circular focusing on ensuring the safe administration of IT chemotherapy.

Most anti-cancer drugs are potentially hazardous substances, since they are mutagenic, teratogenic and carcinogenic. Health care personnel who are involved in the preparation and handling of anti-cancer drugs can, if not adequately protected, absorb potentially harmful quantities of such compounds (Allwood *et al.*, 2002). Protective clothing should be worn at all times when handling cytotoxics. There is evidence to suggest that handling excreta (urine, faeces, sweat, saliva and vomit) from patients having or who have just completed cytotoxic chemotherapy, or laundry contaminated with excreta, puts handlers at risk of exposure to cytotoxic drugs (Allwood *et al.*, 2002). Therefore, protective precautions should be taken and carers similarly advised.

 Case study 8.3

A decision was made for Katie to have a central venous access device inserted to administer the necessary intravenous therapies. As Katie is needle phobic, thorough preparation and psychological support for this was essential. Katie had her central line inserted on week five of treatment as, during induction treatment, the administration of asparaginase interferes with the clotting mechanism, and insertion of a central venous catheter (CVC) at this stage would predispose the patient to thrombus formation. However, due to her phobia and Katie getting extremely distressed with venepunctures, the decision was made with Claire and the multidisciplinary team that a Hickman line would be more suitable than a port-a-cath, as an implanted device would need to be accessed with a needle for use. Due to the risk of infection, Katie cannot continue swimming with the Hickman line in situ. It also may have an impact on body image, as Katie gets older.

Central venous access devices

To administer intensive cytotoxic chemotherapy, withdraw blood samples and deliver supportive products, children with leukaemia usually have a CVC inserted (Sepion, 1990), which reduces the physical and psychological trauma that can be associated with venepuncture (Kegan-Wells & Stewart, 1992).

Central venous access devices (CVADs) have been in use since the early 1970s and have had a great influence on the care and management of children with cancer. However, they are not without risk. Potential complications include septicaemia, catheter occlusion, air embolism, catheter displacement/dislodgement and phlebitis.

Katie had a Hickman line inserted, which is an external silicone tunnelled catheter, made of radio-opaque medical grade silicone. The devices can consist of single, double or triple lumens. Hickman lines are usually inserted for patients receiving aggressive chemotherapy regimens. Patients on ALL protocols usually have the implanted subcutaneous device inserted, due to the lower infection risk with this device (Ingram *et al.*, 1991). Besides the risk of infection, psychosocial issues can also arise. Sanderson (2004) states that a child's response to a CVC could be affected by his/her understanding of the illness, fear of medical procedures, limited coping strategies and impact on body image. Chapter 4 offers a detailed discussion of the psychosocial issues affecting children and young people with a chronic illness.

 Case study 8.4

Katie is currently on week 20 of her treatment undergoing delayed intensification. Since week 17, she has received as paraginase and high oral dexamethasone (a corticosteroid) alongside weekly doses of doxorubicin and vincristine. Up to this time, she has coped well with her treatment, only being admitted once to the unit since diagnosis, with a temperature of 38.1C. She recovered from this after 48 hours on intravenous antibiotics, with no focus of infection found.

Katie has come to the outpatient department (OPD) this morning for a planned FBC. According to her protocol, she is due to commence a block of cytarabine chemotherapy, and her neutrophil count needs to be 1000 cells/mm^3 or above to continue with her treatment.

Claire mentions on arrival at the department that Katie has been complaining of a sore mouth and that she has been lethargic for the past few days. Jess, a senior staff nurse who is familiar with Katie, assesses Katie's oral cavity, which she feels is slightly inflamed, and notices a mouth ulcer developing under her tongue. Claire states that she has commenced Katie on the chlorohexidine mouthwash since the beginning of her intensification treatment as per unit policy. Jess informs Claire that she will get a doctor to assess Katie's mouth and get pain relief prescribed.

Table 8.3   Types and treatment of mouth infections.

Infections in the mouth	Most common type	Treatment
Fungal	Candida albicans	Amphotericin (ambisome) Fluconazole
Viral	Herpes simplex	Acyclovir
Bacterial	Streptococcus	Broad spectrum antibiotics Metronidazole

Mucositis is a general term that refers to an inflammation of the mucous membranes; when it occurs in the oral cavity, is known as stomatitis (Gibson & Evans, 1999). Chemotherapy agents differ in the degree they cause mucositis and the dose also needs to be taken into consideration. Katie received doxorubicin, an anti-tumour antibiotic that is considered to be a highly stomatoxic agent. Other risk factors include pre-existing oral disease and poor oral hygiene. Stomatitis usually occurs 5–10 days post-treatment, commencing with a dry mucosa, tongue and lips and may lead to taste alteration and oral ulceration, which predisposes the patient to infection (types of infection are outlined in Table 8.3). Management is symptom related, the main one being pain. Appropriate care includes ensuring that mouth care is performed and that the patient eats and drinks, to help prevent infection. During times of neutropenia, the mouth is in an ideal condition for microbial growth.

The most common side effect and dose limiting side effect of cytotoxic chemotherapy is myelo-suppression, which is also potentially the most lethal. Myelo-suppression, also known as bone marrow suppression, consists of neutropenia, thrombocytopenia and anaemia.

 Time out

What do you understand by the terms neutropenia, thrombocytopenia and anaemia? Jot your thoughts down.

Bone marrow is the principle haematopoietic tissue, where the continual process of production of blood cells occurs in accordance with the body's requirements. The colony stimulating factors and hormone like glycoproteins, mediate haematopoiesis for all blood cell lines, governing production, cell differentiation and maturation. The granulocyte colony stimulating factor is effective on the white cell lineage. All haematopoietic cells divide rapidly and are vulnerable to cytotoxic chemotherapy. The nadir (decline) is 7–10 days post-chemotherapy, with cell cycle non-specific agents causing the most severe myelo-suppression.

Thrombocytopenia occurs when a platelet count is less than 150 000 per mm^3. The lifespan of a platelet is 7–10 days and its function is haemostasis and fibrinolysis. Claire was given information regarding the signs and symptoms of a low platelet count: fresh bruising, bleeding gums and epistaxis. She was told to avoid administering aspirin and non-steroidal anti-inflammatory drugs to Katie, which may increase the chance of bleeding. When Katie's platelet count dropped below 10 per mm^3 or she was actively bleeding, she received a transfusion of platelets in the OPD.

Claire may have already been familiar with the term 'anaemia' from pregnancy, and the associated signs and symptoms of pallor, lethargy and dizziness. As most oxygen is carried by the red blood cells (RBCs) to the body's tissues, a reduction in the red cell mass causes reduced oxygen supply to body cells (Bryant, 2004). The normal haemoglobin (Hb) of a child is 11–13 g/dl with the lifespan of a RBC being 120 days. According to the policy at Katie's centre, Katie will receive a red blood cell transfusion when her Hb drops below 8 g/dl.

Although all white blood cells are important, the most significant in patients undergoing treatment for cancer are neutrophils. Neutropenia is a deficiency of circulating neutrophils. The function of a neutrophil is phagocytosis. With reduced neutrophils, the normal process of controlling gram positive and negative infections is therefore diminished.

At the commencement of treatment, Claire had been given advice and information regarding how chemotherapy would cause Katie to be susceptible to infection, and the possible signs and symptoms. The family were advised how to protect Katie from infection, including careful handwashing, keeping Katie away from people who have infections, keeping Katie away from crowded areas when she is severely neutropenic and ensuring food is cooked thoroughly. Katie was discharged following her last admission with pyrexia, after it was ensured that Claire had a thermometer at home and she understood that she could contact the unit at any time.

   Key points

- Myelo-suppression consists of neutropenia, thrombocytopenia and anaemia.
- The nurse must advise and educate the family on the signs and symptoms of these side effects and how to minimise the possibility of complications arising by undertaking preventative measures.

🌐 **Case study 8.5**

Jess accesses Katie's Hickman line, known as 'wiggly' to Katie, using the large lumen to obtain the FBC. Katie usually helps to open and close the clamps of her line, but is not interested today. Jess takes blood for an FBC and U/E and sends the sample to the laboratory. As Jess is flushing the line with hepsal, Katie begins to rigor. Jess quickly assesses Katie clinically. Her peripheries are cool and her capillary refill time (CRT) centrally is 2–3 seconds. Her vital signs are taken; temperature 37.6 C, BP 95/45, HR 110, RR 35, oxygen saturations 98%.

Jess informs the medical staff about Katie's condition and the registrar and house officer come to review. They commence her on intravenous fluids via both lumens of her Hickman line and initially prescribe a fluid bolus of 20 mls/kg of 0.9% sodium chloride (NACL). As Katie continues to rigor and her CRT is now 3 seconds centrally, Jess is asked to take blood cultures from both lumens of the Hickman line and then IV antibiotics are commenced: a broad spectrum antibiotic, meropenem, and one to cover gram negative organisms, gentamicin.

Katie's temperature is now 38.1C, BP 88/40, HR 140 and her respiratory status is stable. A swab is taken from Katie's mouth ulcer and her Hickman line insertion site is examined, but shows no obvious inflammation. A creatinine reactive protein test is requested from the U/E sample, which is elevated to 90, suggesting infection. The FBC proves Katie to be neutropenic, with her neutrophils at 600 cells/mm^3, Hb 8.6 and platelets at 40 000 cells/mm^3.

Claire is understandably concerned and anxious and Katie says she is frightened. Jess tries to explain to both of them what is happening and tells Claire that Katie probably has an infection in her Hickman line. Katie is commenced on a strict fluid balance with all her urine measured. Due to her current instability, Katie is transferred to the children's high dependency unit for initial management and observation. Katie responds well to her fluid bolus and, after a period of observation, is transferred back to the oncology ward, for ongoing care and management prior to discharge.

Sepsis

Sepsis is a reasonably common complication of intensive therapies and is a serious systemic response to infection (Ross, 2003), a serious complication that can lead to ongoing morbidity and ultimately mortality. The improvement in survivability of childhood cancers over a number of years has been attributable to an escalation in the intensity of therapy (Attard-Montalto, 2000). Shaw (2002) found that infection was the primary cause of death in eleven non-bone marrow transplant patients; five died due to fungal infection and one due to bacterial infection. Early recognition and commencement of treatment are essential in attempting to reduce mortality and morbidity. If children and young people presenting with sepsis deteriorate to such an extent that paediatric intensive care unit (PICU) admission is required, mortality rates are high at around 53% (Parsons *et al.*, 2001). The goal of PICU treatment is the management of complications, the continuance of commenced therapies and the use of appropriate antibiotic therapy to ensure successful outcomes. If a child or young person requires high dependency or PICU care, a range of issues can have an impact on the family, including possible transfer to lead centres, which may be some distance away from the child's normal in-patient or clinic facility. Issues surrounding family focused care and multidisciplinary working across clinical boundaries can have a major impact on the ongoing treatment and management of the child's underlying condition.

Children's critical care

Across the UK, children's critical care is organised through a series of lead centres supporting local trusts. The decision to transfer a child to a high dependency unit or PICU is dependent on a number of factors, the key factor usually being dependency. Paediatric intensive care units have been described as being low volume, high cost facilities that cannot be provided in all localities but to which all children should have access. Most paediatric intensive care units will care for children at level 2/3 dependency whereas high dependency units will care for children at level 1 (DoH, 1997). Level 1 has been described as delivering closer observation and monitoring than is usually available in a ward environment, level 2 as children who require continuous nursing supervision and are usually ventilated and level 3 as children and young people with two or more body systems requiring support, for example a child suffering from multiple trauma (DoH, 1997). Between 5 and 15% of all district general hospital admissions will require paediatric high dependency care and of these 0.5–1% will require a PICU admission (DoI I, 2001b). As with Katie, most of these children will start and finish their care in clinical environments other than PICU.

 Time out

Think about the children and young people that you have nursed with chronic illness:

- How was their level of dependency assessed clinically?
- What care environments are available on a local and tertiary level to nurse them?
- If they require more intensive nursing, how do the children, young people and their families feel when they are moved from their normal ward environment?

Family focused care

Transfer from acute general children's or specialist children's areas can cause an inordinate amount of stress to parents. Children with a range of chronic conditions will spend protracted periods of time in critical care areas, for example children and young people who require long-term assisted ventilation. A number of these children will experience delays in discharge to their referring hospitals or to their own homes (Noyes, 2000). (See Chapter 7 for a detailed discussion of this issue.) This situation can have a serious impact on family relationships, and on parental ability and confidence to manage ongoing care at home. Parents of children and young people with chronic illness need to develop and sustain trusting relationships with the health professionals caring for their child, but this is often dependent on the attitudes and values of the professionals concerned (Swallow & Jacoby, 2001). Parents of children being cared for in high dependency or critical care areas can experience a range of feelings and emotions. Tomlinson et al. (2002) found that for family centred care to be facilitated, nurses need to recognise the physical, psychological and emotional needs of parents. To meet these needs, staff must appreciate that once a child has been admitted to these areas, there is a profound alteration in the parenting role that needs to be dealt with sensitively (Playfor et al., 2001).

Parents of children with chronic illness are usually experts in the ongoing treatment and care of their child and this often requires some facilitation in critical care areas. It has been found that nurses in critical care areas are technologically proficient but do not always meet the needs and expectations of families (Tomlinson et al., 2002). Parents rely very much on established coping mechanisms in order to fulfil the primary care giver role and this can be compromised in critical care environments. In family centred care, it is important that the needs of parents and siblings are identified in addition to those of the child to ensure that a partnership approach is initiated to facilitate continued parental input into care delivery (Haines & Wolstenholme, 2000). It is essential that parents are able to establish meaning and understanding to the experience of their child being transferred to high dependency and critical care areas. For care to be successful, it is also important that staff communicate well across clinical environments, sharing both knowledge and expertise, whilst maintaining ongoing therapeutic relationships with the child and family in their care.

Multidisciplinary working across different organisations

Professional collaboration is a key issue in ensuring that effective outcomes are achieved in the care, treatment and management of children and young people with a chronic illness. A number of children will be nursed in tertiary centres, particularly during the diagnostic period and when specific interventions are required, for example during Hickman line or port-a-cath insertions. Professional collaboration and access to ongoing support has proved effective in the management of disease processes (Eilertsen et al., 2004). Sloper (1996) found that parents played a particularly active role during diagnosis where information, support and education were provided by a range of professionals.

Due to ongoing changes in the organisation and delivery of both acute and community services, care is often delivered by a range of professionals who may represent a number of health and social care institutions. Children and young people with a chronic illness need to receive care that is integrated and coordinated around their individual needs. National service frameworks have recognised that there is increasing evidence that children with illnesses that are complex, unusually severe or complicated by acute deterioration generally have better outcomes in tertiary centres (DoH, 2003). The development of shared, managed clinical networks has allowed care to be provided in a number of localities and closer to the child's home. Some specialities, such as cardiac, renal and oncology, are unable to provide services in all locations, but access to these services needs to be facilitated. This has been achieved by a number of services providing outreach services and clinics. The coordination of health care disciplines from the primary, secondary and tertiary level is intended to provide closer multi-agency cooperation and closer integration of care environments (DoH, 2004a; WAG, 2005). Care provision should be seamless and based upon the latest evidence. To facilitate this, the NSF for children and young people who are ill (DoH, 2004b) has identified a range of good practice markers to ensure that children and young people with a chronic illness have access to high quality evidence based care delivered by a range of professionals with the relevant skills, knowledge and facilities to provide seamless ongoing care and support.

Parents have recognised the importance of the key worker role in the coordination and facilitation of care (Hall, 1996). This is particularly relevant across professional and geographical boundaries (Eaton, 2000). Cross-boundary working is a key policy objective for the foundation of high quality care across child health services (While *et al.*, 2006). Chapters 2 and 7 discuss the role of the key worker in coordinating the care process. Examples of cross-boundary working can be seen in the provision of nurse specialists in a range of conditions and in the role of the nurse consultant. These roles are often intended to span both primary and secondary environments and can play an important part in the continuation of care, particularly when children experience deterioration in their condition or a complication due to a subsequent pathology. These roles are particularly important to facilitate information sharing and maintenance of already established treatment protocols. A number of these roles require flexibility in the commissioning process (While *et al.*, 2006) to ensure that their roles are able to span a range of health care and multi-agency sectors.

Conclusion

Children and young people with a chronic illness may experience rapid changes in the treatment and management of their condition. Within the case study, we have examined a little girl's journey from diagnosis, through the first phase of treatment to the point of an acute deterioration, which may reflect the illness trajectory experienced by children with a range of conditions. It is important that parents and families are provided with effective, skilled and evidence based care in each of the care environments, whether that be their own homes or tertiary centres. If the aims of the NSF are to be achieved, close cooperation and collaboration across professional and geographical boundaries will need to be achieved, which will ensure that the holistic needs of the individual child, young person and family are met. It is essential that children with existing and chronic medical disorders have a clear plan of action in the event of acute deterioration (DoH, 2004a). This should ensure access to appropriately skilled professionals and care facilities.

> **⚷ Key points**
>
> - A range of acute emergencies may affect the child and young person with a chronic illness.
> - Patterns of service delivery are continually evolving to meet the needs of children and young people with a chronic illness.
> - Children and young people with chronic illness are nursed and often transferred through a range of care environments.
> - Effective intervention by the multidisciplinary team is essential in supporting children, young people and their families through an acute phase of their chronic illness.

Useful websites

www.doh.gov.uk
www.lrf.org.uk/en/1/information.html
www.statistics.gov.uk
www.ukccsg.org.uk

References

Allwood, M., Stanley, A. & Wright, P. (2002) *The Cytotoxics Handbook*. Oxon, Radcliffe Medical Press Ltd.

Attard-Montalto, S.P. (2000) Haematological and oncological problems in paediatric intensive care. In: *Paediatric Intensive Care Nursing* (eds C. Williams & J. Asquith), pp. 293–303. London, Churchill Livingstone.

Bryant, R. (2004) Anemias. In: *Pediatric Oncology Nursing; Advanced Clinical Handbook* (eds D. Tomlinson & N. Kline), pp. 104–130. Berlin, Springer-Verlag.

Department of Health (1997) *Paediatric Intensive Care: a Framework for the Future-National Coordinating Group on Paediatric Intensive Care – Report to the Chief Executive of the NHS Executive*. London, Department of Health.

Department of Health (2001a) *National Guidance on the Safe Administration of Intrathecal Chemotherapy*. London, Department of Health.

Department of Health (2001b) *High Dependency Care for Children – Expert Advisory Group Report for the Department of Health*. London, Department of Health.

Department of Health (2003) *Getting the Right Start: National Service Framework for Children, Young People and Maternity Services: Standard for Hospital Services*. London, Department of Health.

Department of Health (2004a) *National Service Framework for Children, Young People and Maternity Services: Disabled Children and Young People and those with Complex Health Needs*. London, Department of Health.

Department of Health (2004b) *National Service Framework for Children, Young People and Maternity Services: Children and Young People who are Ill*. London, Department of Health.

Dickinson, H. (2005) The causes of childhood leukaemia. *British Medical Journal*, **330**, 1279–1280.

Doll, R. & Wakeford, R. (1997) Risk of childhood cancer from foetal irradiation. *The British Journal of Radiology*, **70**, 130–139.

Dordelmann, M., Schrappe, M., Reiter, A., *et al.* (1998) Down syndrome in childhood acute lymphoblastic leukaemia: clinical characteristics and treatment outcome in four consecutive BFM trials. Berlin-Frankfurt-Munster Group.

Draper, G., Vincent, T., Kroll, M.E. & Swanson, J. (2005) Childhood cancer in relation to distance from high voltage power lines in England and Wales; a case control study. *British Medical Journal*, **330**, 1290–1293.

Eaton, N. (2000) Children's community nursing services: models of care delivery. A review of the United Kingdom literature. *Journal of Advanced Nursing*, **32** (1), 49–56.

Eilertsen, M.E.B., Reinfjell, T. & Vik, T. (2004) Value of professional collaboration in the care of children with cancer and their families. *European Journal of Cancer Care*, **13**, 349–355.

Eiser, C., Davies, H., Jenney, M. & Glasers, A. (2005) Mothers' attitudes to the randomised control trial (RCT); the case of acute lymphoblastic leukaemia (ALL) in children. *Child: Care, Health and Development*, **31** (5), 517–523.

Gibson, F. & Evans, M. (1999) *Paediatric Oncology – Acute Nursing Care.* London, Whurr Publishers.

Gilham, C., Petro, J., Simpson, J. *et al.* (2005) Day care in infancy and risk of childhood acute lymphatic leukaemia: findings from UK case-control study. *British Medical Journal*, **330**, 1294–1299.

Greaves, M.F. (1997) Aetiology of acute lymphatic leukaemia. *Lancet*, **349** (9048), 344–349.

Greaves, M.F. & Alexander, F.E. (1993) An infectious aetiology of common acute lymphatic leukaemia in childhood. *Leukaemia*, **7**, 349–360.

Haines, C. (2005) Acutely ill children within ward areas – care provision and possible development strategies. *Nursing in Critical Care*, **10** (2), 98–104.

Haines, C. & Wolstenholme, M. (2000) Family support in paediatric intensive care. In: *Paediatric Intensive Care Nursing* (eds C. Williams & J. Asquith), pp. 307–316. London, Churchill Livingstone.

Hall, S. (1996) An exploration of parental perception of the nature and level of support needed to care for their child with special needs. *Journal of Advanced Nursing*, **24**, 512–521.

Hann, I., Vora, A., Harrison, G. *et al.* (2001) Determinants of outcome after intensified therapy of childhood lymphatic leukaemia; results from Medical Research Council UKALL XI protocol. *British Journal of Haematology*, **13** (1), 103–114.

Heerema, N.A., Nachman, J.B. & Sather, H.N. (1999) Hypodiploidy with less than 45 chromosomes confers adverse risk in childhood acute lymphoblastic leukaemia; a report from the children's cancer group. *Blood*, **94** (12), 4036–4045.

Hooker, L. & Palmar, S. (1999) Administration of chemotherapy. In: *Paediatric Oncology – Acute Nursing Care* (eds F. Gibson & M. Evans), pp. 22–58. London, Whurr Publishers.

Ingram, J., Weitzman, S. & Greenberg, M. (1991) Complications of indwelling venous access lines in the paediatric haematology patient; a prospective comparison of external venous catheters and subcutaneous ports. *American Journal Paediatric Haematology/Oncology*, **13**, 130–136.

Kegan-Wells, D. & Stewart, J. (1992) The use of venous access devices in pediatric oncology nursing practice. *Journal of Pediatric Oncology Nursing*, **9** (25), 159–169.

Kinlen, L.J. (1995) Epidemiological evidence for an infective basis in childhood leukaemia. *British Journal of Cancer*, **71** (1), 1–5.

Leukaemia Research Foundation (2005) www.lrf.org.uk/en/1/information.html

Margolin, J.F., Steuber, C.P. & Poplack, D.G. (2006) Acute lymphatic leukaemia. In: *Principles and Practice of Pediatric Oncology* (eds P.A. Pizzo & D.G. Poplack) (fifth edition), pp. 538–590. Philadelphia, Lippincott-Williams and Wilkins Publishers.

Morgan, G. (2001) Making sense of cancer. *Cancer Nursing Practice*, **0** (0), 20–24.

National Registry of Childhood Tumours (2003) www.statistics.gov.uk

Noyes, J. (2000) 'Ventilator-dependent children who spend prolonged periods of time in intensive care units when they no longer have a medical need or want to be there. *Journal of Clinical Nursing*, **9**, 774–783.

Parr, M. (2005) Respiratory system. In: *Pediatric Oncology Nursing-Advanced Handbook. Clinical* (eds D. Tomlinson & N. Kline), pp. 291–299. Berlin, Springer-Verlag.

Parsons, S.J., Tomas, K. & Wensley, D.F. (2001) Outcome and predictors of mortality in pediatric oncology patients requiring intensive care. *Journal of Intensive Care Medicine*, **16** (1), 29–34.

Playfor, S.D., Thomas, D.A., Choonara Colliers, J. & Jarvis, A. (2001) Parental perceptions of comfort during mechanical ventilation. *Paediatric Anaesthesia*, **11**, 99–103.

Ross, V. (2003) Uncertainty about the clinical detection of sepsis. *Journal of Infusion Nursing*, **26** (1), 23–28.

Royal College of Nursing (2005) *Competencies: an Integrated Competency Framework for Training Programmes in the Safe Administration of Chemotherapy to Children and Young People*. London, Royal College of Nursing.

Sanderson, L. (2004) The experience of children with central venous catheters. In: *Perspectives in Paediatric Oncology Nursing* (eds F. Gibson, L. Soanes & B. Sepion), pp. 283–310. London, Whurr.

Sepion, B. (1990) Intravenous care for children. *Paediatric Nursing*, **2**, 14–16.

Shaw, P.J. (2002) Suspected infection in children with cancer. *Journal of Antimicrobial Chemotherapy. Ambisone: an International Workshop*, **49** (1), 63–67.

Sloper, P. (1996) Needs and responses of parents following the diagnosis of childhood cancer. *Child: Care Health and Development*, **22** (3), 187–202.

Swallow, V.M. & Jacoby, A. (2001) Mothers' evolving relationships with doctors and nurses during the chronic illness trajectory. *Journal of Advanced Nursing*, **36** (6), 755–764.

Tomlinson, D. (2005) Leukemia. In: *Pediatric Oncology Nursing – Advanced Handbook. Clinical* (eds D. Tomlinson & N. Kline), pp. 2–23. Berlin, Springer-Verlag.

Tomlinson, P.S., Thomlinson, E., Peden-McAlpine, C. & Kirschbaum, M. (2002) Clinical innovation for promoting family centred care in paediatric intensive care: demonstration, role modelling and reflective practice. *Journal of Advanced Nursing*, **38** (2), 161–170.

United Kingdom Children's Cancer Study Group (2005) www.ukccsg.org.uk

Valentine, J.M., Maynard, C., Christakis, D. & Hicks-Thomson, J. (2001) Pediatric hospitalisation patterns for selected health conditions using hospital abstract reporting system data: methods and findings. *Health Services and Outcomes Research Methodology*, **1** (3), 335–350.

Welsh Assembly Government (2005) National Service Framework for Children, Young People and Maternity Service in Wales. Cardiff, Welsh Assembly Government.

While, A., Murgatroyd, B., Ullman, R. & Forbes, A. (2006) Nurses', midwives' and health visitors' involvement in cross-boundary working within child health services. *Child: Care, Health and Development*, **32** (1), 87–89.

Young, G. (1999) Principles of chemotherapy. In: *Paediatric Oncology – Acute Nursing Care* (eds F. Gibson & M. Evans), pp. 3–21. London, Whurr Publishers.

9 Adolescence

Siân Bill and Yvonne Knight

Introduction

Adolescence is a time of rapid growth, development and change, which can be a difficult period for some young people. Any potential difficulties experienced during adolescence can be compounded by the presence of a chronic illness. As advances in medical technology have improved life expectancy, young people with a chronic illness and their families are faced with new challenges. Additionally, health care professionals need to revisit the way in which young people with chronic illness are managed, to ensure that their care meets the holistic needs of the individual.

Aim of the chapter

The purpose of this chapter is to critically examine the issues relating to adolescents with a chronic illness. To examine the pertinent issues, a case study focusing on a young person with chronic renal failure will be used throughout the chapter. However, issues that are raised within this scenario could be applied to young people with different types of chronic illness.

This chapter will not provide an in-depth exploration of adolescent physical or psychosocial development. Neither does this chapter provide an in-depth physiological account of renal failure or the breadth of psychosocial issues that can evolve from this condition. There are a number of available texts that provide comprehensive coverage of adolescent development and paediatric nephrology, and references for these are provided at the end of the chapter. Readers not familiar with these topics, and particularly adolescent growth and development in the context of this chapter, are advised to access these texts (see Recommended reading) to help them understand and apply the information covered in this chapter.

Intended learning outcomes

- To critically examine the impact of chronic illness on adolescent physical and psychosocial development
- To develop an understanding of the associated health risk factors relating to chronic illness and the consequences of these, with particular regard to compliance/non-compliance
- To examine the psychosocial and physical developmental needs of the hospitalised adolescent
- To explore the role of the nurse in facilitating the empowerment of adolescents within the health care setting

Adolescent knowledge

This chapter is written on the assumption that the reader has some prior knowledge and understanding of adolescent physical and psychosocial development. This includes the stages of adolescent development, physical growth patterns, physiological and hormonal changes, sexual development, the development of cognition and the 'conception of self'. As physical and psychosocial development is closely linked with adolescent behaviour, without an understanding of these concepts it will be difficult for the reader to develop an understanding of the way in which young people respond to and cope with a chronic illness. Take some time to try and answer the following questions.

⏲ Time out

- What hormones are responsible for triggering adolescent development?
- How many phases of adolescent development are there?
- What tool is used to monitor adolescent physical development?
- Who leads the way in adolescent developmental milestones: boys or girls?
- What are the first signs of sexual maturation in girls?
- What is the mean age of menarche?
- When does puberty occur?
- At what stage does the peer group become important to adolescents?
- When are adolescents most concerned with their body image?
- At what stage of development is the adolescent capable of abstract thought?

Why nurses need knowledge of adolescence

It is estimated that there are currently approximately 7.7 million young people between the ages of 10 and 19 years living in the UK (Coleman & Schofield, 2005). Over the past ten years, the number of adolescents has risen, while the number of children in the overall population has declined. This has clear implications for policy development and the provision of services for this age group (Coleman & Schofield, 2005). It also sends a clear message that as nurses we need to become more aware of, and develop strategies to meet, the health care needs of young people.

There is no clear consensus regarding definitions of adolescence (Rice, 1999; Santrock, 2001) with a variety of terms used in practice to depict this age range, including youth, teenager, young people and adolescents. The World Health Organization (WHO) advocates that the following definitions should be used: *adolescents* for individuals aged 10–19 years, *youth* for those aged 15–24 years and *young people* when between 10–24 years of age (WHO, 1993), which is in itself confusing, because these definitions overlap considerably.

The word adolescent is derived from the Latin word *adolescere*, meaning 'to grow to maturity' (Rice, 1999) and it is important to keep this translation in mind. Adolescence, therefore, is a transitional period between childhood and adulthood, which involves a great deal of physical, cognitive and psychosocial change (Santrock, 2001).

Since the early 1900s, developmental theorists such as Hall (1846–1924), Gesell (1880–1961), Sigmund Freud (1856–1939), Anna Freud (1895–1982), Piaget (1896–1980) and Erikson (1902–1994) have all theorised on the development of adolescents (Rice, 1999; Griffin, 2005), with diversity of opinion.

Although certain developmental milestones can be followed, adolescent development is unique for each individual. It is difficult, therefore, to categorise adolescents in specific age groups. Also, different cultures have varied markers for determining when adolescence ends and adulthood begins, for example rites of passage, marriage and employment. For the purpose of this chapter, the terms adolescent and young person will be used interchangeably and, unless otherwise stated, will refer to individuals between the ages of 10 and 24 years.

Brief overview of adolescent development

Traditionally, adolescent development has been divided into three stages: early, middle and late adolescence (Rice, 1999). More recently, however, some developmentalists have divided adolescence into two main periods: early adolescence and late adolescence (Santrock, 2001). The main points of development that occur during the stages of adolescence are briefly outlined in Table 9.1. This is only an overview of the topic and further reading in this area is recommended.

Table 9.1　Stages of adolescence.

	Early (11–14 yrs)	Middle (14–17 yrs)	Late (17–20/5 yrs)
Physical growth	Rapid growth Secondary sex characteristics appear	Decelerating growth in girls Reach 95% adult height	Physically mature Reproductive growth almost complete
Cognition	Limited abstract thought Comparisons of 'normal' with same sex peers	Abstract thinking developing Still idealistic in thoughts Concerned with political and social issues	Abstract thought established Can perceive and act on long-term issues Established functional and intellectual identity
Identity	Preoccupied with body changes Conforms to group 'norms' Attractiveness measured by rejection/acceptance by peers	Body image modified Self-centred Idealistic Variable ability to perceive future implications of behaviour	Gender role/body image almost secured Mature sexual identity Self esteem – stable Definition and articulation of social roles
Parental relationships	Defining boundaries for independence Self-conflict – need to remain dependent on parents/desire for more freedom Conflicts with parental control	Conflict-control/ independence Difficulties in parent/adolescent relationship Significant struggle for emancipation/ disengagement with final detachment from parents; period of 'loss' for parents	Emotional/physical separation from family complete Independent with less conflict Emancipation almost secured
Peer relationships	Start of peer identification Mainly same sex friendships Dating and intimacy limited	Stronger peer identification Standards of behaviour set by peer group Acceptance by peers very important/fearful of rejection	Increase in individual relationships Development of intimate relationships Relationships more reciprocal Gender role defined

Source　modified from Hockenberry *et al.*, 2003, p. 804.

Understanding chronic illness from a young person's perspective

The case study referred to in this chapter explores some of the experiences of a young person with kidney disease.

Time out

Write down what you know regarding the normal function of the kidney.

 Case study 9.1

Thomas is a 15-year-old boy, who has chronic renal failure (CRF). He lives at home in a supportive family, with both his parents and his younger brother, Sam. Thomas' father is a lorry driver and works away from home a great deal. Thomas' mother works part time as a cleaner in the local school. At the age of nine years Thomas was investigated for being small for his age, which led to the discovery of his kidney disease. Since this time, Thomas has been managed conservatively. This entails having regular blood tests, such as biochemistry and full blood counts, along with dietary interventions, taking medication and the careful monitoring and managing of symptoms that may further progress the deterioration of his renal function, for example high blood pressure and urinary tract infections (Ward, 2002; Rigden, 2003).

The management of kidney disease is complex, leading to a range of health care professionals being involved with Thomas' care. These include a paediatric nephrologist, children's renal nurse specialist, dietitian, psychologist, social worker, GP and school nurse. Since being diagnosed, Thomas has regularly visited the outpatient department of his regional specialist centre. During one of his recent appointments, the specialist paediatric nephrologist informed Thomas and his family that his condition had further deteriorated and that he would soon require dialysis or a renal transplant. Understandably, Thomas' family are anxious but Thomas himself appears to be unconcerned and refuses to discuss this with his parents or younger brother.

Thomas has always been very close to his parents, but they are becoming concerned that he seems to be spending more and more time with his friends. They believe that this is the reason he refuses to discuss his condition with them and that his friends may be influencing his behaviour. Thomas believes there is no problem with his behaviour or his friends, and he is upset about his parents' negative views towards them.

Chronic renal failure

CRF is an insidious condition, which can present in children and young people at any age. Some contemporary literature also refers to CRF as chronic kidney disease (DoH, 2006). One definition of CRF is 'glomerular filtration rate (GFR) of less than 50 ml/min/1.73m^2 surface area (SA)' (Rigden, 2003, p. 427). CRF is irreversible, usually progressive, associated with metabolic abnormalities and can adversely affect a child's growth (Ward, 2002; Rigden, 2003). Ward (2002) highlights that presenting symptoms of CRF may trigger families to access medical advice and alert health care professionals to refer and investigate the underlying causation. In Thomas' case, his kidney disease lay undetected until he was nine years old, when he presented as small for his age. Potential presentation features of CRF (Rigden, 2003) include:

- Nausea and vomiting
- Failure to thrive
- Short stature
- Urinary tract infections
- Enuresis
- Haematuria
- Hypertension
- Seizures
- Lethargy and pallor

Occasionally, the underlying cause of kidney failure is unknown, but the main causative factors of CRF in children and young people in the UK are congenital abnormalities (Rigden, 2003; DoH, 2006).

As Thomas' renal function continues to deteriorate and progress towards established renal failure, careful consideration is required regarding the choice of renal replacement therapies, such as peritoneal dialysis, haemodialysis or a pre-emptive renal transplant.

 Time out

What do you understand by the terms peritoneal dialysis, haemodialysis and pre-emptive renal transplant?

Peritoneal dialysis (PD) involves instilling dialysis fluid via a PD catheter into the peritoneal cavity. The peritoneal membrane has a good blood supply, large surface area and is semi-permeable. Waste products and excess fluids are filtered from the blood via the semi-permeable membrane by osmosis, diffusion and convection (Wild, 2002).

Haemodialysis (HD) requires venous access, specialist equipment, specialist staff and technical support, so that the patient's blood can be mechanically circulated to a haemodialyser (artificial kidney). The haemodialyser consists of synthetic semi-permeable membranes that separate the patient's blood from the dialysis fluid. The movement of fluid and solutes across the membrane takes place by the processes of diffusion, ultrafiltration and convection (Thomas, 2002).

Pre-emptive renal transplant is a renal transplant that can be performed for children and young people with chronic kidney disease before the necessity of dialysis. Compared to dialysis, renal transplantation may be viewed as the treatment of choice and optimal regarding quality of life (Ward, 2002; Rigden, 2003). However, Ward (2002) indicates that having a pre-emptive renal transplant is dependent upon the status of the patient's health, as well as donor organ availability.

In the UK, the incidence of renal failure in the adolescent population is difficult to ascertain, as some are managed within adult renal services. What is known, though, is that improvements in diagnosis and medical care have seen the survival rates in children and adolescents with a chronic illness improve dramatically (Soanes & Timmons, 2004). It is estimated that during the past 50 years, the number of young people with a chronic illness surviving to their twentieth birthday has risen considerably (Farrant & Watson, 2004). Now, almost 90% of young people with a chronic illness survive to adulthood (Sawyer, 2003). Whilst this can be viewed as a significant improvement in health care overall, it does create some challenges and have lasting implications for adolescents.

Adolescence can be a difficult period for some young people and this is compounded in the presence of chronic illness. In addition to their age-related developmental tasks, young people with a chronic illness have to deal with the demands and challenges of their condition (Meuleners et al., 2002). They need to consider the limitations their condition places upon them (Kyngäs, 2000), the uncertainty of their condition (Suris et al., 2004) and sometimes even need to confront their own mortality. Many young people with a chronic illness need to comply with medication regimes, special diets, exercise programmes (or are faced with immobility problems), regular testing/monitoring and frequent visits to health care providers (Kyngäs, 2000). In cases such as Thomas', nutritional therapy is central to CRF management, requiring the input of a children's dietitian with specialist renal knowledge and experience (Rigden, 2003). Conservative management can potentially prolong renal function, thereby extending the opportunity for normal growth and development and delaying the necessity of dialysis (Ward, 2002). These demands are invasive and affect almost every aspect of the young person's life, including school, recreation, employment, family life, and personal and social life (Kyngäs, 2000).

The psychological implications of chronic illness on children and young people are well documented (Eiser, 1990; Madden et al., 2002; Schmidt et al., 2003; Olsson et al., 2005) and these issues will be discussed later in this chapter. It is not surprising, therefore, that there are times when some adolescents have difficulty communicating their feelings and concerns, or communicating with others in general, including their parents, as highlighted by the case study.

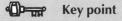 **Key point**

Adolescence can be a difficult period for some young people and this is compounded when they have a chronic illness.

Time out

Reflect on the young people that you have cared for. What potential psycho-social implications could a chronic illness have for them? Write your thoughts down.

Communicating with young people

Good communication is generally viewed as an important aspect of cohesive family functioning (Jackson *et al.*, 1998; Haven, 2001). Communication within families where an adolescent is part of the family is vitally important (Haven, 2001; Carr-Gregg & Shale, 2002). If communication is breaking down in Thomas' family, it is understandable that his parents will be concerned. Communication is key to making adolescents feel 'connected' with their families (or peers) and connectedness is a key factor in building resiliency strategies (Carr-Gregg & Shale, 2002).

In adolescence, communication patterns appear to differ between genders (Haven, 2001). Adolescent girls talk more frequently with their mothers than their fathers whereas, perhaps understandably, adolescent males are more inclined to discuss sexual issues and more generic problems with their fathers (Haven, 2001). Most young people view fathers as judgemental, whilst mothers are perceived as being more open to listening and even instigating conversation when the need arises (Haven, 2001). However, it is not uncommon for adolescents to have difficulty communicating with their families (Carr-Gregg & Shale, 2002) and this lack of communication frequently extends to health care professionals (Beresford & Sloper, 2002). A possible reason for this is that in many situations young people do not believe that their opinions are viewed as being valid by adults or indeed that they are actually listened to (Coleman *et al.*, 2005). As with any other age group, adolescents want to be shown respect, listened to and viewed as valued participants in conversation and discussion (Coleman *et al.*, 2005).

Renal failure can be life threatening, and in order to provide appropriate interventional therapies, communication pathways and information sharing between patients, their families and specialist paediatric renal health care professionals is crucial. The *NSF for Renal Services. Working for Children and Young People* (DoH, 2006) promotes delivery of patient centred services, identifying access to information as one method of achieving this goal. Watson (2003) suggests a range of strategies that may assist in sharing information, including verbal, written, video, CD-ROMs and audio taping consultations. The benefits of providing information concern reducing anxiety, assisting in the development of coping strategies and potentially improving treatment compliance (Watson, 2003).

> **◀▥▦▶ Key point**
>
> The ability to employ effective communication strategies is important in all nurse/client relationships and this is particularly important with young people. If a good rapport is not developed between health care workers and young people, open channels of communication will not be maintained and a trusting relationship will not be formed.

In 1995, Sanci and Young developed some guidelines for communication with young people. Although this was primarily aimed at GPs, the principles within this paper are equally applicable to nurses and other health care providers.

⌚ Time out

Before reading the next section, try this short exercise to help you develop an understanding of your current communication skills.

- Think about the way in which you currently communicate with young people – you may want to make some notes.
- Write a list of the strategies you think would be important when communicating with young people.

The communication strategies outlined in Table 9.2 are predominantly based on the work of Sanci and Young (1995) and the experience of the authors of this chapter, and are given to help you develop your communication skills with young people. However, the importance of developing effective communication strategies when working with young people is highlighted by a number of authors (e.g. Wheal, 1999; Beresford & Sloper, 2002; Christie & Viner, 2005). How do these match with your notes?

> **◀▥▦▶ Key point**
>
> The ability to employ effective communication strategies is particularly important with young people.

Communication issues for Thomas

It would be important to encourage Thomas to discuss his concerns with his parents and try to reach some agreement regarding his friends and his association with them. Parents and adolescents often have disagreements about friendships,

Table 9.2   Useful communication strategies.

Useful communication strategies	
Be yourself	When attempting to develop communication channels with young people, above all you should be yourself. Be friendly, relaxed and responsive but do not try to be something you are not. Adolescents have an ability to 'see through' people and will quickly establish whether the person they are dealing with is the 'real you'. You do not need to try to talk or dress like an adolescent (unless you do normally) and this type of behaviour can actually hamper your ability to communicate effectively with young people.
Be flexible	Although adolescents value consistency, there is also a need to be flexible in your approach to communication. A rigid approach could be viewed as being confrontational and can often make young people 'dig in their heels' and be reluctant to respond to your efforts. This again has the potential to impede effective communication.
Establish confidentiality	Confidentiality is a very important issue for young people and this has been discussed in depth in Chapter 8. It is, however, important to remember that unconditional, complete confidence should not be promised to adolescents, and guidelines should be established, before they disclose anything to you. Therefore, if the adolescent wishes to disclose something, it is better to suggest at the outset that any conversation will be kept confidential providing their (or anyone else's) safety is currently, or potentially, not compromised.
Listen	Always listen to what young people tell you, be attentive and look as if you are listening and interested in what they have to say. As adolescents belong to a group that generally have little attention paid to what they have to say, being listened to is important to them. During your conversation, you may find that the adolescent deviates from the topic or your particular line of questioning. If the adolescent is inclined to talk, it is important to let them identify what is important to them and you can always bring the conversation back to where you would like it to be at a later time.
Be informed	As with all patients/clients, it is vitally important that any information you provide is factual and accurate. However, whether we are clinical nurses or educators, we are not endless vaults of knowledge and there will be times when you may not know the answer to a question the young person may ask. If you do not know the answer, admit it, but ensure that you find out the answer and convey this to the adolescent as soon as you can.
Be consistent	Adolescents value consistency. Therefore, within any area of practice, providing there are no specific contraindications (e.g. changes in medical management or safety issues), what is appropriate today should be appropriate tomorrow and the next day. Any rules and guidelines need to be consistent to enable the young person to establish her/his boundaries. Inconsistent guidelines and rules become confusing and can sometimes lead to confrontational behaviour where the young person may be viewed as being disruptive or non-compliant.

Table 9.2   (*cont'd*)

Useful communication strategies	
Use understandable language	When you need to provide information to adolescents, make sure that it is in easy to follow terms that are free of medical/nursing jargon and presented in a way that is easy for them to follow. Try to present the information in blocks of no more than two sentences at a time, and allow time for the adolescent to ask questions. Patience may be required because, if there is something they are not able to understand, you may need to provide the information a few times and in easier to follow language. This is acceptable practice when dealing with parents and adult patients, and providing information to adolescents should not be any different.
Remember, you are not indispensable	Establishing a good relationship with a young person is not the same as being indispensable. Establishing relationships with adolescents where they/you believe that you are the best person to deliver their care or understand their needs is not conducive to their overall well-being. The management and care of a young person with a chronic illness, regardless of the setting, is continuous and generally undertaken using a multidisciplinary team approach. Although there will always be times when we are able to relate to one person better than another, it is important to remember that the provision of care is a team effort and no 'player' is more important than another.

Source   adapted from Sanci & Young, 1995.

with parents frequently suggesting that friends are a 'bad influence' or blaming the friendship on the changing relationships at home. In some situations, parents can be right and certain friends may be an undesirable influence. There is even suggestion that parents can manipulate their adolescents towards certain friendships and away from others, by organising their social activities (Steinberg, 2001). However, in many situations, disagreements occur because adolescents are passing through the developmental stage where they are testing boundaries, have the desire for more freedom and are expanding their social circle (Rice, 1999; Rew, 2005).

Peer groups

During early adolescence, young people usually begin to develop a wider circle of friends. Although some young people attend the same school from preparatory to senior level, many will change schools at the commencement of secondary education. Young people are exposed to different people who come from a larger geographical area and as a consequence new friendships and peer groups are formed. Peer group formation is an important developmental phase, as during this time young people are developing their ability to interact socially (Carr-Gregg & Shale, 2002). During this phase, young people can also learn to interact with individuals from different regional, societal, religious and ethnic backgrounds. As adolescents are still maturing, they have not fully developed their identities and personalities (Rice, 1999), and this can lead to adolescents becoming anxious and insecure about themselves as individuals. Socialising with a close knit group of peers allows adolescents to learn from each other, form their own identity, increase their self-esteem and develop the social and societal skills that are necessary for them to become part of an adult society (Rice, 1999; Tarrant, 2002).

Adolescents who have a good relationship with their peers have an increased sense of 'well-being' (Tarrant, 2002, p. 110) and those who are unable to achieve acceptance during this developmental stage can become lonely, experience feelings of rejection and in some instances become depressed (Farrant & Watson, 2004). This is of particular significance for young people who have a chronic illness. Some may spend varying amounts of time away from school and/or in hospital and consequently have difficulty maintaining contact with their peer group. This, in conjunction with the presence of a chronic illness, can have a detrimental effect on the young person's overall psychological, social and physical well-being.

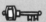 **Key point**

Socialising with a close knit group of peers allows adolescents to learn from each other, form their own identity, increase their self-esteem and develop the social and societal skills that are necessary to enable them to become part of an adult society.

To gain a deeper understanding of the importance of the peer group you may wish to read Tarrant (2002).

The impact of chronic illness on growth and development

 Case study 9.2

Developmental issues

Until recently Thomas has had a good relationship with his peers. However, as an adolescent with a chronic illness, Thomas is not developing physically at the same rate as his peers. As his condition deteriorates, his short stature and small physique is becoming more obvious to his friends and he is unable to keep up with them psychosocially and educationally. It has been noticed that even when in warm environments Thomas, unfashionably, prefers to wear bulky clothes. This, coupled with his moody behaviour and his reluctance to engage in group activities, has led his parents to question whether he is developing poor body image and low self-esteem.

🕐 **Time out**

It is recognised that having a chronic illness has a significant overall impact on the individual. Take some time out to consider the following questions.

- How do you think a chronic illness impacts on the physical growth and development of young people?
- In what way does this have the potential to affect their psychosocial development?

Delayed growth and puberty

Most young people with chronic illness have some degree of delayed growth and puberty (including delayed menstruation in girls). This most commonly occurs when the condition incorporates an element of malnutrition, for example in conditions such as cystic fibrosis (Suris *et al.*, 2004), and inflammatory bowel disease studies show that adolescents with chronic diarrhoea have delayed linear growth (Sawczenko & Sandu, 2003). This situation can result in adolescents being smaller than their peers in height and overall physique. In some situations, the delay may be temporary and the adolescent will 'catch up' with her/his peers over time. However, in adolescents with CRF, this does not always occur and the administration of a growth hormone would be carefully considered (Rigden, 2003).

Inconsistencies between physical and psychological development

As physical and psychosocial development are significantly interrelated, any alteration in the timing of one can have a detrimental effect on the other (Suris *et al.*, 2004). It is important, therefore, that the effects of delayed puberty on the adolescent's psychosocial development are not underestimated. Although delayed pubertal development can affect both boys and girls, it can have a particularly adverse effect on boys (Suris *et al.*, 2004) due to the importance that boys place on their physical (muscular) development. Therefore, in boys, it is not uncommon for delayed puberty to result in low levels of self-esteem and varying degrees of depression.

People's attitudes towards young people who are smaller than their peers can be an issue. It is not uncommon for adolescents with delayed growth/puberty to be treated as less mature than their age, and they may experience difficulty gaining autonomy and independence from their parents, as their outward appearance may suggest immaturity. For older adolescents, this can pose a problem when they try to gain employment as they are frequently viewed as being younger than their chronological age (Suris *et al.*, 2004). It is demeaning for young people to continue to be thought of as children, particularly when they have a far greater level of understanding than children. It is understandable, therefore, that delayed growth/puberty can have an adverse effect on adolescents' overall well-being, particularly regarding body image and self-esteem, which can lead to mental health and behavioural problems. It is not unusual for young people with a chronic illness to be depressed and have suicidal thoughts (Smith *et al.*, 2003; Suris *et al.*, 2004).

Reflection

Reflect on your own adolescence and young people you have cared for.

- What do you understand by body image?
- What can influence people's perceptions of body image?
- What can be the consequences of having a poor body image?

Body image and self-esteem

Body image is defined as the way in which we perceive ourselves and the way in which we believe others perceive us. Individuals can view this in both a positive and a negative way. The importance of body image to adolescents has long been established. With regard to bodily perception, there are certain differences noted between genders, with girls being more dissatisfied than boys, particularly during puberty. This is probably because girls experience a redistribution and increase of fat deposits. Boys, however, tend to be more satisfied with their body image due to an increase in muscle mass as they move through puberty (Santrock, 2001). As we have already noted, this is in direct contrast to the perceptions of adolescent boys who have a chronic illness that is associated with pubertal/growth delay.

During adolescence, young people become preoccupied with their bodies and develop individual perceptions of what their bodies are actually like (Santrock, 2001) and the way they would like them to be. These expectations are often unrealistic and it could be argued that young people's perceptions of what is 'normal' are heavily swayed by the influence of the media (Chow, 2004). Although adolescents' preoccupation with their body continues throughout adolescence, it is at its strongest point during puberty when, generally due to physical changes in bodily shape, they are more dissatisfied with their bodies than towards the end of adolescence (Santrock, 2001).

Any condition that may affect growth, or a disfigurement (e.g. burns, amputations, scarring), which has the potential to alter adolescents' perception of their body image, or how they believe others perceive them, can have an overall detrimental effect on adolescents (Bill, 1999). Being attractive to others is important to adolescents, as they believe this will make them more accepted by their peers. Adolescents believe that if they are viewed as attractive, their peers will think of them in more positive terms, for example friendly, successful and intelligent (Bill, 1999). Although this may seem to be an unrealistic belief, evidence does suggest that there is a direct link between the way adolescents look and the way they are treated by their peers (Koff *et al.*, 1990).

This concept of the perception of attractiveness in adolescence is supported by research undertaken by Koff *et al.* (1990), who found that 'attractive' adolescents are generally more popular than their 'less attractive' peers. Although the work by Koff *et al.* was undertaken a number of years ago, there is no evidence to suggest that adolescents' feelings and beliefs have altered in any way. To the contrary, studies undertaken since Koff *et al.* have continued to demonstrate the damaging effect of chronic illness on adolescents' body image and self-esteem (Sawyer *et al.*, 1995).

Adolescents who are thought of in more positive terms are also found to have higher levels of self-esteem, healthier personalities and achieve a wider variety of social and interpersonal skills. Conversely, adolescents who are thought of in less positive terms and do not enjoy the same level of popularity can experience negative effects on their personality and self-esteem. These include lack of connectedness, social exclusion and depression.

In Thomas' situation, as he is already less physically developed than his peers, it is possible that he has developed a negative body image and low self-esteem. If he is no longer able to keep up with his peers, he may begin to feel socially isolated and depressed. Young people are preoccupied with their 'ideal' body image and if this is altered in any way it can easily lead to feelings of inadequacy. They begin to question the effectiveness of their bodies and, because adolescents are not always comfortable with verbalising their feelings, insecurity can manifest itself through non-compliance with management programmes, experimentation or even risk taking behaviour (Bill, 1999).

Health adjustment can be difficult and some young people and their families may experience periods of depression or behavioural changes (Rigden, 2003). To meet the psychological and social needs of children and adolescents with renal problems and their families, the British Association for Paediatric Nephrology (BAPN) (2003) identified the need for psychosocial services to be available within paediatric renal teams. Maintaining a cohesive and supportive family relationship is vitally important as evidence suggests that a supportive relationship with one or more parents (or other care giver) is crucial to adolescents, as this promotes resilience (Jackson *et al.*, 1997; Smokowski *et al.*, 1999) and an increased ability to cope with their illness (Haase, 2004).

Key point

During adolescence, young people become preoccupied with their bodies and develop individual perceptions concerning what their bodies are actually like.

Compliance and non-compliance

It has already been established that young people experience significant physical and psychosocial changes during adolescence. The presence of a chronic illness is an added pressure that challenges adolescents' ability to eat what they should, take the medication they need, attend medical appointments and adhere to demanding management programmes. At the same time, they are expected to juggle their home, school and social life and be a 'normal' adolescent. It is not surprising, therefore, that some young people are unable to meet the expectations of health care professionals, their families and even themselves regarding the management of their condition.

Reflection

Reflect on young people with chronic illnesses that you have cared for. Can you consider reasons why they may not be compliant with their care management plans?

Without using a general dictionary definition, which suggests that to be 'compliant' is to be 'obedient' (*Oxford Dictionary*, 2002), it is difficult to establish an accepted definition of compliance within a health care setting. As a consequence, terms such as 'adherence', 'cooperation' and 'mutuality' have been used as alternatives (Kyngäs, 2000). Although it is important for young people to adhere to management programmes, compliance within adolescent health care involves more than the individual just obediently following instructions or guidelines (Kyngäs, 2000). In 1995, Blair and Bowes suggested that compliance within the health care setting could be defined as 'the extent to which behaviour coincides with advice' (p. 2037). More recently, Kyngäs (2000) viewed adolescents who are compliant with their management as those who demonstrate an active and responsible approach to managing their care whilst working in collaboration with health care professionals. By definition, this means that adolescents who are non-compliant are not able or willing to achieve this level of approach to managing their care. Although the Kyngäs (2000) view would probably be the preferred definition, it is Blair and Bowes (1995) who possibly more realistically describe the achievement of compliance within adolescent health. Young people are not always compliant with their management and this viewpoint provides a more flexible approach with regard to addressing the issues.

Non-compliance *is* an issue to consider when discussing the management of young people who have a chronic illness. It is difficult to ascertain the exact numbers of adolescents who do not comply with their management programmes as the collection of this sort of data is heavily reliant on self-reporting. However, there are some conditions where compliance can be estimated based on blood test results or lung function tests, which provide an indication of the level of compliance. Generally though, it is suggested that more than 50% of adolescents with a chronic illness are non-compliant (Blair & Bowes, 1995), with no evidence to suggest that compliance has improved since Blair and Bowes undertook their study.

More recently, Kyngäs (2000) undertook a large study of adolescents (n = 1061) with a variety of chronic illnesses, the findings from which suggested that respondents who believed their compliance was 'good' were in the minority (23%). Most respondents believed their compliance to be 'satisfactory' (60%) whilst 17% admitted to 'poor' compliance (Kyngäs, 2000). Again, this study is based on self-reporting and the adolescents' 'honesty' when reporting their level of compliance. Additionally, an individual's perception of what is 'satisfactory' will vary considerably, and it is possible that some adolescents who identified themselves as 'satisfactory' in this study would, if challenged, be deemed less compliant by health care professionals than reported.

Young people with a chronic illness do not set out to be non-compliant. Coping with adolescence and a chronic illness is not easy, and it could be suggested that sometimes it is just too difficult for them to be compliant. Attitudes towards health, the length and complexity of treatment, and culture can all have an effect on individuals' level of compliance (Muscari, 1998). However, there is evidence to suggest that some young people use non-compliance as a manipulative tool, for example to control relationships (Muscari, 1998). As Hentinen and Kyngäs (1996) point out, adolescents may use non-compliance as a way of asserting independence and resisting the authority of parents and health care professionals. Also, young people do not want to be different to their peers (Rice, 1999), an issue that sometimes results in non-compliance, for example drinking alcohol, which in some conditions can cause side effects. Young people desire peer acceptance, which we know is sometimes difficult to achieve for young people with chronic illness (Koff et al., 1990), and the importance of the peer group to adolescents is potentially a significant influencing factor in relation to compliance. Therefore, in some situations, involving peers during an adolescent's hospital admission can improve their acceptance of restrictions.

Just as there are factors that influence non-compliance, there are factors that influence compliance. Family support and motivation have a positive impact and can enhance the adolescent's level of compliance (Kyngäs, 2000; Kyngäs & Rissansen, 2001). Kyngäs (2000) suggests that fear concerning the potential long-term complications associated with a condition is another motivator for compliance, for example diabetes, where non-compliance and subsequent poor glycaemic control increases the risk of developing retinopathy, neuropathy and nephropathy (Robinson et al., 1995). On the other hand, some adolescents 'live for today' and do not see themselves vulnerable to complications, holding the view that 'it will never happen to me' (Timms & Lowes, 1999).

Even when an adolescent is generally well managed and compliant, the potential for non-compliance always exists. Increased stress at school, changes in medical management or an alteration in the adolescent's developmental phase can influence the level of compliance. Although adolescents should be encouraged and trusted to manage their condition, it is important to keep the potential problem of non-compliance in mind when managing their health care needs. This will help ensure that young people are provided with the support and encouragement they need to assist them in their decision making process (Kyngäs & Rissansen, 2001).

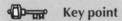 **Key point**

The issue of non-compliance needs to be kept in mind when discussing the management of young people who have a chronic illness.

The social aspects of chronic illness

 Case study 9.3

Currently, Thomas is at a crucial stage in his schooling. Despite his past hospital admissions and numerous visits to the outpatient department, he has been maintaining an average level of academic attainment. A contributing factor to his education has been his parents' diligence in ensuring that he attends school, as Thomas dislikes school and would not attend if he were given the choice.

As Thomas' renal function continued to deteriorate, he presented with some of the clinical symptoms of uraemia, which include nausea and vomiting. As a result, Thomas' renal disease has not only impacted on his time away from school for clinic appointments, but also on his ability to concentrate on academic studies. Lethargy is also a symptom of Thomas' condition, which can adversely affect his ability to participate in his favourite sporting activities.

 Time out

Before reading the next section, take some time out to consider some of the wider social implications of having a chronic illness for young people and their families. You may want to make some notes and then compare them with the content of the next section.

Young people, chronic illness and school

School plays an important part in adolescent development both academically and socially (Haven, 2001). Peer groups are formed and extended during the school years and it is important for all young people to be a part of this. However, not all young people adjust well to school and truancy is a widespread problem throughout the UK (Coles, 2005). For some young people trying to cope with a chronic illness, school can be an added 'stress'. It can be an equally stressful issue for adolescents who have a newly diagnosed illness (e.g. epilepsy/diabetes) when they return to school for the first time, or for young people who have an existing condition.

It is important for young people with a chronic illness to be treated as 'normally' as possible. This includes attending school regularly, but many adolescents with chronic illness do miss varying amounts of school, which disrupts their peer group contact and results in them missing vital educational activities. This potentially impacts on their long-term career goals and financial independence as adults (Suris *et al.*, 2004). In some situations, adolescents with chronic illness are unable to attend school (Suris *et al.*, 2004), which can mean they have additional issues of loneliness and isolation to contend with, which can in turn lead to depression.

Some adolescents with chronic illness miss so much school that they constantly need to play 'catch up' with missed work and have difficulty grasping the new work being taught when they return to school. Where the volume of work needed to 'catch up' is deemed too great, it may be recommended that they repeat a school year. When this occurs, it is understandable that adolescents feel left out, insecure, have low self-esteem and, given the opportunity, would not attend school, so that 'school avoidance' becomes a problem. In Thomas' case, striving to provide educational opportunities for him is challenging. Collier and Watson (1994) offer practical measures to assist adolescents with renal problems maintain their schooling. They suggest that, where possible, hospitalisation is minimised to limit disruption of schooling, there is promotion of continuity of schoolwork through educational liaison between hospital and community school and, where appropriate, the provision of home tutoring services.

Although most hospitals employ teachers, many of these may be primary school teachers (Taylor & Müller, 1995), which emphasises the importance of adolescents maintaining contact with their own schools. In today's technological society, email and facsimile facilities can be used during extended periods of time in hospital (condition permitting) so that young people do not miss too much schoolwork. To optimise career opportunities later in life, young people should be encouraged to continue with their schooling to maximise their potential.

Having a chronic illness does not mean that young people are unable to succeed in life. As the life expectancy of young people with a chronic illness continues to increase, it is important that all aspects of their lifestyle are promoted in a positive way. The writers have known young people with chronic illnesses who have achieved higher degrees and others who have been barely able to read and write. With regard to school and education, young people need support, encouragement and realistic career counselling. The school nurse has an important role to play concerning the care of young people with a chronic illness, and it is vital that nurses caring for adolescents with chronic illness liaise closely with school nurses in an attempt to provide a well balanced level of care.

In the case study, Thomas' continued attendance at school was mainly due to his parents' perseverance and encouragement. This is an important point, because it is recognised that parental support and the way parents communicate with adolescents play a significant role in ensuring that they continue at school (Haven, 2001). However, for many adolescents, the decision to stay on in school is often dependent on a variety of factors, including access to amenities and the level of support and services provided by the school, particularly when young people are physically disabled.

Bullying

 Time out

Before reading the next section, answer the following questions.

- What types of bullying can occur?
- What are the possible effects of bullying on the young person?

It would be negligent to review school issues and not discuss bullying. Bullying is a significant problem throughout schools in the UK. However, this is not a situation unique to UK schools, as both the USA and Australia also have considerable problems with school bullying (Haven, 2001). Bullying presents in a variety of forms and can include physical and verbal abuse, teasing, being taunted and threatened, and name-calling. It is more common for boys to experience physical violence than girls, particularly in the lower school years (Haven, 2001) but violence by girls appears to be occurring more frequently.

It is not uncommon for young people with a chronic illness, or those with physical or cognitive impairment, to experience bullying in school. The inability to 'fit in' with the peer group, being different, needing to take medication in school or just not being able to keep up with their peers is a potential 'reason' for bullying. It is important to recognise that bullying is a reality for some young people with chronic illness, as this can add to the negative issues surrounding body image and self-esteem, in addition to school avoidance.

Key point

Bullying is a significant problem throughout schools in the UK and this is a stark reality for some young people with a chronic illness as this can add to the negative issues surrounding body image and self-esteem, in addition to school avoidance.

 Case study 9.4

Recently, Thomas has been admitted to hospital following further deterioration of his renal function. His parents and health care professionals suspect that this is as a direct result of non-adherence to his conservative management regime. Following assessment by the multidisciplinary team, a number of issues have been identified. In relation to Thomas' CRF, he needs more frequent monitoring of his renal function, which involves additional blood analysis, careful adjustment of his conservative management and open discussions regarding his future renal therapy, for example dialysis and/or renal transplantation. From a psychosocial perspective, Thomas needs further support and encouragement to help him through this difficult phase of his development and medical care. Whilst the whole of the MDT are involved, the youth worker, social worker and clinical psychologist play key roles in his psychosocial care.

⏲ **Time out**

There has been much discussion regarding the appropriate placing of young people within a hospital setting. For this exercise consider:

- The appropriateness of children's and adult wards for adolescent patients
- The facilities that would be important to hospitalised adolescents

The hospitalised adolescent

The debate regarding the most suitable place to care for young people in hospital is long-standing. It is generally suggested that neither adult nor children's wards are appropriate for young people, and adolescents frequently find hospitalisation a restricting, stressful experience (Hutton, 2005). If they are managed on adult wards, they may be placed near dying elderly patients (Taylor & Müller, 1995) and on some children's wards, the age range is far too great to accommodate young people appropriately.

If adolescents are viewed as a distinct group for developmental purposes, then it is important that their development is taken into account when we manage them as patients. The need to care for adolescents as a developmentally distinct group within the health care setting was identified towards the end of the 1950s in the *Platt Report* (Ministry of Health, 1959). However, despite continued evidence (e.g. the Court Report, 1976) supporting this belief, very little appears to have changed in the UK for young people who need to be hospitalised (Miller, 1995; Russell-Johnson, 2000).

In 2003, the Royal College of Paediatricians and Child Health (RCPCH) produced the document: *Bridging the Gaps: Health Care for Adolescents*. It suggested that, despite the many adolescents who use health care services and the recognition of the need to manage them as a distinct group, services for young people are limited. Within the primary care setting, the RCPCH (2003) describe specific general practice facilities for young people as 'rare' (p. 19) and specific outpatient services, where they existed, predominantly focused either on specific conditions (e.g. diabetes) or on the transition from children's to adult services.

The effect of hospitalisation on adolescents has been well documented over many years (Stevens, 1987; MacKenzie, 1988; Gillies & Parry-Jones, 1992; Taylor & Müller, 1995; Kelly & Hewson, 2000). Ultimately, the evidence suggests that adolescents need to be managed within a specialised age appropriate adolescent unit by staff specifically educated in the care of young people (Taylor & Müller, 1995; British Medical Association (BMA) Board of Science, 2003). However, the Royal College of Nursing (2002), in an examination of in-patient services in the UK, only identified 13 dedicated adolescent wards, 16 limited facility units attached to children's wards and 5 adolescent oncology wards.

Issues for young people in hospital

Many of the issues for young people who are hospitalised are purely logistical, particularly when they are cared for on children's wards that are more appropriately targeted towards young children. Children's wards are not always able to provide the facilities that adolescents need and some of the issues raised by young people concerning children's wards are outlined below:

- Small beds and other furniture items
- Décor aimed at children
- Poorly fitting bed curtains that inhibit privacy
- Lack of privacy overall
- Afternoon 'rest' times
- Inflexible rules and regulations
- Being located near small children and crying babies
- Lack of quiet area for young people to study
- Recreation facilities aimed at small children
- Limited opportunity to talk with people of their own age
- Small bathroom facilities, with no locks on doors (Taylor & Muller, 1995; Watson, 2003; Hutton, 2005)

From a child's perspective, it could be suggested that it is also inappropriate for children to be located in close proximity to older adolescents. For example, adolescents, by definition of their age, can watch television programmes and movies that are not suitable for children. Likewise, not all contemporary music enjoyed by adolescents is appropriate for children. Additionally, many adolescents are as physically developed as adults, and as we would not place children and adults on a ward together, careful consideration should also be given to accommodating children and adolescents on the same wards.

In addition to the physical needs of young people, thought also needs to be given to the psychosocial needs of hospitalised adolescents. The importance of the peer group has already been discussed and maintaining peer group contact whilst in hospital is vitally important. Hospitalised adolescents who are unable to maintain contact with their peer group can develop the perception of having lost their status within their peer group and this can be very worrying for them (Hutton, 2005). It should be noted, however, that not all young people with a chronic illness want to be visited by their peers, and many who require frequent admissions often develop a peer group of friends with similar conditions within the hospital setting. It is important, therefore, to assess each situation individually and where appropriate visits by peers should be encouraged.

Young people who are admitted to children's wards frequently complain about a lack of privacy. Adolescent males who may already have facial hair and need to shave do not necessarily want to share a bathroom with a five-year-old (Taylor & Muller, 1995). Lack of privacy raises another important issue – sexuality.

Sexual development is an integral part of adolescent development (Rice, 1999) and young people with chronic illness are no different. Although puberty and sexual development may sometimes be delayed, having a chronic illness does not preclude young people from having an interest in sexual matters. Horseman

(2005) described her 'excruciating embarrassment' (p. 27) when, on two separate occasions on a children's ward, she accidentally encountered adolescent boys masturbating, and cites this issue alone as a reason for adolescents needing extra privacy. In addition to sexuality issues and privacy, nurses caring for adolescents also need to consider the issues of confidentiality (Sanci *et al.*, 2005), negotiating care, promoting autonomy, decision making (Spear & Kulbok, 2004) and managing more 'adult' behaviour, such as smoking, swearing and on occasion the use of alcohol or 'recreational' drugs.

What this situation does highlight, however, is that adolescents clearly have distinctly different needs to children, and what is normal behaviour for them is not necessarily appropriate in the presence of younger children. Furthermore, it emphasises that young people need to be cared for by health professionals who have an understanding of their development needs, issues surrounding confidentiality and privacy and have an interest in and feel comfortable working with them.

 Key point

It is not appropriate to admit young people to adult wards as this can be a distressing experience for them and lead to altered impressions of illness (Taylor & Müller, 1995). Children's wards are also inappropriate to meet adolescents' psychosocial and physical developmental needs. The ideal situation is to admit young people to wards dedicated to this specific age group, where their individual needs can be recognised and met by appropriately qualified staff.

Specialised adolescent units

Adolescent units are wards where the speciality is 'adolescence', and are specifically designed based on young people's needs. Quite often, adolescents are able to have input into the development of these units and the facilities they provide, which is particularly relevant, because understanding the needs of individuals using such units is vital (Hutton, 2005). Although there is considerable debate relating to the current level of in-patient facilities for young people, and whether the focus of adolescent units should be specialist or generic, the UK lags behind the rest of the developed world in the commissioning of adolescent units. Encouragingly, a specialist purpose built Teenage Cancer Trust Unit opened in Wales in 2006, which accommodates young people up to the age of 24 years. Nevertheless, in the USA, there are between 40 and 60 units spaced throughout the country, and in Australia and many European and Scandinavian countries, there is an ever increasing development of adolescent units (RCPCH, 2003).

Generally, the aims of such units are to assist young people to gain autonomy and start to take some responsibility for and make decisions about their care. It is important to facilitate decision making in young people (Miller, 2001) as they will ultimately become responsible for managing their own care. Ward rules and guidelines on adolescent units are flexible and more appropriate to the needs of young people (Women and Children's Hospital, 2004). Additionally, there are usually separate recreation facilities and facilities for adolescents to make themselves drinks or snacks and entertain their friends. The staff would also be well versed in issues surrounding adolescent competency, consent and confidentiality. Health promotion specific to the needs of young people (e.g. smoking and sexual health) can also be undertaken.

⏱ Time out

Please review Chapter 5 regarding the principles of health promotion and education before moving on to the next section of this chapter.

How do you think these principles can be adapted when working in partnership with young people?

Dedicated adolescent units are usually staffed by a multidisciplinary team educated in-house by their employing hospital regarding adolescent health issues to ensure they are responsive to young people's needs. Some staff will hold specific qualifications in adolescent health, but finding appropriately qualified staff to work on adolescent units may pose a problem in the UK, because, as identified at the Trust for the Study of Adolescence (TSA) Conference in June 2005 (personal communication), there is only one physician qualified in adolescent health in the country. Additionally, unlike in Australia, where formal tertiary level courses in adolescent health have existed for some time, there are currently limited formalised courses for nurses specific to adolescent health in the UK.

There has been a long-standing requirement that children aged 16 years and under need to be cared for by children's nurses (Needham, 2000), an undisputed issue, as it is vitally important that appropriately qualified staff care for children and young people. What is questionable, though, is whether there is sufficient adolescent health content in current pre-registration Child Branch courses to provide children's nurses with the knowledge to be able to care for young people appropriately. It could also be questioned whether nurses specialising in condition specific roles (e.g. cystic fibrosis, diabetes) have sufficient opportunity to gain appropriate education in adolescent health. Viner and Keane (1998) promote the development of an adolescent specialist nurse role, and suggest that health care professionals who work with young people need 'core skills' and additional specialist education. Therefore, the development of education programmes for nurses, doctors and allied health professionals should be urgently prioritised to ensure that Britain keeps pace with other countries and meets the needs of adolescents.

Case study 9.5

Conclusion

As part of Thomas' continued management, he will be encouraged to maintain communication and contact with the MDT (multidisciplinary team); this may include the ongoing use of support and counselling services. Thomas will be encouraged to be more proactive in the management of his own health care needs and work closely with his parents to manage his care. A health promotion and education plan is negotiated and agreed with Thomas and his family.

Effective health education for families with children and young people with renal failure is vital to maintain residual renal function and prepare for future health care needs. At Thomas' stage of development it would be important to ensure that he was provided with appropriate information regarding his condition. Involving Thomas in devising his health management plan should enable him to start taking some responsibility for his care, as well as encourage independence and compliance. However, the complexity of renal disease, coupled with the unique experience of adolescence can prove to be challenging. Therefore, health education should be centralised around the needs of Thomas, but take into account the vital, supportive role of his family, thus ensuring the development of a 'family friendly service' (DoH, 2006).

Service delivery and adolescent health

 Time out

For this final exercise:

- Identify the role of the nurse within the MDT specific to the care of young people.
- Consider the role of the children's nurse in facilitating the link between young people and their smooth transition to adult hospital services.

Promoting excellence

Approximately one in five children and young people with chronic illness use health care services but despite this there is limited evidence of involvement of this group in service development (Sloper & Lightfoot, 2003); this has been discussed in Chapter 2. If we are truly to address the needs of young people this is a situation that needs significant revision. A good starting point would be to develop the role of adolescent health nurses, which would send a clear message to young people that health care services are actually interested in addressing their needs.

The document *Guidance for Paediatric Nephrology Nurses* (RCN, 2000) was developed by a working group of children's renal nurses. It identifies that children's renal nurses are striving to promote standards of care, and acknowledges the need to work in a collaborative manner and that nurses working within this specialist field should have access to specialist paediatric renal nursing training (RCN, 2000). The need to provide children, young people and their families with quality renal services and care is also supported within the *NSF for Renal Services* (DoH, 2006).

The role of the nurse

The role of the nurse working with young people, as with all patients, is multi-faceted. Predominantly, though, the adolescent nurse would need to work in the best interest of young people, promoting autonomy and independence, and acting as an advocate by making sure that adolescents' voices are heard within the health care setting. Acting as a liaison between adolescents, their families and the MDT is as important as working comfortably within a MDT setting. The nurse working with young people would need to be committed to and interested in the health of young people, be able to communicate with them effectively and demonstrate a sound knowledge of adolescent physical and psychosocial development (Needham, 2000). Additionally, the adolescent health nurse would promote adherence to a healthy lifestyle and undertake health promotion specifically addressing the needs of young people. The main health promotion themes important to young people are smoking, the use of alcohol and recreational drugs, contraception, sexual health and safeguarding themselves from harm and abuse, and it is vital that they are provided with the correct information about these issues.

Part of the role of the nurse working with young people should also encompass working towards the development or improvement of transitional services, including developing trust wide policies and guidance. Disseminating information, networking and the establishment of research pathways within adolescent health would also be important aspects of this role.

MDT working across agencies and organisations is vital to the care of adolescents, to ensure a cohesive, continuing care approach between health, social care and educational settings. Therefore, a considerable aspect of the adolescent health nurse's role is liaison with staff from these areas to facilitate open communication and enable care pathways to be holistic and to span all areas where the adolescent is based, be it at home, school or in hospital. Working within the MDT, adolescent health nurses could coordinate a smooth transition process for the adolescent from children and young people's services to adult services. They would ensure that adolescents and their families were provided with the appropriate education and information and act as advocates in this area to make sure the needs of adolescents and their families were addressed and their voices heard. Transition of care is reviewed in detail in Chapter 10.

Conclusion

Adolescence is a time of rapid growth and physiological development. Managing a chronic condition during this time is a significant challenge for young people, their family and health care providers (Suris *et al.*, 2004). Adolescents are a distinct group of individuals that require their specific health care needs to be addressed and effectively managed (Needham, 2000) by appropriately educated staff (Viner & Keane, 1998).

Thomas and other young people with a chronic illness have to contend with the developmental changes experienced during adolescence and the constraints placed on them by their condition. This is not easy for many adolescents and there is the potential for stress related conditions and depression to occur. However, with support from families, friends and health care professionals, many young people are generally able to manage their condition, reach their full potential and lead independent and productive lives.

Key points

- Adolescence is a time of rapid growth, development and change, which can be a difficult period for some young people. Any potential difficulties experienced during adolescence can be compounded by the presence of chronic illness.
- Adolescents have distinctly different needs to children, and what is normal behaviour for them is not necessarily appropriate in the presence of children. Therefore, it is inappropriate for them to be cared for on the same ward, and the development of specialised adolescent units is advocated.
- The ability to employ effective communication strategies is particularly important when working with young people to help ensure compliance and facilitate health education, in assessment of psychosocial problems and in enabling their independence.
- The role of the nurse working with young people is important and multi-faceted and needs to be undertaken by individuals who have an interest in adolescent health and a competent level of skill and knowledge in this area.
- Adolescents are a distinct group of individuals that need to have their specific health care needs addressed and effectively managed (Needham, 2000) by appropriately educated staff (Viner & Keane, 1998).

Useful websites

British Medical Association (Adolescent Health Report): www.bma.org.uk
Department of Health: http://www.dh.gov.uk/Home/fs/en
Nephrology at your fingertips: http://www.nephronline.org/
Royal College of Paediatrics and Child Health (*Bridging the Gaps*): www.rcpch.ac.uk

The UK Renal Association: http://www.renal.org/index.html
Trust for the Study of Adolescence: www.tsa.uk.com
UK National Kidney Federation Young Person Group: http://www.kidney.org.uk/ypg/index.html
www.talktofrank.com
www.teenagehealthfreak.org

Recommended reading

Hockenberry, M., Wilson, D., Winklestein, M.L. & Klein, N.E. (2003) *Wong's Nursing Care of Infants and Children* (seventh edition.). St Louis, Mosby.

Rice, F.P. (1999) *The Adolescent: Development, Relationships and Culture* (ninth edition). Boston, Allyn and Bacon.

Santrock, J.W. (2001) *Adolescence* (eighth edition). Boston, McGraw Hill.

Ward, G. (2002) Renal care in childhood and adolescence. In: *Renal Nursing* (ed. N. Thomas) (second edition). London, Baillière Tindall.

Webb, N. & Postelthwaite, R. (eds) (2003) *Clinical Paediatric Nephrology* (third edition). New York, Oxford University Press.

References

Beresford, B.A. & Sloper, P. (2002) Chronically ill adolescents' experiences of communication with doctors: a qualitative study. *Journal of Adolescent Health*, 33, 172–179.

Bill, S. (1999) *Adolescent Health: Module One – Foundations*. Burwood, Deakin University Professional Development Unit, Deakin University Australia.

Blair, S. & Bowes, G. (1995) Compliance issues in adolescence: practical strategies. *Australian Family Physician*, 24 (11) 2037–2040.

British Association for Paediatric Nephrology (2003) *Review of Multi-professional Paediatric Nephrology Services in the United Kingdom – Towards Standards and Equity of Care*. Report of a Working Party of the British Association for Paediatric Nephrology. London, British Association for Paediatric Nephrology.

British Medical Association Board of Science (2003) *Adolescent Health*. London, British Medical Association Publishing.

Carr-Gregg, M. & Shale, E. (2002) *Adolescence: a Guide for Parents*. Sydney, Finch Publishing.

Chow, J. (2004) Adolescents' perceptions of popular teen magazines. *Journal of Advanced Nursing*, 48 (2), 132–139.

Christie, D. & Viner, R. (2005) ABC of adolescence: adolescent development. *British Medical Journal*, 330, 301–304.

Coleman, J. & Schofield, J. (2005) *Key Data on Adolescence* (fifth edition). Brighton, Trust for the Study of Adolescence.

Coleman, J., Catan, L. & Dennison, C. (2005) You're the last person I'd talk to. In: *Youth in Society: Contemporary Theory, Policy and Practice* (eds J. Roche, S. Tucker, R. Flynn & R. Thomson) (second edition), pp. 227–234. London, Sage Publications.

Coles, B. (2005) Welfare services for young people. In: *Youth in Society: Contemporary Theory, Policy and Practice* (eds J. Roche, S. Tucker, R. Flynn & R. Thomson) (second edition), p. 27. London, Sage Publications.

Collier, J. & Watson, A.R. (1994) Renal failure in children: specific considerations in management. In: *Quality of Life Following Renal Failure* (eds H. McGee & C. Bradely). USA, Harwood Academic Publishers.

Court, S.D.M. (1976) *Fit for the Future: Report of the Committee on Child Health Services*. Vols i & ii. London, Her Majesty's Stationery Office.

Department of Health (2006) *The National Service Framework for Renal Services. Working for Children and Young People*. London, Department of Health.

Eiser, C. (1990) *Chronic Childhood Disease: an Introduction to Psychological Theory and Research*. Cambridge, Cambridge University Press.

Farrant, B. & Watson, P.D. (2004) Health care delivery: perspectives of young people with chronic illness and their parents. *Journal of Paediatrics and Child Health*, **40**, 175–179.

Gillies, M.L. & Parry-Jones, W.L. (1992) Suitability of the hospital setting for hospitalised adolescents. *Archives of Diseases in Childhood*, **67**, 1506–1509.

Griffin, C. (2005) Representations of the young. In: *Youth in Society: Contemporary Theory, Policy and Practice* (eds J. Roche, S. Tucker, R. Flynn & R. Thomson) (second edition), pp. 10–18. London, Sage Publications.

Haase, J.E. (2004) The adolescent resilience model as a guide to interventions. *Journal of Pediatric Oncology Nursing*, **21** (5), 289–299.

Haven, P.C.L. (2001) *The Social Psychology of Adolescence*. Basingstoke, Palgrave.

Hentinen, M. & Kyngäs, H. (1996) Diabetic adolescents' compliance with health regimens and associated factors. *International Journal of Nursing Studies*, **33** (3), 325–337.

Hockenberry, M., Wilson, D., Winklestein, M.L. & Klein, N.E. (2003) *Wong's Nursing Care of Infants and Children* (seventh edition). St Louis, Mosby.

Horseman, W. (2005) Sexuality in the hospital setting. *Paediatric Nursing*, **17** (8), 27–29.

Hutton, A. (2005) Consumer perspectives on adolescent ward design. *Journal of Clinical Nursing*, **14**, 537–545.

Jackson, S., Bijstra, J., Oostra, L. & Bosma, H. (1998) Adolescents' perceptions of communication with parents relative to specific aspects of relationships with parents and personal development. *Journal of Adolescence*, **21**, 305–322.

Jackson, S., Born, M. & Jacob M.N. (1997) Reflections on risk and resilience. *Journal of Adolescence*, **20**, 606–609.

Kelly, A.F. & Hewson, P.H. (2000) Factors associated with recurrent hospitalisation in chronically ill children and adolescents. *Australian College of Paediatrics*, **36** (1), 13–18.

Koff, E., Rierden, J. & Stubbs, M.L. (1990) Gender, body image and self-concept in early adolescence. *Journal of Early Adolescence*, **10**, 56–68.

Kyngäs, H. (2000) Compliance of adolescents with chronic disease. *Journal of Clinical Nursing*, **9**, 549–556.

Kyngäs, H. & Rissansen, M. (2001) Support as a crucial predictor of good compliance of adolescents with a chronic disease. *Journal of Clinical Nursing*, **10** (6), 767–774.

MacKenzie, H. (1988) Teenagers in hospital. *Nursing Times*, **84** (35), 55–58.

Madden, S.J., Hastings, R.P. & V'ant Hoff, W. (2002) Psychological adjustment in children with end stage renal disease: the impact of maternal stress and coping. *Child Care Health and Development*, **28** (4), 323–330.

Meuleners, L.B., Binns, C.W., Lee, A.H. & Lower, A. (2002) Perceptions of the quality of life for the adolescent with a chronic illness by the teachers, parents and health professionals: a Delphi study. *Child: Health, Care and Development*, **28** (5), 341–349.

Miller, S. (1995) Adolescents' views of outpatient services. *Nursing Standard*, **9** (17), 30–32.

Miller, S. (2001) Facilitating decision making in young people. *Paediatric Nursing*, **13** (5), 31–35.

Ministry of Health (Central Health Services Council) (1959) *The Welfare of Children in Hospital. Report of the Committee (The Platt Report)*. London, Her Majesty's Stationery Office.

Muscari, M.E. (1998) Rebels with a cause: when adolescents won't follow medical advice. *American Journal of Nursing*, **98** (12), 26–30.

Needham, J. (2000) The nurse specialist role in adolescent health. *Paediatric Nursing*, **12** (8), 28–30.

Olsson, C.A., Boyce, M.F., Toumbourou, J.W. & Sawyer, S.M. (2005) The role of peer support in facilitating psychosocial adjustment to chronic illness in adolescence. *Clinical Child Psychology and Psychiatry*, **10** (1), 78–87.

Oxford Dictionary (2002) *Oxford Dictionary, Thesaurus and Word Power Guide*. Oxford, Oxford University Press.

Rew, L. (2005) *Adolescent Health: a Multidisciplinary Approach to Theory, Research and Intervention*. London, Sage Publications.

Rice, F.P. (1999) *The Adolescent: Development, Relationships and Culture* (ninth edition). Boston, Allyn & Bacon.

Rigden, S.P.A. (2003) The management of chronic and end stage renal failure in children: In: *Clinical Paediatric Nephrology* (eds N. Webb & R. Postelthwaite) (third edition). New York, Oxford University Press.

Robinson, J.J.A., Sowden, J.A. & Tattersall, R.B. (1995) The management of diabetes in young adults: a preliminary case study. *Journal of Clinical Nursing*, **4** (4), 257–265.

Royal College of Nursing (2000) *Guidance for Paediatric Nephrology Nurses*. London, Royal College of Nursing.

Royal College of Nursing (2002) *Getting it Right for Teenagers in Your Practice*. London, Royal College of Nursing.

Royal College of Paediatrics and Child Health (2003) *Bridging the Gaps: Health Care for Adolescents*. London, Royal College of Paediatrics and Child Health.

Russell-Johnson, H. (2000) Adolescent survey. *Paediatric Nursing*, **12** (6), 15–19.

Sanci, L. & Young, D. (1995) Engaging the adolescent patient. *Australian Family Physician*, **24** (11), 2031–2127.

Sanci, L.A., Sawyer, S.M., Kang, M.S.L., Haller, D.M. & Patton G.C. (2005) Confidential health care for adolescents: reconciling clinical evidence with family values. *Medical Journal of Australia*, **183** (8), 410–414.

Santrock, J.W. (2001) *Adolescence* (eighth edition). Boston, McGraw Hill.

Sawczenko, A. & Sandu, B.K. (2003) Presenting features of inflammatory bowel disease in Great Britain and Ireland. *Archives of Disease in Childhood*, **88**, 995–1000.

Sawyer, S.M. (2003) Developmentally appropriate health care for young people with chronic illness: questions of philosophy, policy and practice. *Pediatric Pulmonology*, **36** (363), 35–65.

Sawyer, S.M., Rosier, M.J., Phelan, P.D. & Bowes, G. (1995) The self-image of adolescents with cystic fibrosis. *Journal of Adolescent Health*, **16**, 204–208.

Schmidt, S., Petersen, C. & Bullinger, M. (2003) Coping with chronic disease from the perspective of children and adolescents – a conceptual framework and its implications for participation. *Child: Care, Health and Development*, **29** (1), 63–75.

Sloper, P. & Lightfoot, J. (2003) Involving disabled and chronically ill children and young people in health service development. *Child: Care, Health and Development*, **29** (1), 15–20.

Smith, M.S., Martin-Herz, S.P., Womack, W.M. & Marsigan, J.L. (2003) Comparative study of anxiety, depression, somatization, functional disability and illness attribution in adolescents with chronic fatigue or migraine. *Pediatrics*, **111** (4), 376–381.

Smokowski, P.R., Reynolds, A.J. & Bezruczko, N. (1999) Resilience and protective factors in adolescence: an autobiographical perspective from disadvantaged youth. *Journal of School Psychology*, **37** (4), 425–448.

Soanes, C. & Timmons, S. (2004) Improving transition: a qualitative study examining the attitudes of young people with chronic illness transferring to adult care. *Journal of Child Health Care*, **8** (2), 102–112.

Spear, H.J. & Kulbok, P. (2004) Autonomy and adolescence: a concept analysis. *Public Health Nursing*, **21** (2), 144–152.

Steinberg, L. (2001) We know some things: parent-adolescent relationships in retrospect and prospect. *Journal of Research on Adolescence*, **11** (1), 1–19.

Stevens, M.S. (1987) Which adolescents breeze through surgery? *American Journal of Nursing*, **87** (12), 1564–1565.

Suris, J.C., Michud, P.A. & Viner, R. (2004) The adolescent with a chronic condition: part 1 developmental issues. *Archives of Disease in Childhood*, **89**, 938–942.

Tarrant, M. (2002) Adolescent peer groups and social identity. *Social Development*, **11** (1), 110–123.

Taylor, J. & Müller, D. (1995) *Nursing Adolescence, Research and Psychological Perspectives*. Oxford, Blackwell Science.

Thomas, N. (2002) Haemodialysis. In: *Renal Nursing* (ed. N. Thomas) (second edition). London, Baillière Tindall.

Timms, N. & Lowes, L. (1999) Autonomy or non-compliance in adolescent diabetes? *British Journal of Nursing*, **8** (12), 794–800.

Viner, R. & Keane, M. (1998) *Youth Matters: Evidence Based Practice for the Care of Young People in Hospital*. London, Caring for Children in the Health Services.

Ward, G. (2002) Renal care in childhood and adolescence. In: *Renal Nursing* (ed. N. Thomas) (second edition). London, Baillière Tindall.

Watson, A.R. (2003) Meeting the information needs of children and their families. In: *Clinical Paediatric Nephrology* (eds N. Webb & R. Postelthwaite) (third edition). New York, Oxford University Press.

Webb, N. & Postelthwaite, R. (eds) (2003) *Clinical Paediatric Nephrology* (third edition). New York, Oxford University Press.

Wheal, A. (1999) *Adolescence: Positive Approaches for Working with Young People*. Trowbridge, Russel House Publishing.

Wild, J. (2002) Peritoneal dialysis. In: *Renal Nursing* (ed. N. Thomas) (second edition). London, Baillière Tindall.

Women and Children's Hospital (2004) *Adolescent Ward: Addressing the Health Needs of Teenagers in Hospital*. Adelaide, Women & Children's Hospital.

World Health Organization (1993) *The Health of Young People*. Geneva, World Health Organization.

10 Transitional Care

Siân Bill and Beverly Hodges

Introduction

Improvements in health care have seen increased numbers of children and young people with chronic illness surviving into adulthood. Therefore, the seamless transition between child and adult services should be viewed as a priority for all health care professionals working with children and young people. Currently, there are inequalities in the provision of transitional care, which has the potential to lead to a fragmented provision of services.

Aim of the chapter

The purpose of this chapter is to critically examine the transitional issues faced by young people with chronic illness and their families. The discussion surrounding these issues will highlight the need for, and the importance of, a seamless transitional service. Although a scenario of a young person with cystic fibrosis will be used to explore in detail the issues raised within this chapter, these will be applicable to many other young people with chronic illness moving through the transitional phase. As this chapter specifically relates to young people, it is suggested that you first read Chapter 9, which provides a discussion on many issues that arise for adolescents with a chronic illness and an overview of adolescent development, to give you an insight into the topics covered in this chapter.

Intended learning outcomes

- To develop an awareness of the issues surrounding adolescents with chronic illness related to the transitional phase

- To explore the differences between transitional care and transfer
- To examine the psychosocial and physical developmental needs of the adolescent in the transitional phase
- To critically analyse the current evidence to demonstrate the benefits of providing an adolescent transitional service
- To outline the role of the nurse in facilitating the transition process for young people and their families

Overview of cystic fibrosis

Cystic fibrosis (CF) is the most common life-limiting inherited condition in the Caucasian population (Hockenberry *et al.*, 2003). The incidence of CF appears to be reducing over time, with estimations of 1:2500, 1:3300 or 1:4000 live births cited by various authors (Cunningham & Taussig, 1994; James *et al.*, 2002; Hockenberry *et al.*, 2003; Winter, 2006). The reducing numbers are possibly due to the availability of antenatal screening, leading to elective termination of pregnancies. Although it does occur, CF is relatively uncommon in individuals of South American, African and Asian descent (James *et al.*, 2002). In the Caucasian population, approximately 1:28 people are carriers of this condition (Winter, 2006).

 Case study 10.1

Background information

Sophie is a 17-year-old girl who has CF and lives at home with her father and younger sister Sally, aged 14 years who does not have CF. Sally is very supportive of her sister and they get on well together. When Sophie was six years old, her mother died in a car accident and, since then, her father has been the main carer for Sophie and Sally, with some support from both sets of grandparents. Sophie's father works full time as a civil engineer and occasionally works away. Sophie recently left school and works in the local supermarket. Although she achieved good results in her end of school exams, Sophie decided that she did not want to stay on at school.

Sophie was diagnosed at birth as she developed a meconium ileus. Sophie has the most common form of CF, which is the ΔF508 deletion (Hockenberry *et al.*, 2003). She has both respiratory and digestive problems and needs to undertake daily physiotherapy and exercise regimes, as well as eating a high fat, high calorie diet.

Since starting her new job, Sophie is finding it difficult to maintain her usual physiotherapy and dietary programme. She has acquired a new social circle of friends whom she has not informed that she has CF, as she is concerned that she will not be able to maintain these friendships if she discloses her diagnosis. Sophie believes that by requesting time off to visit the hospital, her new friends will find out about her condition. Currently, Sophie is losing weight and has developed another chest infection. Her father believes that she needs a hospital admission for reassessment. Sophie is reluctant to visit the hospital and, although her father has made some appointments with Sophie's GP, she has not attended them.

Sophie is currently a patient at the local children's hospital where she attends clinic regularly and is admitted for antibiotic therapy as required. She is managed by a multidisciplinary team (referred to as the CF team), which generally includes a paediatric respiratory consultant, a CF children's nurse specialist, a paediatric physiotherapist and a paediatric dietitian. The suggestion has been made that Sophie needs to be transferred to the adult hospital, which manages patients with CF. However, this is further away from Sophie's home and working environment.

Time out

This may be a good time to recap what you have learned from Chapter 9 and review your current knowledge regarding CF by answering the following questions.

- What impact does chronic illness have on young people? Consider this from a physical and psychosocial perspective.
- What is the aetiology of CF? (Refer to Chapter 1.)
- How is CF diagnosed?
- What are the main symptoms of CF and their underlying rationale?

CF is an inherited autosomal recessive disorder caused by a defect on chromosome 7 (Velasco-Whetsell *et al.*, 2000) and approximately 1 in 28 people are unaffected carriers of this condition (James *et al.*, 2002). CF occurs when the infant inherits a defective gene from both parents (Hockenberry *et al.*, 2003) and with each pregnancy there is a one in four chance of producing a child with CF (James *et al.*, 2002). The ΔF508 is the most common gene mutation found in CF as this accounts for 70% of diagnosed cases (Hockenberry *et al.*, 2003). In addition to the ΔF508, there are approximately 700 other types of mutations, which account for most of the remaining cases, although a very small percentage (2%) are unable to be genetically matched (Hockenberry *et al.*, 2003). Chapter 1 describes the genetic implications of an autosomal recessive disease such as CF.

Generally, CF is diagnosed in infancy either by neonatal screening or by the presence of a meconium ileus within the first few days of life (Velasco-Whetsell *et al.*, 2000; Hockenberry *et al.*, 2003). However, approximately 10% of individuals with CF are not diagnosed until childhood or adolescence (James *et al.*, 2002), usually when their condition is caused by one of the more unusual mutations. When this occurs, the individual may present with repeated chest infections, digestive problems and/or failure to thrive, and diagnosis may need to be confirmed with a sweat test (Winter, 2006).

CF is a multi-system disorder caused by dysfunction of the exocrine glands (James *et al.*, 2002) and is characterised by the presence of abnormally thick mucus secretions that block the ducts of the respiratory system, pancreas, liver and reproductive system (Velasco-Whetsell, 2000). Symptom severity varies between individuals and can change as the condition progresses (Hockenberry *et al.*, 2003). Difficulty digesting food (leading to malabsorption), pancreatic insufficiency, diabetes, cirrhosis of the liver and male infertility are common manifestations of CF (Cunningham & Taussig, 1994; Velasco-Whetsell *et al.*, 2000; James *et al.*, 2002; Hockenberry *et al.*, 2003). Eventually, most children and young people affected by CF colonise a variety of pathogens in the lungs, the most common being *Pseudomonas aeruginosa* and *Burkholderia cepecia* (Hockenberry *et al.*, 2003) and as the condition deteriorates over time, the symptoms will worsen. Predominantly, however, the main cause of morbidity and mortality are repeated lung infections, leading to progressive lung damage, atelectasis, emphysema and respiratory failure (Hockenberry *et al.*, 2003; Winter, 2006).

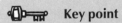 **Key point**

Cystic fibrosis is a multi-system disorder caused by a defect on chromosome 7. It is an autosomal recessive disorder and is life limiting.

Management

A multidisciplinary team generally manages individuals with CF. The focus of care is multifaceted, aimed at reducing symptoms and maintaining as healthy a lifestyle as possible. Promoting airway clearance through a regime of physiotherapy, which aids in expectorating mucus from the lungs, along with the use of antibiotics, aims to prevent repeated lung infections (Esmond, 2000; Velasco-Whetsell *et al.*, 2000). Pancreatic enzymes and nutritional supplements are given to prevent malabsorption, alongside a high protein, high calorie diet to reduce malnutrition and minimise growth delay (Velasco-Whetsell *et al.*, 2000). As the inability to absorb fat-soluble vitamins (A, D, E & K) is inhibited, vitamin supplements are also necessary (James *et al.*, 2002). However, it is suggested that most patients with CF will still have some level of malabsorption and failure to thrive regardless of their dietary and enzyme intake (James *et al.*, 2002). Additionally, in approximately 2.5–12% of individuals with CF, there is the possibility that diabetes mellitus caused by pancreatic insufficiency will also develop (James *et al.*, 2002). This type of diabetes is known as cystic fibrosis related diabetes (CFRD).

To gain more information regarding CF and its management, please refer to the further reading section at the end of this chapter.

Adolescents with a chronic illness

The effect of chronic illness on adolescents was discussed at length in Chapter 9 and readers may want to revisit this chapter before continuing further. One of the main issues regarding chronic illness and young people is that advances in management have increased the overall survival rates for children (Beresford, 2004) and young people (Carson & Heiber, 2001) with life-limiting conditions, and CF is no exception. Fifty years ago, most infants born with CF died within the first year of life, whereas infants born with CF in the twenty-first century can expect to live to approximately 30 to 40 years of age (Esmond, 2000; Cowlard, 2003). It is currently estimated that 30% of individuals with CF are over 18 years of age (Por *et al.*, 2004). Consequently, the focus of care is changing and greater emphasis now needs to be placed on the development of an appropriate, supportive transition process between children and young people's services to more adult focused services (McDonagh, 2004).

Transitional care

The need for a supportive transition between children and young people's services to more adult focused services has been a recognised health care need for some time (DoH, 1991; Betz, 2004; McDonagh, 2004; While *et al.*, 2004). However, the development and provision of such services appears to be fragmented and inconsistent.

Despite concern being expressed regarding the current level of transition services, few strategies are presented to make improvements in this area (Soanes & Timmons, 2004), possibly because the development of such services is a challenge for health care providers (McDonagh, 2004) to implement effectively due to budget and staffing issues. The issue of transition is also an area of adolescent health care that is surprisingly under-researched (Soanes & Timmons, 2004) and there is a lack of contemporary literature in this area.

The philosophy of transitional care

Transitional care has been described as a multifaceted active process that attends to the medical, psychosocial and educational/vocational needs of young people as they move from child to adult centred care (Blum *et al.*, 1993; Soanes & Timmons, 2004). This recognises that the issue of transition is far more involved than transferring a patient from one hospital to another.

Models of transition

There are several identified models of transition care, for example transition based on chronological age or specific conditions. However, there is little evidence to demonstrate that one transition model is more effective than another (Conway, 1998; Rosen *et al.*, 2003) and more research is clearly needed in this area. Regardless of which model is used, it is clear that transition needs to be informal and flexible, with young people and their families being involved in any decision making regarding transfer to adult services (Conway, 1998; Rosen *et al.*, 2003).

What has been noted is that transition is likely to be more successful when it is coordinated by a designated health care professional who, in conjunction with the needs of young people and their families, is responsible for the transition process.

 Key point

As more young people with chronic illness survive into adulthood, the transition from child to adult services becomes a significant issue (Soanes & Timmons, 2004).

Reflection

Transition is a major step for many young people. Before continuing with the rest of the scenario, pause a minute to think about the issues you consider may be of concern to Sophie as she contemplates moving to adult services.

 Case study 10.2

As Sophie has been attending the children's hospital since birth, she is familiar with both the outpatient and ward MDT and is reluctant to transfer to a new service where she may not trust the staff as she currently does. She feels that, at the new hospital, she will have to relate her history all over again, which is often the case. As one of her friends, who also had CF, died not long after being transferred to the adult services, Sophie is concerned about transferring and worries that this only happens 'when the doctors think that you are going to die'. She is also afraid that she will be left with strangers at the 'new hospital' and that it will be full of old and dying people. Although she has not discussed this with the medical staff, she has mentioned it to the CF specialist nurse who recently visited her at home. Additionally, the adult hospital is further away, and it will be difficult for her to get time off work to travel to her clinic appointments as she cannot drive a car.

Sophie's father is her sole carer, with help from both sets of grandparents. Since her diagnosis, Sophie's father or one of her grandparents has probably been encouraged to stay with her when she is in hospital. Although parents do not usually tend to stay with hospitalised adolescents, it is still an option for them. It is issues such as this, which young people are aware of, that help to make them feel comfortable with their surroundings. Lack of knowledge about what is available for them in the adult setting is another example of the way in which the adolescent can be made to feel vulnerable.

There are several key issues that are raised within the case study that have implications for nursing practice. This part of the chapter will focus on issues regarding transition for young people, vulnerability, advocacy, managing chronic illness, and support and decision making.

  Time out

What are the possible reasons that adolescents may be anxious or concerned about moving to adult services?

Issues regarding transition for adolescents

Transferring from children's to adult services can be problematic and stressful for adolescents (Cowlard, 2003; While *et al.*, 2004), particularly when they are not prepared appropriately for the move (Viner, 2003). Consequently, young people may be frightened of moving to adult services for a variety of reasons, including:

- Fear of the unknown
- Moving away from familiar surroundings and familiar staff they have known for many years
- A lack confidence and trust in the new service
- Not feeling ready
- Need for more preparation
- Too much change at one time, because it may coincide with other changes that are occurring in their lives, for example leaving school, starting a new job
- Negative perceptions given by children's services staff regarding adult services
- Parental views of the transition process
- Having to provide information about themselves to the new service providers
- Being cared for by health care professionals with limited knowledge of their condition
- Coming into contact with older people with CF who may be more ill, which increases the adolescent's awareness that CF is a life-limiting condition
- Facing their own mortality
- Previous experience of adult services, for example have had adult relatives hospitalised

In children's nursing, where the concept of family centred care is fostered, parents are encouraged to stay overnight and the focus is on making the hospital environment more like home (Carson & Hieber, 2001). This can be in stark contrast to the services and philosophies of an adult focused service (Carson & Hieber, 2001). Facing the transition from children's services, with which they feel familiar, comfortable and safe (Viner, 2003) to an adult service that is new and unknown to them, is an additional challenge. This has the potential to increase their overall vulnerability (Fleming *et al.*, 2002).

It is not uncommon for young people to express concern with the new services that they will be offered. This is particularly concerning clinics in adult hospitals, as many adolescents fear that services will be 'impersonal' and staff 'unfriendly' (Viner, 2003). Young people who have had a chronic illness since birth or early childhood are familiar with staff who have been caring for them. Viner (2003) identifies that transition can be a major event for adolescents as they are forced away from people they trust and respect, towards people they do not know and consequently will have difficulty trusting. This can often lead to a lack of confidence in the service by both adolescents and their families. Viner (2003) suggests that some parents may even 'sabotage' the transition process if they do not understand the need for transition or are not included in any decisions regarding transition. Therefore transition should be a well coordinated, planned and unhurried process (Cowlard, 2003) and although there is no specific fixed time for transition (Viner, 2003) young people and their families need to be ready for the move.

Young people experience significant changes in developmental transition as they move though the life continuum from childhood to adulthood (Newacheck *et al.*, 2003). This is often a difficult time for them as they come to terms with the final years of their education, move to higher education or employment and form new relationships (Cowlard, 2003). Adding a chronic illness to this developmental stage increases the factors that adolescents need to cope with, and the stress that young people can experience at this time should not be underestimated.

During the transition between services, it is important to share any appropriate information. Where there is an insufficient exchange of knowledge between health care professionals regarding the young person's past history, the adolescent needs to keep providing information about themselves and in some situations tests and investigations are repeated unnecessarily (Viner, 2003).

Viner (2003) identifies that many adult consultants have had a limited interest in what were perceived to be children's conditions. Although Viner (2003) discusses this issue in the context of caring for young people who have survived childhood cancer, there is no evidence to suggest that this is different for any other perceived childhood condition. To a certain extent this is understandable. When children with chronic illnesses or disabilities died in childhood, there was no need for adult medical staff to concern themselves with managing conditions such as CF, muscular dystrophy, cerebral palsy or congenital heart disease. However, as has been noted, young people with a chronic condition are surviving longer (While *et al.*, 2004); staff providing adult focused care do not appear to have kept in step with this changing situation, and many lack knowledge about some conditions. Additionally, for both medical and nursing staff, there are limited opportunities to gain further education regarding adolescent health as the concept of adolescent health as a speciality is new (Michaud *et al.*, 2004), particularly in Britain.

Although improvements have been made to potential life expectancy, with the average life expectancy of a person with CF now estimated at 30 to 40 years (Esmond, 2000; Cowlard, 2003), young people still die at an early age. Therefore, it is possible that many young people with CF will have had friends within their peer group who have already died (Cowlard, 2003). When young people move to adult hospitals it can be expected that they will come into contact with older people who have CF. Potentially, these individuals could be at a more advanced stage of the disease process and as a consequence of this young people may be forced to confront their own mortality, even if they are not ready to do so, causing them some distress. This is recognised as an important issue by the Cystic Fibrosis Trust, and is addressed in their information booklet *Growing up with CF* (Cystic Fibrosis Trust, 2001a).

> **Key point**
>
> Adolescents with a chronic illness have much to cope with and this can increase their overall vulnerability.

Gaining autonomy

Autonomy is an important part of adolescent development (Spear & Kulbok, 2004) and excessive dependence on the family, particularly where a chronic ill-ness is present, can result in a lack of autonomy (Carson & Hieber, 2001). Recently, Sophie has left school and is working part time. It is sometimes difficult for young people with a chronic illness to achieve independence and starting work is one way of trying to achieve this. Transferring to the adult hospital, which is further away from Sophie's home, has the potential to impact on her job and therefore her autonomy. Taking time off work for hospital appointments may lose Sophie any 'good will' she has with her employer, although there is limited literature regarding this issue in relation to young people. There is, however, growing evidence to suggest that this occurs with parents of children who have a chronic illness (Callery, 1997) and it would be easy to transfer this situation from parents to working adolescents who have a chronic illness.

Managing a chronic illness

Maintaining a physiotherapy and exercise programme whilst trying to work is difficult, as demonstrated in the case study. It is important that this should be as flexible and manageable as possible to make it easy for the adolescent to comply with their management, including attendance at outpatient appointments. The issue of adolescent compliance and the ability to cope with a chronic illness has been discussed in Chapter 9.

Another issue highlighted in the scenario is Sophie's reluctance to disclose her condition to new friends. This is not unusual because, above all, adolescents want to be the same as their peers as the peer group becomes very important to adoles-cents (Carr-Gregg & Shale, 2002). Whilst they are still maturing and developing their personalities, adolescents can often feel insecure about themselves (Rice, 1999). By socialising with their peers, adolescents are learning from each other and developing their ability to interact socially on a wider scale (Rice, 1999). The presence of a chronic illness has the potential to inhibit this. Where adolescents have had a long-standing illness, it is likely that their 'old' school-friends are aware of this. However, many young people have concerns about meeting 'new' friends (Cystic Fibrosis Trust, 2001a) either through changing schools or starting work. Understandably, no one would want to say, 'Hi, I'm Sophie and I have CF' (or diabetes or any other condition) on first meeting someone, and the issue for many young people is at what point is the disclosure made? Some young people are very concerned that a disclosure of chronic illness will prevent new friendships being made. This is another area where the Cystic Fibrosis Trust is able to provide information and advice for young people (Cystic Fibrosis Trust, 2001a).

Support and decision making

Within the scenario, Sophie has raised concerns regarding her transfer to the adult services. She is feeling frightened, which can be a natural reaction for any young person with a chronic illness facing the prospect of moving from child to adult care. Such a transition is a life-changing event that needs to be managed in a sensitive manner for the transition phase to be effective (Por *et al.*, 2004).

The move from child to adult services can coincide with a period of developmental transition for young people, a stage where they are maturing and want to be recognised as individuals and accepted by their peer group (Soanes & Timmons, 2004). Not only are they adapting to growing up with a chronic illness, but they are also confronting the same issues as many other young people, such as finding their independence and discovering where they fit into the wider context of society. This could include exploring their sexuality and being involved in the misuse of alcohol and other substances. It is a stage where young people want to be respected and gain more responsibility. All these issues need to be considered within the transition process, particularly as young people like Sophie, with a chronic illness, may be frightened of moving to adult care.

   Key point

Young people with a chronic illness need to be recognised as individuals. They have the same needs as their peer group but often have additional needs related to living with a chronic illness.

Case study 10.3

Sophie has continued to lose weight and her chest infection has worsened. With much persuasion from her family and the CF team, she has finally agreed to be admitted to the children's hospital for assessment and management. Sophie is really unhappy as she has recently met a new boyfriend and feels she is being 'forced' to tell people about her condition because she has to be admitted to hospital.

During the admission process, Sophie was noted to have diabetes, caused by pancreatic insufficiency, which is fairly common in young people who have CF (James *et al.*, 2002). Understandably, Sophie was shocked and distressed by the new diagnosis as she feels that she has enough to cope with already.

While Sophie has been in hospital, the CF specialist nurse has been visiting her on a daily basis. She has a good rapport with Sophie and has identified a number of issues of concern to Sophie. These include her fear of transfer to adult services, her ability to form relationships, to be accepted as an individual, to cope with the additional diagnosis of CF related diabetes and trying to juggle her home, work and social life within her current management regime. Sophie has met with the diabetes nurse consultant who will now be part of the MDT caring for her.

The CF team has identified a plan of action including the support needed relating to the issues outlined above.

(clock icon) **Time out**

- What key factors do you consider ought to be included in a plan of action?
- Provide the rationale to support your choice.

The role of the nurse

It is important to remember that not only do adolescents and their families experience concerns about the transition process, but so, too, can health care professionals. Many staff will have known the young people in their care for some time and it can be difficult for them to let go (Conway, 1998). It is possible, therefore, that staff could send out non-verbal messages to young people causing them increased anxiety regarding the transition to adult services, thereby hindering the process (Viner, 2003).

The nurse, whether a children's nurse, adult nurse, CF or adolescent specialist nurse, has an important role to play in facilitating transition. It is imperative that nurses build good relationships and maintain open channels of communication with young people and their families. It is important, however, that young people and their families do not become overly dependent on the nurse, and any relationship forged should maintain professional boundaries as set out by their *Code of Professional Conduct* (NMC, 2004). Further suggestions regarding ways in which nurses can facilitate the transition process are outlined later in the chapter.

As the CF specialist nurse described in the case study has already built up a good rapport with Sophie, she is ideally placed to act as an advocate within the transition process. To ensure a meaningful, involved transition, the CF specialist nurse will need to identify the needs of Sophie and her family through exploration of their views, values and beliefs, and past experiences. It is essential to find out what is important to young people in relation to their chronic illness, as well as exploring their aspirations and goals in life. This will allow options to be considered before the transition, as well as anticipating future needs.

> ### Key point
>
> To promote a purposeful transition, the children's nurse/CF specialist nurse should identify the needs of young people and their families, through exploration of their views, values and experiences.

Beresford (2004) recommends the consideration of individual needs because transition does not occur in a single step. Flexibility and the gathering of appropriate information enable effective planning of a supportive network. This includes multidisciplinary and multi-agency involvement in the transitional process as the CF nurse does not work in isolation. An MDT approach will allow thorough preparation, greater continuity of care, a communication network and enhancement of trust within the therapeutic relationship. Facilitation of the transition should aim to meet the expectations of young people and their families, which will help alleviate any apprehension regarding the move to adult services. If expectations are not met, it could impact on the outcomes of transition planning.

To enable a more seamless transition, it is essential that the CF nurse and the MDT involve young people with a chronic illness (like Sophie) and their families in the decision making process. Involvement in decision making allows a more 'person centred' approach to care (Beresford, 2004), which focuses on the young person's preferences, goals and outlook for the future.

> ### Key point
>
> It is during the transition period that there is a 'locus of control' shift in the amount of involvement in decision making between the parent/carer and the young person.

Time out

Consider why there may be changes in the amount of involvement in decision making for young people and their parents and how this may impact on their relationship?

Due to their increasing level of maturity and need for independence, young people will be more involved in decisions about their care and treatment, and

the CF team will encourage this process. Some young people may be apprehens-
ive initially regarding their level of involvement in decision making, but by
including them at an early stage, they will begin to understand the relevance
of their participation. This will impact on their understanding of their health,
well-being and treatment regimen, encouraging them to take responsibility for
themselves. Many young people who have been involved in their care and decision making from an early age become experts in their own condition and its
management. This has the potential to influence their ability to adapt to living
with their chronic illness, reduce the potential problem of non-compliance, and
be comfortable with balancing their lifestyle in terms of education, social relationships, work life and home life (CF Trust, 2003). Consideration of all of these issues
is important when planning the transition process with any young person with
chronic illness.

Whilst the young person is establishing independence and having greater
involvement in decision making, the role of the parent/carer cannot be ignored.
The parental role in decision making is now changing. Potentially, this can be a
difficult time of adjustment as previously the parent would have worked closely
with the CF team, often taking full responsibility for decisions about their child's
care and treatment. This may have included involvement in learning about all
aspects of care in order to manage their child's CF appropriately. The young
person is now seeking independence and will take centre stage in decisions made.
Parents' views may be consulted and considered in decision making, but their
role will not be in the forefront as it has been previously. This can leave parents
feeling a sense of loss and helplessness. The CF team can help promote this shift in
the parental role as parents move to a more supportive/advisory role, enabling
them to engage with their adolescents and actively encourage their new found
responsibility.

In the earlier part of the case study, Sophie did not want to go to hospital
despite her father's concerns. Conflict can occur during the transitional phase, as
the young person and parent may have differences of opinions relating to aspects
of changes in care. Some young people may actively rebel against their treatment
as they adjust within the period of adolescent development, as well as with their
chronic illness, whereas others may embrace this transitional time.

The CF team needs to support parents and young people through this process
in a sensitive manner, offering guidance and reassurance throughout to enhance
positive outcomes. Such support is demonstrated within the scenario. Members
of the CF team will have built up a relationship with young people and their
families over several years. They will have become familiar with their patients,
building strong attachments along the way. Thus, this can also be a difficult time
for the staff involved in the care of young people, because they have protected
and nurtured their patients. Having watched young people with chronic illness
grow up, it may not be easy for the health professional to 'let go' of their care
(Viner, 2003). Health professionals need to be mindful of their role in supporting
young people and involve them in decisions about their care to increase their
confidence and their self-esteem. This can promote the development of their identity, allowing them to feel in control, and give them the ability to cope with the
transition process and beyond.

Lack of involvement in decision making and inadequate transitional support can disadvantage the young person. It could create developmental difficulties in terms of self-concept and autonomy (Blum *et al.*, 1993) and may hinder the evolvement of their identity and movement towards adulthood. Additionally, this has the potential to impact on their ability to integrate into the wider social world because, as a consequence, they may lack confidence, feel lonely and have low expectations of their illness and future outlook. This can have a negative influence on their ability to establish new relationships, their career choice and ability to become economically viable and independent.

Lack of involvement in decision making and inadequate transitional support also has a counter-impact on the family, as the young person with chronic illness may be more dependent and over-reliant upon them. This can be a worrying, anxious time, putting an added strain on the family emotionally and financially. Parents may need to support the young person for a longer period of time.

 Case study 10.4

Whilst in hospital, Sophie's condition improved, her chest infection subsided and she gained some weight. As she feels better in herself, she is able to think more rationally about her present situation. During her hospital admission, her boyfriend and a few work friends visited her and to her surprise were more accepting than she had expected they would be. This has helped her feel more secure.

During Sophie's hospital admission, the CF team have taken the opportunity to provide her with some education about her overall condition and the process of moving to another hospital. She has been informed that transition is not a sudden process and that she will be transferred via a transition clinic where she will get the opportunity to visit the new hospital and the staff, but still be predominantly under the care of the children's hospital. Due to the structure of the transition protocol, Sophie will be able to choose her own timing for transfer and thus have an element of control in deciding when it is right for her to move on. Consequently, Sophie feels much happier in herself and with the transition process.

 Time out

What are the benefits of involving young people and their families in decision making?

Promoting the paradigm shift

Young people have previously been disadvantaged in relation to transitional service provision (RCPCH, 2003). The specific needs of young people and their families have been insufficiently met, potentially due to a variety of reasons, including:

- An overall lack of understanding of adolescent transitional care issues
- Lack of provision of staff training regarding understanding the needs of young people and their families during the transition phase
- Clinical areas being too focused on children's health care issues and not acknowledging the growing independence of young people
- Clinical areas too focused on adult issues, valuing autonomy, but not acknowledging concerns of the family and young people's state of readiness in the move towards independence
- Insufficient specialist staff to offer appropriate support
- Poor communication and collaboration between children, young people and adult services (RCPCH, 2003)

 Time out

Outline the consequences of inadequate transitional support for the young people and their families.

Poor transitional support has led to rapid transfer of some young people to adult services without any planning, leaving them and their families feeling isolated and rejected (Conway, 1998). Additionally, it has resulted in some young people remaining under the care of children's services for a greater period of time, possibly due to a lack of appropriately experienced adult physicians. Historically, as previously mentioned, the survival rate of children with chronic illness was poor and specialist training for adult physicians in what were perceived to be childhood conditions was not necessary. Facilities for specialist medical training do not appear to have been put in place at a national level and it is evident that this is an area of inequality that needs addressing (Viner, 2003). However, there is now recognition of the importance of transition service provision. The RCPCH (2003), *National Service Framework* (DoH, 2004) and the Royal College of Nursing (2004) are aiming to promote the paradigm shift that will inform, guide and educate health care professionals in this process. MDT working is essential to enable a seamless transition and continuing education can add to the development of knowledge and skills in this area.

The principles of successful transitional care

 Time out

What do you think should be included in transitional care training programmes?

The RCPCH (2003) and Hancock (1998) have outlined recommendations for multi-disciplinary training, which should include:

- Transitional care
- Young people's perspectives
- Mental health issues and problems
- Communication and leadership
- MDT working

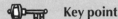 **Key point**

It is essential that health care professionals collaborate and share their expertise to ensure a smooth transition between child and adult services.

Once staff have enhanced their knowledge by undertaking further training, they need to bridge the gap between child and adult services by ensuring a multi-agency approach to care, whereby expertise is shared and appropriate resources are provided to support the young person and their family. Out-of-hours clinics and collaborative joint clinics can be more suitable for the young person in the transition phase. Young people may or may not wish to have their parents present at their clinic consultation. As they become more involved in their own decision making and geared towards self-care they should be supported in their preference. Whilst the multidisciplinary approach is essential, the role of the children's nurse is paramount.

Key points

- Young people need to be allocated a key worker to coordinate, involve, guide and educate them and their families through the process of transition. The CF nurse may take on this role.
- The transition from child to adult services does not need to occur during a fixed timeframe but can take place when it is felt that the adult hospital would be more appropriate in meeting the young person's needs (Beresford, 2004).

The transition phase may begin as early as 12 years of age and continue until the young person is aged 16 years or above. The complex issues surrounding adolescent development determine that adolescents of the same age are not all at the same level of physical and cognitive development (Rice, 1999; While *et al.*, 2004). Consequently, it would not be appropriate to suggest that chronological age alone should be the major determining factor in adolescent transition. The transition from child to adult services does, however, need to be planned and well coordinated. The RCN has suggested the need for three stages of transition. These

Table 10.1   Stages of transition.

Early stage (12–14 years)
At this stage, the young people can be introduced to the idea of transition and move towards independence with support from their family. The young people should be encouraged to develop an awareness of their chronic illness and care needs, and future implications of their condition. Assessment of their understanding of their illness at this stage is essential to support them.
Middle stage (14–15 years)
Young people and their families should be introduced to the process of transition. They should be informed about what they can expect from adult-led services. The children's nurse can encourage the young person to participate in goal setting.
Late stage (15–16 years)
At this stage, young people may feel more confident regarding their move to adult care. Young people may have adopted a self-caring approach to dealing with their chronic illness.

Source   RCN, 2004.

stages are outlined in Table 10.1. The RCN makes further recommendations about the ways in which nurses can facilitate the transition process. It is recommended that at each transitional stage, the children's nurse or allocated key worker can assist the young person in six key areas. These are outlined in Table 10.2.

Whilst the main focus of adolescent health is to promote autonomy and decision making, it is important to maintain a close relationship with parents throughout the transition process. Therefore, it is recommended that young people are encouraged to include their parents in the information sharing process. This will ensure that the health and lifestyle needs of young people are addressed, helping them to develop and feel respected as individuals.

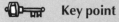   **Key point**

Children's nurses/specialist nurses should start talking about the move to adult services at least one year prior to transfer. This will allow time for questions and discussion with young people and their families.

To enable a seamless transition, the role of the children's nurse/specialist nurse during this time will involve:

- The coordination of joint clinics
- Provision of adequate information and support

Table 10.2 Guidelines for nurses in facilitating the transition process.

Self-advocacy

The nurse can:

- Provide education regarding the condition
- Encourage them to ask questions
- Ensure they know how and where to access health care information

Independent health care behaviour

The nurse can:

- Provide them with a personal health care record book
- Assess their level of understanding regarding their medication
- Discuss the principles of confidentiality

Sexual health

The nurse should be able to discuss:

- Changes associated with puberty
- Safe sex practices and general sexual well-being
- Issues regarding fertility and provide basic genetic counselling
- Their concerns and allow them to ask questions

Psychosocial support

The nurse will encourage:

- The adolescent to talk about their friends and supportive relationships
- The adolescent to join social groups
- The adolescent to set positive and realistic goals
- Autonomy and decision making

Education and vocational planning

The nurse should:

- Discuss the responsibilities and restrictions affecting education and recreational activities
- Have an awareness of health care entitlements and benefits and guide the adolescent appropriately

Health and lifestyle

The nurse should be able to discuss and advise young people on:

- Smoking, alcohol consumption, drug use and overall general well-being
- Weight gain and weight loss related to their condition
- Issues related to body image

Source   RCN 2004.

- Liaison with school, college or areas of employment to ensure appropriate support
- Support to parents
- Promotion of self-care

The CF Trust (2001b) provides a checklist for care for the young person:

- Early discussion about moving
- Time to talk and ask questions
- Full involvement in plans and transfer
- Meeting the adult team
- Visiting the adult centre/joint transition clinic

- Allocating a key person
- Providing an information booklet
- Reassurance about patient care

It is recommended that care is audited to monitor its effectiveness. It has already been noted that the transition from children's to adult services does not always occur in a seamless manner, although every effort should be made to ensure that it does. The children's nurse has a vital role to play with regard to evaluating the progress of the transitional process. If children's nurses are able to monitor the progress of transition they will be able to address any identified problems early and renegotiate goals and timescales where appropriate.

 Time out

You can now use these next questions to test your knowledge on the content of this chapter:

- What is the most common gene mutation in CF?
- What is the philosophy of transitional care?
- Why is it important for young people to be involved in decision making?

Outline the role of the nurse in the transition process.

Conclusion

This chapter has clearly identified that there are ongoing needs for young people and their families as they move through the transition process. However, transition is currently often a neglected dimension of health care provision, which clearly needs to be addressed. An MDT and multi-agency approach is required to accomplish this, and further education for health care providers is required if they are to deliver an enhanced level of care and a seamless transition between child and adult services. Nurses working with young people with a chronic illness play a key role in the transition process, promoting autonomy and self-actualisation, which will enable adolescents to make a successful transition between service providers.

> **Key points**
>
> - As more young people with chronic illness survive into adulthood, the transition from child to adult services becomes a significant issue (Soanes & Timmons, 2004) and poor transitional support can have a detrimental affect on young people.
> - Transitional care is a multifaceted active process that attends to the medical, social and educational/vocational needs of young people as they move from

child to adult centred care (Blum *et al.*, 1993; Soanes & Timmons, 2004). However, research in this area is limited.

- The nurse working with young people has an important role to play in facilitating the transition process.
- During the transition period, there is a 'locus of control' shift in the amount of involvement in decision making between the parent/carer and the young person. With increased autonomy, the young person will have greater involvement in the decision making process.
- Regardless of the evidence to support the importance of a smooth and coordinated transition process, transition remains a frequently neglected area of health care provision.

Useful websites

www.likeitis.org.uk
www.teenagehealthfreak.com
www.youngminds.org.uk
www.cf.org.uk

Recommended reading

Hockenberry, M., Wilson, D., Winkelstein, M.L. & Kline, N.E. (2003) *Wong's Nursing Care of Infants and Children* (seventh edition). St Louis, Mosby.
Glasper, E.A. & Richardson, J. (eds) (2006) *A Textbook of Children's and Young People's Nursing*. Edinburgh, Churchill Livingstone.

References

Beresford, B. (2004) On the road to nowhere? Young disabled people and transition. *Child: Care, Health and Development*, **30** (6), 581–587.
Betz, C.L. (2004) Transition of adolescents with special health care needs: review and analysis of the literature. *Issues in Comprehensive Pediatric Nursing*, **27**, 179–241.
Blum, R., Garrell, D. & Hodgman, C. (1993) Transition from child-centred to adult health care systems for adolescents with chronic conditions: a position paper of the Society for Adolescent Medicine. *Journal of Adolescent Health*, **14**, 570–576.
Callery, P. (1997) Paying to participate: financial, social and personal costs to parents of involvement in their child's care in hospital. *Journal of Advanced Nursing*, **25** (4), 746–752.
Carr-Gregg, M. & Shale, E. (2002) *Adolescence: a Guide for Parents*. Sydney, Finch Publishing.
Carson, A.R. & Hieber, K.V. (2001) Adult paediatric patients. *American Journal of Nursing*, **101** (3), 46–54.
Conway, S.P. (1998) Transition from paediatric to adult-oriented care for adolescents with cystic fibrosis. *Disability and Rehabilitation*, **20** (6–7), 209–216.

Cowlard, J. (2003) Cystic fibrosis: transition from paediatric to adult care. *Nursing Standard*, **18** (4), 39–41.

Cunningham, J.C. & Taussig, L.M. (1994) *An Introduction to Cystic Fibrosis for Patients and Families*. Maryland, Cystic Fibrosis Foundation.

Cystic Fibrosis Trust (2001a) *Growing up with CF*. Kent, Cystic Fibrosis Trust.

Cystic Fibrosis Trust (2001b) Transition. A guide for young people moving from paediatric to adult care. Fact sheet: www.cftrust.org.uk Accessed 11/11/05.

Cystic Fibrosis Trust (2003) Transition. A guide for parents. Fact sheet: www.cftrust.org.uk Accessed 11/11/05.

Department of Health (1991) *The Welfare of Children and Young People in Hospital*. London, HMSO.

Department of Health (2004) *National Service Framework for Children, Young People and Maternity Services. Core Standards. Change for Children – Every Child Matters*. London, Department of Health.

Esmond, G. (2000) Cystic fibrosis: adolescent care. *Nursing Standard*, **14** (52), 47–52, 54–55, 57.

Fleming, E., Carter, B. & Gillibrand, W. (2002) The transition of adolescents with diabetes from the children's health care service to the adult health care service: a review of the literature. *Journal of Clinical Nursing*, **11** (5), 560–567.

Hancock, C. (1998) Time to stand up and be counted. *RCN Magazine*, Summer, 8–9.

Hockenberry, M., Wilson, D., Winklestein, M.L. & Klein, N.E. (2003) *Wong's Nursing Care of Infants and Children* (seventh edition). St Louis, Mosby.

James, S.R., Ashwill, J.W. & Droske, S.C. (2002) *Nursing Care of Children*. Philadelphia, W.B. Saunders.

McDonagh, J.E. (2004) Growing up and moving on: transition from pediatric to adult care. *Pediatric Transplantation*, 10, 1–9.

Michaud, P.A., Suris, J.C. & Viner, R. (2004) The adolescent with a chronic condition. Part II: health care provision. *Archives of Disease in Childhood*, **89**, 943–949.

Newacheck, P.W., Hung, Y.Y., Park, J.M., Brindis, C.D. & Irwin, C.E. Jr (2003) Disparities in adolescent health and health care: does socio-economic status matter? *Health Services Research*, **38** (5), 1235–1252.

Nursing and Midwifery Council (2004) *The NMC Code of Conduct: Standards for Conduct, Performance and Ethics*. London, Nursing and Midwifery Council.

Por, J., Golderg, B., Lennox, V., Burr, P., Barrow, J. & Dennard, L. (2004) Transition care: health professionals' view. *Journal of Nursing Management*, **12** (5), 354–361.

Rosen, S.D., Blum, R.W., Britto, M., Sawyer, S.M. & Siegel, D.M. (2003) Transition to adult health care for adolescents and young adults with chronic conditions. *Journal of Adolescent Health*, **33**, 309–311.

Rice, F.P. (1999) *The Adolescent, Development Relationships and Culture* (ninth edition). Boston, Allyn and Bacon.

Royal College of Nursing (2004) *Adolescent Transition Care. Guidance for Nursing Staff*. London, Royal College of Nursing.

Royal College of Paediatrics and Child Health (2003) *Bridging the Gaps: Health Care for Adolescents*. London, Royal College of Paediatrics and Child Health.

Soanes, C. & Timmons, S. (2004) Improving transition: a qualitative study examining the attitudes of young people with chronic illness transferring to adult care. *Journal of Child Health Care*, **8** (2), 102–112.

Spear, H.J. & Kulbok, P. (2004) Autonomy and adolescence: a concept analysis. *Public Health Nursing*, **21** (2), 144–152.

Velasco-Whetsell, M., Coffin, D.A., Lizardo, L.M. *et al.* (2000) *Pediatric Nursing*. New York, McGraw-Hill.

Viner, R. (2003) Bridging the gaps: transition for young people with cancer. *European Journal of Cancer*, **39**, 2684–2687.

While, A., Forbes, A., Ullman, R., Lewis, S., Mathes, L. & Griffiths, P. (2004) Good practices that address continuity during transition from child to adult care: synthesis of the evidence. *Child: Care, Health and Development*, **30** (5), 439–452.

Winter, J.M. (2006) Caring for children with gastrointestinal problems. In: *A Textbook of Children's and Young People's Nursing* (eds A. Glasper & J. Richardson). Edinburgh: Churchill Livingstone.

Index